Framing and Imagining Disease in Cultural History

Also by G.S. Rousseau

THIS LONG DISEASE MY LIFE: Alexander Pope and the Sciences (*with Marjorie Hope Nicolson*)

ENGLISH POETIC SATIRE (*with N. Rudenstine*)

THE AUGUSTAN MILIEU (*with others*)

TOBIAS SMOLLETT (*with P.-G. Boucé*)

ORGANIC FORM: The Life of an Idea

GOLDSMITH: The Critical Heritage

THE FERMENT OF KNOWLEDGE: Studies in the Historiography of Science (*with Roy Porter*)

THE LETTERS AND PRIVATE PAPERS OF SIR JOHN HILL

TOBIAS SMOLLETT: Essays of Two Decades

SCIENCE AND THE IMAGINATION: Thr Berkeley Conference

SEXUAL UNDERWORLDS OF THE ENLIGHTENMENT (*with Roy Porter*)

THE ENDURING LEGACY: ALEXANDER POPE TERCENTENARY ESSAYS (*with Pat Rogers*)

EXOTICISM IN THE ENLIGHTENMENT (*with Roy Porter*)

THE LANGUAGES OF PSYCHE: Mind and Body in Enlightenment Thought

PERILOUS ENLIGHTENMENT: Pre- and Post-Modern Discourses – Sexual, Historical

ENLIGHTENMENT CROSSINGS: Pre- and Post-Modern Discourses – Anthropological

ENLIGHTENMENT BORDERS: Pre- and Post-Modern Discourses – Medical, Scientific

MEDICINE AND THE MUSES (*translated into Italian*)

HYSTERIA BEYOND FREUD (*with Sander Gilman, Roy Porter, Helen King and Elaine Showalter*)

GOUT: The Patrican Malady (*with Roy Porter*)

Framing and Imagining Disease in Cultural History

Edited by

George Sebastian Rousseau

with

Miranda Gill
David Haycock
Malte Herwig

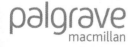

First published 2003 by
PALGRAVE MACMILLAN
Houndmills, Basingstoke, Hampshire RG21 6XS and
175 Fifth Avenue, New York, N.Y. 10010
Companies and representatives throughout the world

PALGRAVE MACMILLAN is the global academic imprint of the Palgrave
Macmillan division of St. Martin's Press, LLC and of Palgrave Macmillan Ltd.
Macmillan® is a registered trademark in the United States, United
Kingdom and other countries. Palgrave is a registered trademark in the
European Union and other countries.

ISBN 1–4039–1292–0

This book is printed on paper suitable for recycling and made from fully
managed and sustained forest sources.

A catalogue record for this book is available from the British Library.

Library of Congress Cataloging-in-Publication Data

Framing and imagining disease in cultural history / edited by George
    Sebastian Rousseau, with Miranda Gill, David Haycock, Malte Herwig.
        p. cm.
    Includes bibliographical references and index.
    ISBN 1-4039-1292-0
    1.Medicine–Philosophy–History. 2. Health–Philosophy–History.
3. Diseases–Social aspects–History. I. Rousseau, G. S. (George Sebastian)
II. Gill, Miranda. III. Haycock, David Boyd, 1968-

R723.F725 2003
610'.1–dc21   2003040537

10   9   8   7   6   5   4   3   2   1
12 11 10 09 08 07 06 05 04 03

Printed and bound in Great Britain by
Antony Rowe Ltd, Chippenham and Eastbourne

Contents

List of Illustrations

Acknowledgements

Varia: First and foremost to Leverhulme Trust large institutional grant F793A, thanks for sustaining some of this enterprise; in Leicester to Professor Judy Simons, Pro-Vice-Chancellor of De Montfort University, who continued to encourage George Rousseau and the Framing Disease Workshop to present their programmes at De Montfort University, which they did over several years while George Rousseau was a professor there; in London to the Wellcome Trust Centre for the History of Medicine at University College which hosted our meeting in December 2001 in Euston House, at which this volume was actually launched; in Toronto Canada to Adam Budd, formerly at the Wellcome Centre in London, who had organized our 2001 meeting in London and was its most confident lynchpin, triumphantly assuring us that there was matter here of interest to *both* the literary and medical communities we so much wanted to reach; in Paris to Sophie Vasset, who further encouraged us by inviting us to come to 'her country' and test our largely Anglo-American theories on a French academic audience, an idea we implemented and which produced brilliant results, as the Gallican content of this book attests; in Oxford to two ancient colleges – Merton College and New College – which awarded Visiting Research Fellowships to George Rousseau, where he was able to ponder some of framing's theoretical riddles, and, beyond this generosity, to New College for its hospitality in hosting the 2002 meeting of the Framing Disease Workshop where all these chapters, apart from chapter 11, were first delivered as conference papers; finally, but not least, in Basingstoke, to our remarkable editorial team – especially Luciana O'Flaherty, Daniel Bunyard, Tim Kapp and Nick Brock – who did everything humanly possible to ensure that this book would be published by 4 July 2003 – American Independence Day – on which day some of our group, especially those who have written here, would brace themselves again for the theoretical hurdles of framing and imagining disease at the international Anglo-American Conference on the Body in London. We have not, of course, solved any of the problems. We have merely initiated a dialogue about them – a broad interdisciplinary conversation we hope will continue for a very long time.

George Rousseau
Oxford, England

Notes on the Contributors

Caterina Albano holds a PhD in Renaissance Studies. She has focused her research primarily on the cultural significance of food and its denial in the early-modern period, publishing various articles on the subject. She has also edited the volume by Hannah Woolley, *The Gentlewoman's Companion* (2001). She is currently working for the art consultancy Wallace /Kemp Artakt, and has worked on various exhibition projects exploring the links been the art and science, including 'Spectacular Bodies: the Art and Science of the Human Body from Leonardo to Now' (Hayward Gallery, 2000–1), 'Head On: Art with the Brain in Mind' (Wellcome Trust/Science Museum, 2002), 'The Genius of Genetics' (St Thomas Abbey, Brno, 2002).

Stephan Besser has studied German Literature and History in Marburg, Amsterdam and Berlin. As a PhD candidate at the Amsterdam School for Cultural Analysis (University of Amsterdam) he is currently preparing a dissertation on the imagery of tropical diseases in German culture at the turn of the twentieth century, provisionally entitled *Pathographie der Tropen. Kolonialismus, Medizin und Literatur um 1900.* His interest lies in the interdiscursive circulation of medical knowledge in imperial contexts (see most recently 'Germanin. Pharmazeutische Signaturen des deutschen (Post)Kolonialismus', in Alexander Honold and Oliver Simons (eds), *Kolonialismus als Kultur. Literatur, Medien, Wissenschaft in der deutschen Gründerzeit des Fremden* (Tübingen: Francke, 2002) 167–96). He also contributes to a research project on the cultural history of German colonialism at Humboldt University, Berlin.

Kirstie Blair is a Research Fellow and Tutor in English at Keble College, Oxford. She has recently completed a PhD on nineteenth-century poetry and the heart, and also works and publishes on Victorian religion, George Eliot and her circle, and twentieth-century poetry.

Michael R. Finn is Professor of French at Ryerson University in Toronto. His 1999 study of Marcel Proust (*Proust, the Body and Literary Form*) attempted to situate the author in the context of *fin-de-siècle* medicalized nervousness and to analyse how neurasthenia and hysteria act as figures that condition the Proustian notion of style and fictional structure. His current research foci are the interplay between science, medicine and literature and issues of gender, censorship and pornography at the French *fin-de-siècle*. Recent publications include

Rachilde–Maurice Barrès: Correspondance inédite 1885–1914 (2002), an edition of love correspondence from the decadent 1880s. He is presently working on two projects – a monograph on the novelist Rachilde and a broader-based study dealing with the fictional representation of the debate over hysteria and neurasthenia, gender and abnormal sexuality in late nineteenth- and early twentieth-century French fiction.

Pamela K. Gilbert is Associate Professor of English at the University of Florida and editor of the series, Studies in the Long Nineteenth Century. Her work has appeared in several journals, including *Nineteenth Century Studies, Nineteenth Century Prose, Women and Performance, English, LIT: Literature/Interpretation/Theory, Essays in Arts and Sciences, Essays in Literature, Victorian Newsletter* and others. Her book, *Disease, Desire and the Body in Victorian Women's Popular Novels*, was published in 1997. *Beyond Sensation, Mary Elizabeth Braddon in Context*, a collection co-edited with Marlene Tromp and Aeron Haynie, appeared in 2000. She has also edited the collection *Imagined Londons* (2002). *Visible at a Glance*, a book tracing the mapping of the social body and cholera epidemics in London and India in the mid-nineteenth century, is forthcoming.

Miranda Gill is a Senior Scholar at Christ Church, University of Oxford, having previously studied at St John's College and New College, Oxford, and the University of Geneva. She is currently working on her doctoral thesis, a cultural history of eccentricity in nineteenth-century France. In addition to the history of psychiatry, research interests related to her thesis include the relationship between contemporary hermeneutics and the history of enigma in nineteenth-century French culture; dandyism; monstrosity; and the methodology of cultural history. She has presented various conference papers on these topics.

David Boyd Haycock read Modern History at St John's College, Oxford, and Art History at the University of Sussex. His doctorate on the eighteenth-century antiquary and Newtonian scholar Dr William Stukeley was undertaken at Birkbeck College, University of London, and completed in 1998. Between 1998 and 2002 he was a Junior Research Fellow at Wolfson College, Oxford, during which time he also held a Leverhulme Research Fellowship working on the cultural histories of disease with Professor George S. Rousseau. He is the author of *William Stukeley: Science, Archaeology and Religion in Eighteenth-Century England* (2002) and *Paul Nash* (2002).

Malte Herwig is Junior Research Fellow in German Literature and History of Science at Merton College, University of Oxford. He has studied at the University of Mainz and The Queen's College, Oxford, and spent a year as Visiting Research Fellow at Harvard University. He received his DPhil at the University of Oxford with a dissertation on science in Thomas Mann's work, which will be published by Klostermann in the Monograph Series *Thomas-Mann-Studies* later this year (*Bildungsbürger auf Abwegen. Die Naturwissenschaften im Werk Thomas Manns*). He has given conference papers throughout Europe and has published articles in American, British and German learned journals (most recently 'The Unwitting Muse: Jakob von Uexküll's Theory of Umwelt and Twentieth-century Literature', *Semiotica* 2001). In 1999 he was awarded the Goethe Prize of the English Goethe Society in London and he is currently Gundolf Fellow at the Institute of Germanic Studies in London. He is assistant editor of the new critical edition of Thomas Mann's early stories. In his current research on the *Cultural Roots of Modernism in German Literature and Science* he brings together literary historiography with recent approaches in the history of science in order to investigate the parallel development of modern thought in both German science and art between 1890 and 1930.

Emese Lafferton is a PhD candidate in History at the Central European University, Budapest, completing her doctoral dissertation on nineteenth-century Hungarian psychiatry, a topic that has hitherto received little attention from modern social sciences. She has received a Wellcome Research Fellowship at the Department of History and Philosophy of Science, University of Cambridge, to start in the Summer 2003. During her Wellcome Fellowship she will work on the history of Hungarian psychiatry in a European context, 1850–1918. She has edited and translated books in Hungary, and for many years was the editor and then editor-in-chief of the Budapest-based but internationally circulated social science journal *Replika*. She is currently working on a book in Hungarian, provisionally titled *Hipnózis, hisztéria, és pszichiátria a századfordulós Monarchiában* ('Hypnosis, Hysteria and Psychiatry in the Austro-Hungarian Monarchy at the Turn of the Century') to be published in 2003. She completed her MPhil thesis on a case of hysteria and hypnosis in the Austro-Hungarian Monarchy focussing on the doctor–patient negotiation, part of which was published in the *History of Psychiatry* (2002).

George Rousseau received his PhD at Princeton University and has taught at the universities of Harvard, UCLA, Cambridge, Oxford, Leiden, Lausanne, and Aberdeen. He is Emeritus Professor of the Humanities at De Montfort University and is now attached to the Faculty of Modern History at Oxford University. He has been Professor of Eighteenth-Century Studies at UCLA and Regius Professor of English at King's College Aberdeen in Scotland. His primary interest lies in the interface of literature and medicine, for which his work has been internationally acclaimed, most recently in the award of a three-year Leverhulme Trust Fellowship (1999–2001). His often-cited 1981 article, 'Literature and Medicine: the State of the Field', *Isis*, vol. LXXII (September 1981): 406–24, is often said to have charted a new academic field. He is the author of numerous articles and books dealing with medicine and the humanities, his most recent book, written jointly with Roy Porter, is *Gout: The Patrician Malady* (1998; 1999). He is based in Oxford, England.

David E. Shuttleton lectures in English Literature at the University of Wales, Aberystwyth, and has teaching and interdisciplinary research interests in the relationship between literary representations, medical culture and embodiment. He has published many essays, largely on eighteenth-century themes, and is co-editor of *Women and Poetry, 1660–1750*. He is currently editing the letters of the fashionable early-Georgian physician George Cheyne for *The Cambridge Edition of the Correspondence of Samuel Richardson* and writing a monograph on the literary representation of smallpox 1660–1830 for which he held a Clark Library fellowship in 2001.

Agnieszka Steczowicz is currently a doctoral student in the Modern Languages Faculty at the University of Oxford, and is writing a thesis on the use of the genre of paradox in the Renaissance disciplines of medicine, theology, law, natural philosophy, and the 'practical sciences' (ethics, politics, and economics). Before she came to Oxford she studied at the École Normale Supérieure (Fontenay) in France. Her academic interests are centred upon medieval and Renaissance intellectual and cultural history, and include the literature, art and science of the period.

Jane Weiss is an Assistant Professor in English Language Studies at the State University of New York College at Old Westbury. She received her doctorate in English and American Literature from the City University of New York Graduate Center in 1995. She has published articles on nineteenth-century domestic literature and the culture of domesticity, and is editing the journals of Susan Warner, a novelist who lived in New York and the Hudson Valley between 1819 and 1885. She has also worked as a researcher and consultant at two museums of nineteenth-century American culture, the Warner House at Constitution Island, and the Mount Vernon Hotel Museum and Garden in New York City. Her current scholarship includes a study of gardens and farms in nineteenth-century domestic culture, and an article examining the impact of the corporatization of the academy on scholarship and critical theory.

1
Introduction

George Sebastian Rousseau

Frames and framing

Frames hold many things but familiarly visual images. By doing so the frame shapes the picture inside it and gives it another form, or at least – once we begin to think about pictures in relation to frames – changes the meaning of its interior. Framing assumes pictures and – if extended by analogy to areas other than the visual – assumes that those subjects or objects can be understood in pictorial terms through a type of translation. Frames also serve to exhibit and display pictures, and – if the analogy is extended yet again – framing encourages viewers of pictures to ponder what it is that is occurring to the picture at its top and bottom and on its sides; at the rim where the picture meets the frame and inside the core at the perceived dead centre of the picture. The frame thus opens up all sorts of possibilities, even for absent, imaginary frames, for even bare pictures have borders whether or not we can actually see the frame. This point of juncture of the parts occurs on the margins. In our time margins – literal and imagined – have taken on a theoretical life of their own, as in the expressions we have generated about life on the margins and discourse on the borders of this or that perimeter.

Frames thus exist to delimit and confine and contextualize: especially to define the object in terms of diverse types of relevant constituent elements. The frame permits understanding, for example, of how the object is situated and evaluated. As Jacques Derrida claimed in 'The Parergon,' a famous theoretical essay about borders and margins, 'no theory or practice can be effective if it does not rest on the frame.'[1] The passage is worth citing at length:

No 'theory', no 'practice', no 'theoretical practice' can be effective here if it does not rest on the frame, the invisible limit of (between) the interiority of meaning (protected by the entire hermeneutic, semiotic, phenomenological, and formalist tradition) *and* (of) all the extrinsic empiricals which, blind and illiterate, dodge the question . . . Every analytic of aesthetic judgment presupposes that we can rigorously distinguish between the intrinsic and the extrinsic.

This 'resting' permits us to distinguish between the intrinsic and extrinsic of an object, in the case to hand – illness – the inside and outside of disease. And it further suggests that everything excluded in the process of moving from inside to outside contains the conditions of the possibilities for constructing contexts for disease and sickness. Hence frames contain pictures or images to the extent that they define perimeters and prevent pictures, or subjects, from expanding. Pictures without physical frames open up in ways unknown to those inside frames. Thus frames exist in relation to pictures as boxes serve to confine their contents.

Linguists, cognitive psychologists, anthropologists, psychoanalysts and a wide range of other types of other practitioners have resorted to the frame as their essential unit of measure, and it is by now common coinage to refer idiomatically to 'the way something is framed' as a shorthand for the kind of context that has been constructed around the object of attention. For example, linguist Deborah Tannen has divided frames into two essential categories: the first a 'frame of interpretation,' the other, a 'schema', amounting to the basic unit of knowledge structures themselves.[2] Tannen explains the difference and what is at stake in the two categories:

> The interactive notion of frame refers to a definition of what is going on in interaction, without which no utterance (or movement or gesture) could be interpreted. To use Bateson's classic example, a monkey needs to know whether a bite from another monkey is intended within the frame of play or the frame of fighting. People are continually confronted with the same interpretive task. In order to comprehend any utterance, a listener (and a speaker) must know within which frame it is intended: for example, is this joking? Is it fighting? Something intended as a joke but interpreted as an insult (it could of course be both) can trigger a fight.[3]

Hence frames are also contexts without which meaning can never be derived. So long as interpretations continue to be made frame interaction will occur: the juncture of meanings happening at the point where the competing interpretations exist or eventually will be contested. But frames are not secure objects. No matter how seemingly durable their material contents – whatever is inside the frame – they are tested at the point where image (the picture) meets the frame's border. All this suggests violence done to framing, as if the meeting points exert tension and friction on each other. It makes sense therefore to consider the degree of security of any frame, even if some frames are clearly firmer than others. Each case is different: no way exists to generalize from one instance to another.

Frames and the act of framing can also be contested on other grounds, not least for their degrees of efficiency. Tests can be made of the degree of security in confining the picture, but also bearing in mind the way the frame holds the picture or changes it. But even the efficiency of frames is less secure than meets the eye. The tests applied to distinguish degrees of efficiency are themselves subject to scrutiny and interrogation. In their discussion of 'frame shifting' and 'juggling frames', Deborah Tannen and Cynthia Wallat shrewdly demonstrate that the complexity of framing depends upon the number of audiences being reached and the timing of each interaction.[4] Their dissection of what happens, for example, in a paediatric examination – a simple medical encounter between mother, child and doctor – demonstrates the types of shifting and juggling that occur. Similar, if more complex, shifting and juggling occur in the medico-linguistic encounters we describe in the chapters of this collection. If anything, our translation of codes between written texts – past and present – and living persons makes the task more fraught.

So far we have been speaking of the frame primarily in the singular, as if each picture is permitted one and *only* one frame. But picture frames are plural; they always exist with the potential of a plurality of frames in mind. Every picture is a candidate for any number of frames, and it is less than clear what we mean when we claim that 'this frame is the best, or most appropriate, frame for this picture.' Do we mean best on the grounds of efficiency, security, lack of contestation by viewers, or by the application of other tests not yet devised or described?

Framing is also an abstract notion, bounded by a set of metaphors that endow both picture and frame with greater meaning than either could have without the other, just as a disease constellation is enlarged by viewing it in relation to its frame or frames, as this book aims to demonstrate. A disease without a frame has no boundaries or borders. It cannot sustain itself and possesses no interior domain. It rests or leans on nothing, yet it spills out everywhere, knows no limits, is both small and large by virtue of the lack of containment.[5]

No theory or practice can be effective if it does not lean in some way on the frame to provide its containment. Without the frame it contains neither inside or outside, nor can be seen for the object – the theory or practice – it is. In medicine, such pictures without frames would amount, as it were, to disease classifications without words and things, contexts and cultures. This resting, or leaning, is precisely what permits the possibility of distinguishing the object's intrinsic from its qualities. Diseases without frames possess neither insides or outsides nor limits or borders beyond which they retain their differences from other disease conditions. The history of medicine can be read – in one sense – as the progressive perfecting of tight-fitting frames: those which fit the empirical facts of observation without violating laws of logic and reason.

The suggestion therefore is that pictures, or diseases, without frames would fall apart or collapse; or at least be so loosely defined as to be virtually indistinguishable from other disease constellations. An unframed picture on a wall is bounded by the wall – a frame of sorts – but remains ambiguous in many ways it would not have been with the security of a specially constructed frame, no matter how unstable or unpredictable. If this fitting is the best the frame maker can have made, there probably was a reason.[6]

Yet if framing is a notion about the way the mind confronts reality – the direction in which this line of reason seems to be moving – it can be approached both in historical and transhistorical modes. The latter transhistorical mode collapses time – all diachronic components evaporate, as it were – and proceeds as if the metaphors of framing are sufficient to carry out all of its work. Language in medicine becomes sufficient in and of itself. The former framing – the historical – proceeds by demonstrating that the metaphors themselves are generated under specific local circumstances and socio-economic conditions that play a part in shaping the metaphors. How large that share was becomes a question of paramount significance for the students of framing. Therefore it makes all the difference whether one approaches these acts of framing in historical or transhistorical terms.

Collectively we invoke the former – the historical versions – in part because our diseases were themselves historically constructed, as were the diverse discourses treated below representing these disease constellations and, in turn, shaping them through reverse reciprocity. That is, the perceptions of doctors, patients, participants, observers and commentators, involved in these transactions and cultural negotiations were themselves produced by historically contingent situations. What would it mean, for example, to dislodge a person – a patient – from her era? To disembody language from its historically situated speakers? To dislocate symptoms and their semiological interpretations from the flesh-and-blood bodies that were themselves bounded by diachronic time and space? To wrench texts encoding and representing these medical subjects from the circumstances, no matter how bizarre or eccentric, in which they were generated? To construe medical representations as if they had evolved outside history: beyond the pale of individual lives – happy and sad, healthy and pathological – which constitute biographies? Apart from the vast annals of autobiographical literature and outside the small groups who add up to what social historians call a society, and so forth? In brief, to frame disease as if its *métier* were transhistorical without any need to provide evidence?

Imagining disease

We hope the essays collected in this volume will persuade readers of (at least some of) the virtues of an historical approach, standing in opposition in large part to the theoretical gaze cast by such recent synthesizers as Michel Foucault.[7] If this is the case, this historical, as distinct from transhistorical, imperative may nevertheless have less utility for the categories implicated in the imagining of illness. Even in analogous forms, as we have developed them above, the two activities – framing and imagining – seem to be divided by a gap between them. The matter addresses the nature of the divide and what sorts of bearing this divide has for the framing of disease within cultural history.

The imagining of pictures would seem to be an altogether different activity, existing in counterpoint to framing them. This subject is, of course, vast and cannot be treated here. Still, a few basics begin to focus on the differences: the imagined picture does not yet exist, is not drawn or painted, except within the imagination of particular minds. An undrawn picture has no frame, almost by definition, not even in the mind – the imagined picture is thus at least as unstable and insecure as the painted image. It too resides in the mind in the sense that the mind slowly endows it with form and is nonetheless real than the fully-drawn canvas; but its ontological status would seem to be different. It is the picture one *will* draw; the picture one *can* paint. Even in its imaginary state its borders are more vulnerable than the already painted picture while it still lacks frames. The imagination may not visualize it as existing inside concrete frames at all, and this lack is one of the main differences from its representation when a finished canvas. The point of this analogizing for imagining disease is our *raison d'être*.[8]

It is not merely that the analogy throws light on the latter, especially on medical conditions that have not, as yet, been born. It has also begun to lead the way to the pathologizing and medicalization of types of human behaviour in history which forms much of the heart of Parts II and III of this book. The point of these distinctions is that the imagining of disease has much in common with imagining pictures, especially undrawn pictures in the mind. Fred Hoyle, the noted contemporary astronomer, may have drawn (unconsciously?) on these processes in his book *Diseases from Space* (New York: Harper & Row, 1979). Less fabulously, the doctor pronounces a name which will become the label of a disease: AIDS, cancer, dementia, diabetes, gout, insanity, stroke. He has probably learned it in a medical school; the name of a human malady which was once imagined and did not as yet exist, just as Johannes Hofer, a now obscure Alsatian army surgeon of the late seventeenth century, invented the condition of nostalgia (from the Greek root *nostos*, meaning home, and *algia*, the disease of longing for).[9] Once named and defined the name became the label for a malady: a shorthand for all sorts of relationships and associations, and, in turn, began to conjure pictures in the imagination of both doctor (surgeon or physician) and patient. Hence label and picture existed in sets of historical relationships. But these pictures in the mind also had internalized frames, whether or not doctors – and, eventually through transmission, patients – were aware of them. Pictures were sometimes self-contained, at other times spilling over and overflowing, to the rest of the patient's body beyond the insides of the head, as in images of disease as battle or warfare. These are idiosyncratic pictures – of turmoil, fire, flames, the apocalypse of life – and partake of images forming part of a coherent pictorial language: the language of imagining illness. They include the patient's imagining of disease: the psychotic's pictures, for example, in *art brut*; the neurotic's seemingly unintelligible and incoherent verbal discourse which itself needs to be framed – to lean on something else – to be decoded; the cancer patient's ruminations on a bleak future visualized as barren, leafless seacoast stretching for miles with pounding waves that gradually engulf him, or as a pyre with gigantic flames in which she will be burned to a crisp.[10]

Names and labels also participate in these acts of imagining. But however different this imagining of disease is from conceptualizing it as malady containing *pre-existing* frames – such as the tuberculosis that entails a wasting away but that is nevertheless not the more invasive ravishment of cancer – it nonetheless bears similarities to framing disease.[11] Framed diseases and imagined diseases are not entirely opposed, nor do they lie in total counterpoint: they exist on a spectrum of contingency in which the imagination always plays a large role.[12] The parallels of the two types of disease-forming overlap at the margins and on the rims of their imaginary worlds, riddled both by core insides and by marginal outsides. Both are obsessed by inclusions and exclusions within their figuration of disease – on the practical level by the ravages malady will bring, or – if fortunate – the havoc illness may not play. So let us imagine: the patient has been diagnosed with cancer of the pancreas, has given it a label. The physician has named the disease. The patient engages in no conscious notions of framing his cancer – that is, rationally conjecturing at what points and in what ways it will impinge on his life – but, instead, begins to imagine it. What pictures will he imagine? What scenes of devastation? What rises before him in the conflagration of his final illness when this smallest of hidden organs burns up the rest of his body? Or is it they – the other organs – which will eventually consume the pancreas?

A context for frames

The serious framing of categories generally – in philosophy and science – has by now had a venerable history. In this context one means by categories subjects, or topics, under careful scrutiny, such as life, death, liberty, freedom and – more specifically – subjects or topics within recognizable discourses or academic disciplines. The more self-conscious the subject of study, the more rigorous, it seems, the applications applied in relation to the frame, as in art history, where framing has practically been elevated into a science by now.[13]

That framing as a self-conscious reflective process should have loomed so large in recent history is unsurprising. As the social sciences, especially anthropology, introduced a new relativism into the exploration of the humanities historically viewed, new forms of self-reflexivity were required. If tropes of the savage and civilized, for example, could frame each other and thereby prevent the other from collapse (that is, the civilized transformed almost by sleight of hand into the savage and vice-versa), it soon became apparent that discourse about language also implied the vocabulary of the other: coherent discourse implying its other as incoherent discourse and vice-versa. Hence the language of the psychotic was said to be as coherently organized, albeit according to different norms, as that of so-called healthy persons.[14]

ll rigorous thought is, of course, self-reflective to a degree: weary about itself and fretting about its ontological status and truth claims; framed thought perhaps doubly so in that it construes the categories it studies with rigour and subjugates them (the categories) to different kinds of contextualization and problematization. In our generation frames have been tested through diverse approaches ranging from the epistemological and ontological to the anthropological and broadly cultural – this gamut partly in response to the challenge of postmodern methodologies which have themselves been under unusually tense scrutiny. In medicine, the interaction between patients and doctors in the so-called 'medical interview' has been shown to be far more coded, if also confusing and in need of close scrutiny, than was previously thought.[15] Hitherto medical writing proved to be the site of ambiguity as literary critics of diverse persuasions analyzed its form and content. But now historical-medical treatises have found competitors in other linguistic interchanges.

Theorizing about frames has also become an especially active field in our time as the result of a widespread preoccupation with methodology at large. Sensuous, spontaneous, unreflective approaches seem to have been decreasing since the 1970s. Researchers in all fields are routinely requested to reflect on their methodologies and, then, to justify their approaches to particular topics depending on an array of local and global factors. These must in turn be explained along the lines of established method. By the time we spiral downward to the framing of disease we discover a topic embedded inside no one subject or discipline but simultaneously within medicine, culture, history and representation. A whole series of negotiations must occur before we can even begin to understand how the framing occurred; and most of these are far more culture-bound and socially determined than so-called pure, medical theory – whatever that could be.

Hence it is becoming increasingly clear that no single discipline is adequate to explain how diseases – especially diseases in history – attained their current profiles. How cancer, for example, developed its particular sets of cultural codes and pictures to the mind, or depression the widespread embrace it has received today in all western societies (and perhaps eastern too if the studies of depression in China and Japan are accurate[16]) without comprehending how it evolved in this way. How consumption progressed from the sixteenth century, being later transformed into phthisis and tuberculosis, and then cementing itself to the most bizarre, lingering images and metaphors common in the high Romanticism of the nineteenth century; images swept by notions of social class, heroism, nationalism, romance, destiny. Or, alternatively, why madness has continued to be the least stable of the framed maladies. Whatever these processes of framing amounted to historically – and, as a group of expositors, we would probably concur that our work comes early rather than late in this self-reflective development of framing – they cannot have been entirely, or even pre-eminently, *medical*. They have also been – perhaps more prominently – visual, narrative, rhetorical, moral, political, mythic, religious, and allegorical (if loosely construed as the representation within disease of something standing in for something else: illness as the substitute for moral defect). The Jobean framing of disease, where illness is interpreted according to the severity of types Job suffered, would fill a book in itself. And for a major portion of western human history Job-the-comforter was a guide in the early-modern world for patients' framing of disease: according to his sufferings they could measure their own gradation.[17]

Jobean morality was merely one of several kinds of framing: another type is found in Defoe. In *Robinson Crusoe* (1719) Robinson recognizes, by his near encounter with death through fatal illness, that all along he has been a sinner. At the time of malady he is already far removed from society, having by this time been shipwrecked on the deserted island for almost twenty years. In the fictions of Tobias Smollett, a ship surgeon who secured overnight literary success with his first bestselling novel *Roderick Random* (1747), sickness also plays a major thematic role.[18] Literally dozens of doctors who populate these Smollettian pages are satirized, and the actual medicine of the epoch is framed in ways that must have appeared extraordinary to the mid-eighteenth-century reading public. Smollett frames his ideas by appealing to greed as the most interesting of the passions and dissects every aspect of – what he calls – 'the medical knot': an intricate set of relationships among practitioners all vying for economic gain with little regard for care or cure. He could be called an early sociologist of medicine. But this merely tags him; surely, it is more accurate to extract from his framings a passionate adherence to the persistence of the economic motive in all medical transactions.[19] He remained an experimental novelist throughout his career without ever surrendering the primacy of the medical motif, which renders him a primary candidate for framing in our sense, and he could well have been the subject of one of the below chapters. Even his last work, widely considered to be his masterpiece – *The Adventures of Humphry Clinker* (1771) – is the comic journey of five characters in search of different kinds of health.

Nineteenth-century literature embroidered these incorporations and embodied medicine as a lynchpin to understanding its main characters through the status of their bodies. Some authors appealed to physiognomy and phrenology, others to craniology and the brain, still others – like Coleridge and de Quincey and the opium prophets – explored mind–body consciousness as revealed in dreams.[20] In the words of George Eliot disease both protects and removes her protagonists from society, rendering the author Eliot (and her hero, Dr Lydgate in *Middlemarch*) a free-floating agent unaccountable to society's exigencies. Charles Darwin's chronic illness – forever sick to ensure that he could pamper himself and get on with his work largely by functioning outside society – was the daytime reality of this fictive Otherworld of malady: yet another species of behaviour he had observed in himself. At least in Victorian and Edwardian literature down through D. H. Lawrence, where the sexual body in both its healthy and pathological states still holds the keys to revelation, these frames have figured pre-eminently. If there is a general point that all these fictions reveal it is that sickness guarantees the imagined removal from society – the chance to go it alone. In these post-Romantic versions sickness is imagined as the guarantor of solitude, social apartheid, individualism, the ultimate freedom so many nineteenth-century heroes and heroines craved. Their maladies may be conjured rather than real, yet they serve primary functions in the novel.[21]

Yet fiction is only one of several contexts for framing disease. There are many others, and we would not wish to imply otherwise. But fiction, and in particular the novel, was in fact the most popular form of literature in the western world after the great European Revolution of 1848. The uses it made of medicine are so diverse that they could be distilled into a taxonomy of frames, in the way we saw Tannen and Wallat construct a classification of linguistic frames. Fiction itself is obviously a type of 'context' (something *con*, or with, the *text*). Our point is rather that disease has multiple contexts: some more appropriate, some less, for particular conditions and that we need to take stock of how diseases acquired the diverse profiles we take for granted. In some instances – depression, for example – we are utterly baffled about how we arrived at the point we find ourselves in today, a strange, almost Shandean trajectory from the old Renaissance melancholy.[22]

Framing disease

The framing of disease began to preoccupy academic medical historians in the United States during the 1970s. They did not proffer their research in this way – framing again – but this is what their peregrinations in search of method amounted to.[23] Then, in the 1980s when the wave in attention given to the body crested, cultural historians followed suit. Around that time (although the moment itself is difficult to pinpoint), diverse groups began to ask hard questions about the status and profile of medical conditions in relation to the body, even as generalized affliction, pain and suffering outside narrow disease constellations. The mountain of work on these subjects was so large, and impressive, it would impossible to survey. Suffice it to say that disease and malady was elevated to a new threshold – one asking hard ontological questions about the objects themselves. Resistance emerged from hardliners, who claimed that the history of medicine should not range so widely: these were the internalists whose gaze was fixed to the craft or *techne* of their subject. But even they proved vulnerable to the waves of interdisciplinarity sweeping over all the humanities during this period. Besides, they found themselves outnumbered by those asserting that the time had come to be more reflective about contexts. As interdisciplinary methodologies were triumphing and the new cultural history began to embrace the discourses of the body that included illness, pain, suffering, death, indeed, all the forms of body derangement, these 'internalists' lost out.

Set the dials to 1985, for example, and it was clear that those academics serious about the study of the body – healthy and pathological – were equally vigilant to the types of contexts they would need to construct. These included the historical, medical, ethical and metaphorical, as in the body of the text, the body politic, and many other types of bodies. Sufficient attention was to legitimate a large conference on the framing of disease held in 1988 at the College of Physicians in Philadelphia under the expert direction of Professors Charles E. Rosenberg and Janet Golden: historians with a wide net and democratic gaze at the recent development of their field who could hardly be considered internalists. The talks at this conference were delivered almost exclusively by medical historians who later collected (some of) their papers and published them four years later in an important book edited by the conference organizers: Charles E. Rosenberg and Janet Golden (eds), *Framing Disease: Studies in Cultural History* (New Brunswick, NJ: Rutgers University Press, 1992).[24]

This landmark volume, published a decade ago and a companion to an earlier collection edited by Edward Clarke, *Modern Methods in the History of Medicine*,[25] construed its task in chronological terms and according to social categories. That is, it divided and classified the various approaches of its members into two basic formations: 1. historical eras and 2. socio-institutional categories. The divisions made pre-eminent sense, especially in light of the contributors' background, and advanced the state of the history of medicine, as some reviewers acknowledged.[26] In this sense *Framing Disease: Studies in Cultural History* was to prove in time an important and influential academic book, and any young scholars overlooked it at their peril. But it was actually less interdisciplinary than it seemed, and its authors dealt a sleight of hand to private voices and their literary embodiments. Rosenberg and Golden fixed their attention on the historical period – Renaissance, Enlightenment, Romantic, Victorian – in relation to disease formation. Literature as the great purveyor of knowledge and disseminator of information – high and low, serious and comic – hardly figured at all.[27] Susan Sontag had already opened up everyone's eyes to the metaphoric possibilities of illness in this heyday of AIDS, but the academic community was slow to take up her gauntlet.[28] By contrast, the approach adopted in our volume minimizes historical periods and social factors (important as these factors have been in social history) and aims to frame instead with language and narrative categories in mind; especially the strategies of persuasion used by narrators, whether sufferers or healers or gazers, and the range of narrative modes sought by those eager to express their thought about states of health or illness.[29]

The differences between the Rosenbergian enterprise and the Rousseavian – if one may group the former for the purposes of brevity into a shorthand of the Rosenbergian and the latter into the Rousseauvian without suggesting that either set of contributors was in the least influenced by their organizer – are noteworthy. Where Rosenberg and his team turn to society – its collective voice in social arrangements and public institutions – Rousseau and his fellow contributors gravitate to individual voices; in particular, those of poets, novelists, philosophers, diarists, memoirists, all those who are recording, the mind's wreckage on the body rather than merely vice-versa. Literature, more than any other domain, contains this massive annals of the private voice. Literature may be unreliable in all sorts of ways, and it may be too vast a territory for historians of medicine to tackle (since no one can learn everything), but as the repository of the solitary expressive voice it has no competitor, especially in the face of pain, malady, suffering, death, and the annihilation of the self.[30]

These Rousseavian acts of framing also require the active participation of a category such as imagination: hence the imagining, as well as the framing, of disease. The addition is not fanciful or rhetorical or resurrected here because historically it was medical theory that pathologized the imagination and paved the way for the late Enlightenment discourses of 'diseased imagination' that nurtured a theory of insanity. Rather, it appears, even in the title of our book, because imagination plays a main role in the cognitive processes and epistemological models generated by the dual acts of framing and imagining. If anything, we ought to have paid more attention to the differences. We should have stated more emphatically than we do when one of us – or some obscure figure of the past – is framing rather than imagining and what the overlaps and reciprocities are. Finally, where Rosenberg and his group mentalize according to disease conditions (the disease label is more often than not their frame), Rousseau's group tends to internalize the frame in terms of the imaginary: the unseen, the invisible, the unheard, the barely expressed.

Moreover, Rosenberg's frames are generally embedded in public discourse, their cerebral dimensions outstripping any private emotional ones; in contrast, Rousseau's framed discourses are idiosyncratic, private, and solitary, and they court fear and terror. They assume that the individual voice is as valid as the public, collective one. Everywhere in the Rousseavian endeavour are traces of an arduous process of coping with death by somehow imagining it and giving it a language, even imagining it as death-in-life. Given that mortals have no more highly developed equipment with which to formulate complex thoughts than language broadly construed (for example, the language of music), and have no higher capacity than the linguistic, it is not surprising that words should feature so prominently in the Rousseavian frames. In brief, we think – to the degree we can agree – that the language used to frame historical illness and disease is as significant as the malady itself.

By vesting so much in language we do not mean to lend an impression that we are in any way idiosyncratic in our views of people in the past and the suffering they endured. Of course, we acknowledge the history of pain and – institutionally – the history of medicine as a discrete discipline, entitled, as it is, to its own professional needs and codes. As moderns – and postmoderns – living in a world in which the cost of medical provision grows exponentially, we accept that medical realism is a fact of life: the diurnal reality of doctors, hospitals, diagnoses, patients, illness infectious and genetic, and – of course – the huge cost of supporting all this. But by elevating the ante, as it were, of the representational in framing, our approach also assumes that medicine is now too important (and expensive) a component of the human story to be left entirely to medical experts and specialists whose gaze may be narrowly focused: certainly they cannot tell the whole story of suffering.[31]

We need to complement their work with the record of private voices and solitary texts, but always keeping an empirical history of medicine in the foreground of our imagination.[32] Until recently the history of medicine has largely focused on disease as seen from the top down (this was certainly true until the last generation), generally without listening to private voices. This state of affairs is changing, we know, and we hope that approaches of the sort found here will accelerate the pace. Furthermore, it has become clear that medicine has played a larger role in shaping cultural history than has been conceded previously. The modes of expression through which the life of the body has been configured remains a large and demanding agenda. This wider cultural understanding of medicine includes discussion of the frames and forms of imagination through which, and inside which, disease is constructed. The strands of argument are diverse, and the processes complex. There is a need to embrace multiple layers of pain, suffering, deprivation, and death, as well as the all too necessary illness diagnoses offered by medical practitioners.

This version of *framing and imagining disease* construes language and discourse as inherent in the process. Language was, of course, crucial in the formation of medical and scientific theory itself over the centuries – how could it not be? But that consideration of language is more literal than the versions treated here in terms of narrative, rhetoric, genre, and especially metaphor, and – for those imagining poems or fictions with deep-layer medical content the way they moved from the other to the other. Tone, voice and literary form must be included in these considerations. The genre into which a speaker – and also a writer – deposits thoughts, as if in a box which itself frames a set of objects, is often a singular clue to intention and desire. But genres, no less than medical theories, also possess contexts and histories; a transhistorical view of them may be as delimiting as synchronic histories without time lines.[33]

The 'frame', then, is inherently interdisciplinary in the sense that it belongs to no single discourse or academic discipline. However, ownership and its implications must not be minimized even in postdisciplinary life. The fact that most scholars who conceptualize disease and frame illness in this linguistically charged way continue to be students of language and literature is not without effect. Literary scholars apprize themselves about the facts of disease in history no less than healthcare professionals read – indeed consume – literature and make the time to read about the lives of its writers. It would be the rare approach within our enterprise (the below essays) that wilfully ignored the facts of – for example – plague, tuberculosis, cholera, influenza, AIDS. Hence it needs emphasizing yet again that while we are not prejudiced towards tran-shistorical approaches or purely theoretical formulations privileging themes and tropes, we have nevertheless given preference in this vol-ume to scholars whose method is primarily empirical and historical.[34]

This leaves the historical imperative: *what type of history?* Many scholars today number themselves among the ranks of cultural historians, yet we perceive that some of their interfaces differ from ours. Collectively we emphasize, of course, different threads in the historical enterprise and harbour different senses of the domains of literature and medicine. But most of us would concur in the belief that we must know *both* areas in depth: not merely each as labels or metaphors for something else (the old issue of realism again and its forms of evidence) but for the role they played within literary and medical history. Beyond this point it is a fea-ture of almost every one of these essays that they continue to reflect the author's wonder about the appearance of each domain in the heartland of the other. It is probably impossible to affirm when, or how, medicine was discovered in, or recovered for, literature – its traces are so inherent in the human condition that it may have been there from the earliest-known oral literature. It can certainly be clearly detected in the Homeric poems, which start with a dream as the sign of troubled mind in dis-turbed body; throughout biblical scripture (Job's narrative remains the greatest story ever told about the sufferer reproaching his God); in sev-eral of the Platonic dialogues. Every subsequent civilization, Medieval or Renaissance, eastern or western, learned – sooner or later – that it could not omit medicine and the body from the categories of its domi-nant concerns. Why then should it not be inscribed in its imaginative literature? Each description acted as if it were reinventing the world anew: explaining how patient-sufferers conceptualized their experience of violation done to their bodies in the terms of sickness or illness. Patients often aimed to capture – in our conceptualization unwittingly to frame – their experience of suffering in literature. It was more essen-tial to be a sufferer than a trained doctor when describing the kingdom of sickness. In extreme cases writers had themselves not sufferered but nonetheless described and commented on others' pain. What differ-ences were these?[35]

We glimpse what is at stake in a long didactic poem of the early eight-eenth century by William Thompson (1712–66), one of the lengthiest explicit poetic pronouncements about illness over the whole course of that century. David Shuttleton has discussed this work in his chapter below and I will not repeat his comments here except to draw out their further ramifications for the framing of disease. Historically, the 1740s proved to be a crucial watershed for the rapid development of the Romantic strain in poetry as well as the incorporation of health into literature. It is probably no accident that several long poems of this period were then devoted to this subject. In 1744 the long didactic poems of two physicians appeared: John Armstrong's *Art of Preserving Health*, versifying wisdom about staying well and growing old, and Mark Akenside's *Pleasures of Imagination*, permeated with fantasies about the role played by the body's anatomical nerves, spirits and fibres in the imaginative act.[36] These were followed by Thompson's *Sickness: A Poem* (1745) and, a year later, Malcolm Flemyng's epic *Neuropathia*, or the pathway of the nerves. Flemyng's grand epic poem was composed in Latin hexameter verse (never translated into English) over hundreds of lines displaying the post-Newtonian confidence that wondrous physiological fibres pulsate on the inner highways of the bloodstream – a type of busy Enlightenment anatomical Internet.[37] These sprawling poems seemed to blend into each other and lurked, as it were, under the 1747 umbrella of Thomas Warton's *Pleasures of Melancholy*, as if to suggest that poets are chemically deranged melancholics whose bodily humours are out of kilter through a surfeit of black bile.[38]

But *Sickness's* three-canto structure extending to approximately 2,000 lines is perhaps unique among these poems of the 1740s for its focus on illness as a central theme. It was written – as the author claims – after his recovery from a near-fatal smallpox. Thompson, unlike most of these other poets of the 1740s, was not a trained doctor (although neither was Warton). He had read Classics at Queen's College Oxford and succeeded to a vicarage in Hampton Poyle, Oxfordshire. Here, in rural semi-seclusion and enjoying the gift of his sinecure, he pursued his primary passion, poetry. A close call with death around the time of Pope's and Swift's deaths (respectively 1744 and 1745) brought his intimations on mortality to the foreground and gave him the confidence that illness was a fit subject for high heroic poetry. Otherwise, he had no role models for this incorporation of illness into literature and took his creative chances: as he says, 'I don't remember to have seen any poem on the same subject to lead me on the way.'[39]

Thompson's other poetic concerns in *Sickness* also touch on framing. He had read widely in the ancient classical literature and was steeped in canonical poetry in English, especially Spenser, whose diction and syntax he often imitated. The recent deaths of Pope and Swift further prompted him to reflect on the immensity of their influence on him. But his launching into a new province of poetry – the versification of illness – made him to take stock of his own physical and poetic resources. For one thing he was profoundly worried that readers would neither understand medical terminology nor be able to stomach his explicit descriptions of illness: 'it cannot be suppos'd that I should treat upon sickness in a medicinal, but only in a descriptive, moral and religious manner'. Medical realism appeared potentially perilous to him because it had not yet been widely adopted as an appropriate subject for long poems – hence my point about the framing of illness in the poetry of the 1740s. As a result Thompson omitted the gory details, nor did he allegorize or generalize them – a mainstay of his framing: 'I have just taken such notice of the progress of the Smallpox as may give the reader some small idea of it, *without offending his imagination* [my emphasis].'[40]

Thompson's approach frames both poetry and sickness. First, despite the recognition that health and its opposites are mighty subjects for literature the poet must not indulge a habit to provide too much detail or the reader will pause.[41] Secondly, Thompson settles on the metaphor of war or battle rather than (for example) the stage of disease – illness as theatre – for his dominant image. Sickness is frequently compared to the fires of hell that engulf him; force him to fight on as 'Aetna rages here. . . with her fury and furies.'[42] Over time war and theatre have been the two dominant images in the metaphorical representation of sickness: entire books could be written on the spectacle of each. Thirdly, Thompson frames his own illness by claiming – and here he anticipated the school of Romantic poets who celebrated the joys of melancholy as 'Ah what ails thee knight at arms alone and palely loitering' – that those who ail have heightened sensibilities. It is something of a *quid pro quo*: poetic art in return for ill health. Thompson's long eulogy to Alexander Pope in Book II is not merely appropriate (Pope had just died) but also serves to frame the homology between sickness and writing:

> With pain embarras'd, all his tedious days,
> and head-achs acked, the boundless sea of wit
> Spread o'er the world.[43]

Pope, a lifelong invalid despite holding to a hectic routine, claimed that his body never enjoyed three days of consecutive health, and he was obsessed by his aches and pains. His poetry contains many references to his ailments, but never as the main theme or centrepiece (his *Epistle to Dr Arbuthnot*, for example, written to a physician who is himself remarkably literary, includes medical content only to the degree that it has larger moral and artistic significance).[44] Finally, Thompson positions his ideas around two main moral frames (frames in our sense) lodged in God and friendship: these are the Jobean beliefs that the deity has created doctors and potions as an act of benevolence to mankind, and, secondly, the (again Jobean) view that friends count for more than anything during illness: 'Health is disease, life death, without a friend.'[45] Having carved out his kingdom of illness, Thompson continues by drawing on the old paradoxical tradition in medicine, which Agnieszka Steczowicz will expound in her chapter, that 'Health's the disease of morals: few in health/ Turn o'er the volumes which will make us wise.'[46]

The months it took Thompson to execute his poem also forced him to reconsider providence's benignity in sparing him. Hence his tributes to Mercy and Hygeia (the goddess of health). The particular malady, as Shuttleton shows, was smallpox but Thompson devotes only a fraction of his attention to the onset and progress of this disease. He is more concerned to 'frame' his experience in other ways: especially by arguing that sickness is a fit subject for poetry; conversely, that it is foolish to waste time on ephemera – trifling themes – when great subjects like health are available. A poem like Thomas Gray's 'Ode on the death of a favourite cat', for example, which would appear just two years later in 1748, makes the case, even if it is structurally and rhetorically far more accomplished than any lines Thompson ever wrote.[47] High-mindedness energizes the new framing precisely because the state of health is not something that can be taken for granted: hence the invocation to Urania (muse of astronomy and scientific phenomena), the dramatic descriptions of the onset of a great illness and its first sudden attacks, and the extended allegory of the 'Palace of Disease' (I: 252–380) in which all major diseases are enumerated as if in an epic catalogue.

I have lingered over these poetic frames of the 1740s in order to make the point about an important moment in the evolution of English poetry at a time when it brushes closely with illness.[48] Suffice it to say here that some of Thompson's anxiety was his – and other poets' – doubt about the way forward in the immediate aftermath of Pope's death in 1744. These writers (Armstrong, Akenside, Flemyng, Thompson et al.) felt they had to move away from Pope's poetic forms and versify in other ways. But the explanation is insufficient in itself: they were also turning to fresh fields as the route to human improvement. They hoped to gain greater entry into their souls – a deeper self-knowledge – through the experience of fleshly suffering. For decades autobiographers and memoirists had recounted their illnesses, so why shouldn't take poets themselves?[49] Thompson, however, is comparatively silent about the poet's melancholy and the generic solitude of illness. Briefly he mentions spleen and – of course – the smallpox from which he had recovered, but he omits to acknowledge how the patient suffers *alone* (one thinks, in contrast, of the later post-Romantic ethic that each of us dies alone). And he appears oblivious, in turn, to the compensatory pleasures of malady: the possibility that such shoring up of the self in times of bodily crisis, and the ensuing spiritual warfare, was somehow salutary. For Thompson, Armstrong, Flemyng and most of their poetic contemporaries of the 1740s melancholy's web – spleen, vapours, all the low spirits – necessitated solitude as a precondition of the malady. But the huge range of pleasures such solitariness conferred had not yet been imagined. Nor did their poetic contemporaries of the 1740s – Edward Young, William Collins, and Thomas Gray (whose morbidly depressive personality should have alerted him to the pleasures of melancholy rather more than they did[50]) – explicitly celebrate or extol these pleasures. That would come a generation later, by which time illness of every type had become established as proper subject for literature. But the explicit portion of the foregrounding entails the point here about framing and imagining illness.

Those poets cited above happened to be writing in the English language; they could as well have been composing in French or German, and it was in France in the next century – the nineteenth – that the pleasures of melancholy would be elevated almost to the status of a verbal science.[51] On both sides of the Channel new concerns for self and ego in a troubled post-1789, and then post-1815, political milieu combined to produce a new psychology. Concurrently, the institutionalization of psychiatry – first in England on a small scale and then on a grander scale in the Paris medical schools under the tutelage of doctors Pinel and Esquirol – changed the pathway of melancholy's future. In an increasingly secular world, in which religious inspiration was receding, derangement was increasingly ascribed to socio-economic causation. Here too was another type of framing, as we shall see below.

Organization of the volume

The chapters in this volume amount to a series of explorations of the appropriateness of diverse frames. In an ideal world in which we could have first imagined contributions and then commanded them there would have been greater plenitude and diversity, as well as a larger number and different ordering of sections. For example, we can imagine sections on framing disease in non-western cultures and in other historical periods; imagine illness in pictures exclusive of words except for the words needed to describe these images; conceptualize frames for disease along economic class lines in different societies. But this has not happened and we have been delighted instead to work with what we were fortunate enough to find. Collectively we are all too aware that our approach is eclectic, and can only respond to the criticisms it will inevitably elicit that our contributors, however excellent, are comparatively few and work in narrow periods of cultural history or in the long-distance trajectories of disciplinary histories (i.e., the history of psychiatry, the history of madness and so forth).

Our contributors also work in different disciplines and are united by their consuming interest in literary discourse and its representations in texts, genres, and word patterns. Even the historians among us will concede the major role played by literature in the versions of framing given below: a different state of affairs from approaches in which history – especially the history of medicine – assumes the lion's share. In those framings within the history of medicine (Rosenbergian) literature seems strangely absent; in these (Rousseauvian) it may appear that we are deaf to class distinctions, political and economic structures, the social arrangements of societies, and the integral dependence of sickness on religious belief. We acknowledge these gaps in advance and can only hope that subsequent volumes on framing disease will include them as we continue to refine our eclectic approaches.

But none of these caveats should suggest that we have been cavalier about our methodology. Each of us has been vigilant to, and reflective about, the nature of our enterprise. Each of us is immersed one way or another in the fine detail of our topics – Clifford Geertz's resonating phrase 'thick-description' in *The Interpretation of Cultures* (1973) comes to mind. In another academic identity each of us is a specialist, or expert, in the subject we write about here, whether smallpox in the eighteenth century or the development of Tropenkoller (tropical fever in German colonies at the end of the nineteenth century), and we hope to have penetrated so thoroughly to the heart of our specialism that each of the chapters presented here holds up in its own right. That is, each of the contributions sustains itself to the degree that any other expert without our penchant for framing disease would think it breaks new ground purely by dint of its relation to the narrow internal field – for example, the new research presented here on the reception of Thomas Mann's *The Magic Mountain* (1924) among medical practitioners, or the extensive accumulations of allusion and reference to heart disease in Victorian literary culture.

This said, all of our chapters have been conceived also as if they were trial-runs executed for the generation of a discursive frame: each is situated within a defined era or epoch and then contextualized in particular cultures. We are fortunate to be able to cover a broad expanse of chronology, from the early-modern world to the present, since this ensures that our frames are not repetitive within one society, although we are the first to concede that even within small groups sickness is diversely framed. Despite the limited number of case studies presented here, the diversity of figures, national settings, and historical eras ensures a sufficiently broad repertoire from which to develop a feel for transhistorical frames. Our goal is to buttress the belief that we can only understand the insides and outsides, as it were, of disease conditions if our frames are sufficiently developed.

Each of our four sections – framing and imagining disease, framing and imagining madness, the patient's narratives and images, a poetics and metaphorics of disease – possesses a historical context and historiography, and each has already evolved to an advanced degree in the current interdisciplinary debates about the historical body and its healthy and pathological productions. If the first (framing and imagining disease) represents the bread-and-butter of our approach – the selection of a category and its discourse representations in the attempt to explicate its contours at a historical moment – the second dealing with madness is somewhat different. It demonstrates that madness, at least relatively recent versions that have been reframed since the rise of psychiatry in the late eighteenth century, has had a closer affinity with literature than other forms of written cultural artifact. Whether this is because the mad are more prone to write or because their writing has proved their best therapy (at least as valid as art therapy), the fact remains that insanity has relied more intensely on language than other types of medical pathology.[52]

The patient's own narratives captured in his own voice (Part III) flourishes today as the study of pathographesis and few literary historians will be surprised that self-analysis has made such strides in our time, to the extent that writing classes all over the world encourage their students therapeutically to write themselves out of anguish and pain. Both chapters in Part III make specific contributions to the debate: one looks at the role of naming in the patient's cosmology of illness, while the other considers mistaken self-diagnosis and its consequences for recovery in the future. Part IV focuses on the poetics and metaphorics of disease. Like pathographesis, this is an established area for those immersed in the interfaces of medicine and literature. This is a proliferating field, unsurprisingly when we recall that even the most basic concepts of medicine – contagion, pollution, communicability, to seize only on the fundamental words in English used for the transmission of illness – are thickly metaphoric. The significance of our fourth section (Part IV), we think, is that it breaks ground by being *overtly* historical. Whether in Renaissance Italy, as in Agnieszka Steczowicz's chapter, or Kirstie Blair's new approach to the clichés about the heart and head in nineteenth-century England, it is important to note the degree to which each author had to steep herself in the core centre of the philosophical ideas studied. We can well think of other sections – for example, the doctor's first-person narratives on subjects *other than* his case histories or medical pronouncements, or patients' responses to rationed medicine in history – but we hope that the four sections included here are sufficiently representative to indicate the range of methodologies invoked to frame and imagine illness.

Approaches to framing and imagining disease

Caterina Albano starts our collection by offering a series of frames for the phenomenon of self-starvation, which she resists labelling anorexia, instead focusing her gaze on the late-seventeenth-century English case study of one Martha Taylor, the modernity of which is compelling. Albano asks how starvation has been a mirror *as well as* a lamp of the local cultures producing it: a double-bind enabling Albano to contemplate the ways that self-starvation has itself been a metaphor for the processes by which it was enculturated (her word).

But is self-starvation an illness and, if so, under what circumstances? How did self-starvers become objects of desire, or the converse, in their local (rather than global) cultures? Idealized Renaissance women were ordinarily rotund in their supine *maja nuda* poses, especially as framed on Rubensesque canvases by swelling pillows and plush fabrics, indicating no lack of protein nourishment as enhancements to erotic pleasure. How then was the notion of the eroticized female transformed from substantial junoesque *corpora fabrica* into the Twiggy-thin ribs-and-bones bodies of the present day? Albano's focus is firmly genderized on women, in line with the practices of early-modern western cultural history. Self-starving male hermits of the early modern world, for instance, fasted for different reasons from these maidens who had deprived themselves of nourishment for all sorts of reasons other than religious ones.[53] But – by the late eighteenth century – male dandies were routinely squeezing themselves into foppish lace-trousers so tightly fitted that they may as

well have been girdled corsets. This was a practice ridiculed by the pictorial satirists of the age (Rowlandson, Gillray and company) who eventually accustomed the eyes of Regency men to be prepared by 1825
for one Claude Seurat, perhaps the thinnest man of his epoch who
practiced the arts of self-starvation to reduce his *corpora fabrica* to just
five kilos! – a counterpoint to the sebaceous Doctor George Cheyne who
had swelled, one hundred years earlier, to 22 stones, about 300
pounds.[54]

This long record of gendered eating patterns has a central position in
Albano's notion of framing, as she inquires into its cultural history from
the late Renaissance to the present day. The gender consequences of her
story remain foregrounded: what were the profiles of self-starving
males? Have they been idealized – more recently – and then eroticized,
in circumstances even remotely resembling Albano's early-modern
women? Albano's framing surmounts the narrow limits of historical
explanation usually offered for this phenomenon and, in parallel, opens
up an examination of new pathways for contemporary anorexia: a transition of self-starvation from cultural practice to medical condition.

In contrast, David Shuttleton's treatment seems to resist metaphor-
ization to this degree, appearing instead as the natural revenge on
mankind of an English political system running amok in the aftermath
of the seventeenth-century Revolution. But the chimera cannot endure:
rhetorical and metaphorical smallpox better describes Shuttleton's subject, a corrective to Raymond C. Anselment's position that somehow
smallpox the malady resisted figuration.[55] Of course, smallpox had
existed for centuries before the 1660s but was then becoming more visible, if also rhetorically handy, for those wishing to deface others with
its mortal blemishes. One political faction after another in Britain (the
situation abroad was different) was castigated with the dirty pox-label,
proof of a fallen morality. Yet if the historical rise of smallpox (the variola) was framed in this pre-eminently political way, revolution and turmoil were not its only historical contexts. It was also useful to stir the
imagination through shock and disfigurement: the disfiguring that
occurs when a body has surpassed the point of recognition as in leprosy
and – more recently – AIDS.

The history of science also contributed to this dramatic new awareness of smallpox. The faculty of imagination – then almost a palpable
anatomical organ in the generations after the effects of Cartesian dualism were felt – assumed new prominence in this heyday of competing
mechanistic methodologies as the mother's ability to imprint her foetus
was being hotly debated. Shuttleton demonstrates how diverse types of

subjective voices – poets, writers, commentators, ephemeral scribblers, bluestockings, male and female – recorded their responses to the new disfigurement as having been conferred through the wreckage of diseased imagination. It is an intriguing story. Histories of smallpox are not usually presented in this rounded way. They are more routinely described in monochrome colours of the appearance and disappearance of a disease condition – as if illness were as colour insensitive as that.

The political dimension of Shuttleton's reframing can be expanded chronologically backwards and forward to enlarge the contexts of accepted political history. We might pose the question: What – in this vein pushing his heuristic methodology – has been the effect of smallpox on political leaders in different epochs? The disfigurement of the youthful Hal, for example, suggests one possibility: he had contracted smallpox in 1514 and so far emerged unscathed. Later on, his tantrums of the 1530s, leading to swollen rage, paranoia, and lust, may have been the result of syphilis, but they too seem not to have disfigured his body. Then he ruled as Henry VIII: the medically disordered leader but not through the routine disfigurement associated with maladies like smallpox. But smallpox was also rhetorical and metaphorical, as the deaths of several seventeenth-century English princes and princesses made evident. Moving forward to the last two centuries, would any western nation have been able to endure a leader thus marked and tarnished in the disfigurement of smallpox? F. D. Roosevelt served as a distinguished American president while suffering from poliomyelitis – could he have done so with smallpox? What has been the cultural genealogy of this particular disfigurement almost in the Foucaldian sense?[56]

Jane Weiss moves forwards two centuries – from the seventeenth to the nineteenth – across the ocean to America and from smallpox to cholera. It is not surprising that 1832 should figure as the great year in her story about the city on its way to becoming America's largest: New York. What is new is her framing in terms of communities and their locally coded rhetorics. And her stunning demonstration that all parties were manipulated by a single dominant media – newspapers – is noteworthy and has not yet been analysed in previous discussions of the first crest of cholera in America. Here is medicine in deference to the press: it may cause readers to pause and ponder the degree to which it remains in the grip of that influential media almost two centuries later.

Historically New York City was riveted by the invasive illness which ravaged it and punctured its daily rhythms. The infected were quickly brandished immoral by (so far) uninfected groups claiming to be the proud possessors of purity. This anti-Jobean mentality swiftly altered as segment upon segment, community after community, succumbed. Who, if any, were the genuinely pure and untainted in this hierarchy of moral dirt crowned by implied sexual excess? None, but it soon became evident that cholera was shattering all social norms and smashing its frames: it stopped at no borders in the march to expose the underlying enmity among social groups. Amidst this welter of abuse how were any medical facts of the epidemic established? Who could be trusted for any information – Weiss shows how today's fact was savaged as tomorrow's fiction. Medical reality (that glaring category again) altered daily: nothing, no one, could be relied on. Here then was another reframing caught in the inability of those in the dead heat of the moment to ascertain what was happening. If Weiss' approach suggests a generalized cultural pattern it is this: disease is almost never framed in terms of conditions of certainty about the knowable; rather, it demonstrates the opposite – an inability to frame it adequately for lack of facts.

Pamela Gilbert's treatment of the same malady occurs two decades later in the 1850s and 15,000 miles away on the Indian subcontinent. Yet it assumes shapes of a different sort in maps and, perhaps unexpectedly, maps of life under the soil; demonstrating that frames for disease conditions are inherently open-ended, yielding to new approaches and refined interpretations and partaking of the plenitude commensurate with the human condition. Gilbert decodes this abundance of Victorian maps – literal, fantastic, utopian – to show how they projected a vision of civilized and savage places. Maps were thus an inherent part of the colonial enterprise: grafting, inculcating, projecting notions of British superiority measured against Bengali barbarism. But maps were not merely visual representations of suprasea-level life: they also charted the unseen, that which was below the earth. And it is in this subterranean domain of the unseen that Gilbert reveals an unknown chapter in the long evolution of cholera: its colonial mapping.[57]

A *leitmotif* also plays along in her chapter suggesting that every map of distant parts assumes one closer to home (i.e., the all-important home of the mapmaker). For Gilbert demonstrates how British metropolitan mapping of the entry of the cholera into London contrasts with the colonial mapping of it in the Indian cities. Here then – on maps – were coded representations of the differences between familiar urban and remote colonial spaces. This contrast may seem more pertinent to cholera's anthropology and geography than to its medical history. But only if we accept the idea that medicine exists on discrete islands – apart, as it were, from the mainland of culture. Nineteenth-century cholera eventually came to imply many cultural codes among which was one presided over by the notion of the battleground: those fields where cultural wars would be fought out in different contexts: political, racial, colonial, sexual. Construed as companion chapters, those by Weiss and Gilbert could be viewed as aiming to describe something akin to 'cultural cholera': that is, diseases almost removed from their medical components.

Malte Herwig tests the limits of some of these boundaries. He pushes further forward in time to the twentieth century and the reception of Thomas Mann's *The Magic Mountain* (1924; English 1927). No previous epic-scale novel, in any language, had been so firmly grounded in medical content: an alpine sanatorium whose patients, doctors, staff, guests and quondam visitors form the main characters of the book. Everyone has some stake or other in the fate of tuberculosis. The conception and execution of the book, especially the imposition of medicine on this stratospheric world high up in the Alps (so high that the characters live in fog), was daring beyond most readers' expectations. Add to this leap Mann's degree of satire – particularly in his portrayal of doctors and their incredibly lucrative asylums for the rich – and you can see why his early readers were surprised by what they found, his medical readers often shocked or enraged. Herwig isolates this reading community after 1925 and shows that part of their response was grounded in self-interest rather than any aesthetic merits of one of the books for which Mann was awarded a Nobel Prize.

His chapter constitutes important work: in considering the first thoroughly medical novel you want to know what contemporary doctors made of it. Compare *The Magic Mountain* with Tobias Smollett's experimental medical novels (especially *Roderick Random*), Sterne's *Tristram Shandy* where medical themes are exploited for the purposes of bawdry and ribaldry, and George Eliot's *Middlemarch* which weaves Dr Lydgate's career into Eliot's vision of the fabric of a society, and you see the differences with the German work. Hitherto physician-readers of Mann's book have posed as learned antiquarians or amateur historians of medicine: annotating medical procedures and explicating how this or that medical topic (e.g. pneumothorax) would have appeared in the 1920s or 1930s when the book was first being read. But Herwig shows how the book itself stimulated a medical debate about tuberculosis during the thirty years (1925–55) when there was still no guaranteed cure (streptomycin and other antibiotics were not administered until well after the end of the Second World War). Even more pertinently to the theme of framing at hand, he shows in which ways the book framed the malady. Usually cultural forces and institutions frame a malady: pumping life into it as a breathing organism rather than as a medical classification. In Herwig's estimate *The Magic Mountain* acts a cultural force framing the illness: the arrows of influence have been, as it were, reversed. Only a philosopher of medicine could rise to this challenge and Herwig comes close to claiming Mann was one. Mann the philosopher of humanism and humanist heritage for western civilization has already been studied in great detail.[58] But Mann the philosopher of framing – framing medicine in one of the greatest novels ever written – has only just begun to receive the attention he deserves.

No one could reasonably assert that these first five frames are identical. Each scholar dwells on, or teases out, something else inside the frame. Each would compose the frame of another chapter in a slightly different way, emphasizing this or that nuance. This is as it should be: no matter how empirically grounded in the real world of facts and historical events, the framing of disease is no more monolithically uniform than the diagnosis of individual illness. All share a belief, however, that frames require contexts; houses of cultural history that must be adequately built. Without these, frames are bogus: they become edifices of words that lack all substance. Framing acts become more cumbersome than they were found to be in this first section when their interiors – the points where insides meet integuments – are themselves irrational. When you frame *madness*, to which our second section is devoted, something else happens. This topic we approach eclectically again, but not, we hope, without making the general point, common to all three chapters in this second section, that madness is itself culturally constructed to a very large degree.

Framing and imagining madness

This had been, of course, one of Foucault's fundamental projects which spurred a generation of cultural and medical historians in the aftermath of the first English translation, in 1965, of *Madness and Civilization: a History of Insanity in the Age of Reason*. Even here, though, the majestic contributions of imaginative literature were largely omitted. Writers who foregrounded madness were either unread or deemed too unreliable in their imagined fictions of despair to figure in – all the more so for second- and third-rank writers. Such foregrounding, however, is what the scholars in our second part accomplish, each focusing on a component of, or moment in, the development of the 'mad-trade'. Their approaches are each so different from one another that the three form salutary companions for the methodology of framing.

Miranda Gill turns to a subject – eccentricity – that many have pondered, usually without an awareness of its historical contours. She frames eccentricity on the axis of sanity by gazing back at the continuum of Western European mental health since the mid-eighteenth century. Yet much that would impinge on post-Enlightenment theories of madness had changed since then: Newtonianism had risen and fallen, challenged by scientists more curious about the terraqueous globe than stars and planets, and replaced by the neo-Lamarckian life sciences, especially biological growth and the evolution of forms. Personal mood and mentality seem to have slipped out of the net of their concerns. A theory of insanity, developed in Britain by physicians such as William Battie and the Monro brothers, stirred debate about the sanity continuum, and within two generations (by 1830) a new science of psychiatry found itself being established as a valid field for medical research. Concurrently, a new sub-genre of writing about one's own madness arose (in England, for example, the popular diaries of invalids in the Regency), which soon mushroomed into a small library of works by doctors and sufferers observing the compromised states of mind of the strange.[59] The genuine leaders in theory, however, were French rather than British, especially in their famous medical schools in Paris where doctors such as Pinel, Esquirol, and eventually the illustrious Charcot in the 1830s, installed psychiatry as a major branch of the new medical science.[60]

In this march to medicalize and pathologize the mind, borders – shared with other medical discourses, other medical specialties, other maladies – remained contested zones. Here in this murky lagoon between healthy and sick minds, functional and dysfunctional, the battle over the definition of lunacy was waged. Where in this continuum did one sphere end and the other start? Where indeed were the exact boundaries? The meeting point – to extend this image of the biogeography of mental states – between picture and frame soon became the contested site for interpretation as all sorts of intermediate states were described in detail. Neurotic, hysteric, anxious, compulsive and depressive types became as intriguing to inquisitive doctors as the polarized healthy and sick patients. Somewhere among these, as Gill shows, was the eccentric, who existed on the tantalizing continuum of 'a little bit mad/almost mad, not quite mad'.

If eccentricity became a national British trait by the time Victoria ascended to the throne, it also developed a life and discourse of its own in nineteenth-century France, the country that led the way in establishing it as a pathological category. Across the Channel, in Britain, the 'original' had been its counterpart since the seventeeth century but was rarely medicalized. The English 'original' character type was attributed to odd British manners, morals, climate, even bogs and fogs, but not to biophysiological causes; and when it was, briefly in the mid to late eighteenth century, it was without the authority and funding of the powerful French academic-university hospitals. Gill traces the development of eccentricity as an intermediate characteristic moving from moral and social framing towards an organicist and biological frame. For her Claude Bernard plays an important role, as do the theories of degeneration, positivism, and physical equilibrium.

Michael Finn continues, chronologically and geographically, into the next generation within France, demonstrating some of the consequences of such framing for French literature at the end of the century. He re-frames hysteria as the crowning culmination of nineteenth-century psychiatric science, a non-contested gesture to be sure, but Finn goes on to claim that both doctors and writers in the last quarter of the century set out to rewrite the history of the possessed – the hysterics of earlier epochs. Ecstatics, demoniacs, mystics, many of the possessed and dispossessed of a pre-Sadean Gallican past, were merely the hysterics of today, especially incurable patients of the *fin-de-siècle*. It should have been predictable that two groups in particular – medical and literary – would frame their (not our) present-day hysteria in this way: by locating it exclusively in a French past prone to give rise to such wretches. Finn recognizes that it remains to be shown how the French reading public – composed of ordinary educated readers – was persuaded to embrace this dark, revisionary view of history.[61]

Finn's approach dissolves conventional genres (prose, poetry, drama, and their sub-groups) in an attempt to situate explanations for possession in high literature and low journalism. The main stories – about the devils of Loudun, the convulsionaries of Saint-Médard, the incredible excesses of the Marquis de Sade himself – are still renowned today, more than one hundred years later. But most are accounts of demoniacs and the possessed within monastic settings whose protagonists have long since disappeared from secular consciousness. Freud's sexually frustrated hysterics wiped the slate clean and replaced them as more credible Viennese burghers; others have disappeared from our cultural memory by virtue of the decline of clerical institutions of ascetic retreat. Sorcerers, witches, exorcists, demented priests and their gyrating concubinical nuns: these are the types of possessed lunatics some of our contemporaries today claim as the counterparts of fundamentalist born-again Christians deranged by late capitalism. Finn retrieves this jungle of narratives, literary and medical, to demonstrate how they composed the patterned tiles of a cultural mosaic. And he gives a clear account of how the practices of magnetism and hypnotism fed into the development of the female hysteric as *le grande névrose* of her epoch. Imaginative literature in this version of framing contributed much to expose (so-called respectable) medicine's masculine dominion.

Emese Lafferton also focuses on this late-nineteenth-century European culture, but now in case studies occurring on the banks of the Hungarian Danube; as glosses not on Freud's Vienna but on Laufenauer's Budapest. Laufenauer *who*? The obscurity marks the drift of Lafferton's framework as a lack of referents constitute one of the main virtues of her focus. Readers familiar with the French psychiatry of this period (1850–1900), or even Austro-Germanic, will continue to impose their associations of those traditions on this 'No Man's Land' between Central Europe and the Ottoman lands. Lafferton's first task is to frame Hungarian psychiatry itself – the whole story – as it has not been subjected to any systematic treatment. In this sense she is the only member of our present company who frames a territory for the very first time. The others have all had precedents; are re-framing their existing pictures, as it were, as revisionists who both refocus a field and chart its boundaries and borders. But for Lafferton neither field or border exist. So the frame itself must be constructed as part of the act of conceptualizing and drawing the picture itself. There may be in-depth histories of Austro-Hungarian psychiatry in German or Hungarian (a doubtful prospect) but they are not to be found in English.

As part of her task Lafferton also struggles to elicit what is *different* about the Hungarian development. Her conclusion lies within private and public institutions rather than discourses, genres or metaphors. If she is keen to demonstrate that in the developing national psychiatry the Hungarians were late-bloomers and derivative, imitating the Germanic traditions and trying to establish them on Magyar soil, she also frames by placing great value on the role of academic research. She finds a progression from private clinics to large university asylums among her major institutional shifts in these developments. University physicians are running the show by the early twentieth century. The historian wonders what difference – if any – these institutional shifts and sites of power made to the incapacitated or demented patient. Or to current ephemeral literature – short stories, novels, low-life plays – incorporating themes and tropes of madness.

Did the different types of institution define the quantum of knowledge the patient could have about her condition? Most deranged patients craved treatment, whether privately or in a university setting, and were largely uninterested in the institutional arrangements of the available therapies. Of all the national cultures presented in this book, the Hungarian picture vis-à-vis 'framing madness' appears most to isolate medical theory from lay writing. Is this a fantasy or an instance of retrieval catching up with reality?

The patient's narratives and illnesses

It is still unclear why so many patients who do not consider themselves to be mad write out (pathographesis) their illnesses. Do they do so (bearing in mind Lafferton's retrievals) out of frustration that they have not been listened to or understood? Or – if heard – then not helped? Or is it that sickness itself is a more complicated component of human experience than has been explained hitherto?[62] Philip Rieder offers an approach through the perspective of the patient, one that used to be called doing medical history from the patient up. Rieder's argument focuses on names, diagnoses, and the kinds of language embodied in the knowledge patients have of their own conditions.[63]

He shows that in a fundamental sense names – the labels and labelling so inherent to the medical transaction and so crucial to the human condition that it functions as one of its great consolations – these are unimportant to the stories patients tell themselves, and perhaps others, about their maladies. Such a claim almost reverses the Rosenbergian position that diseases do not exist as social phenomena until they are named.[64] Drawing his material largely from Swiss-Romande sources in the period of the eighteenth-century Enlightenment, Rieder mounts a case against these invasive medical labels, to the extent that patients who resisted them actually improved. It could be salutary, even beneficial, to dismiss them, or at least to doubt the doctor's interpretation. Still, the doctor–patient interaction was a negotiation conducted largely, if not wholly, through language organized into units of discourse: Discourse inherently and necessarily ambiguous, fragmented, chaotic, often misunderstood. The patient's search for the so-called 'reality' of the condition was based on a diagnosis she (the lay patient) had to comprehend in language composed of few name-tags. Lay patients (those with a minimum of medical know-how) employed language that lagged far behind the doctor's specialized vocabulary. Much has been written about the discourse of mental patients, especially psychotic patients, but little about the speech acts of ordinary interchanges in the consulting rooms past and present.[65]

Rieder also seems to be reaching for a fuller medical history: more rather than less historical, one taking its energy from the implied religio-moral spheres of the Genevese (or at least Suisse-Romande) patients he retrieves. In particular, the tenor of this chapter is informed by the sense of a local *geist* crying out to be heard in that world of Jean-Jacques Rousseau and Samuel Tissot. Rieder's patients have unique voices that speak idiopathic – but not necessarily learned – languages. How salutary then to contrast his patients with Rousseau's and Haycock's solitary drug addict: the inimitable Samuel Taylor Coleridge, poet, philosopher, literary critic, Romantic, revolutionary, traveller, wanderer, biologist, psychologist, polymath, polyglot, spiritualist – and chronic patient. So ingrained in the pleasures of addiction, despite his protestations, that his particular type of malady may require a new name (here also bearing in mind Rieder's names and labels). Coleridge may accurately be described, as Rousseau–Haycock suggest, as the hypochondriac par excellence in the recent history of English poetry. Somehow, though, the empty label – hypochondriac – cannot begin to explain what is important about the Coleridgean variety.

Coleridge's biographical case history is less straightforward than it at first appears: he was fascinated with his own body, in particular his stomach and bowels. In one sense these sites occupied the centre of his attention, the object of his boundless curiosity (if only he could have been aware of the degree to which the middle-class Königsberg misogynist – Kant – he had read and idealized stood at the opposite end of the corporal spectrum, denigrating and repressing his own body). But what did this anatomical zone of the midriff, typically a purgatory for Coleridge, signify to a man of sensibility of the new post-Mackenzean variety?[66] What role did chronic sickness play in the development of the type of man of feeling Coleridge imagined so crucial to his actual practice of sensibility? And what was the role of health, anyway, among philosophers of Nature on both sides of the English Channel, in the England and Germany in whose rapidly changing science the young Coleridge was so immersed? These are not questions that can be answered easily, not least because the human role of illness and suffering has only recently entered into biography. Even so, there is more to his maladies than this: Coleridge seems to have been half in love with illness despite its nagging demons. If Death-in-Life remains one of the visionary conceits for which his poetry is remembered, Illness-in-Life could have been his semi-serious biographical epitaph. Around the same time that Coleridge was enduring these nocturnal demons, during the first decade of the nineteenth century, Blake was writing, in *Jerusalem*, that 'We who dwell on earth can do nothing of ourselves, every thing is conducted by spirits, no less than Digestion or Sleep'. How Coleridge would have consented!

How then do we define someone – a great Romantic visionary – who pursues malady in this way? Obsessed with its effects on his body; compulsively curious about the relation of medical terms and diagnoses – he was ready to compose celebratory poems on medical heroes including Beddoes, Jenner, and even German doctors; compulsively drawn to the physicians he repeatedly consulted. Is this not a type of purist intellectual hypochondria? The answers to these questions plot the starting point of Rousseau–Haycock: first to understand the myriad ways the biographical Coleridge ailed and – having charted that – to frame as their main task his hypochondria within a context that could be seen to open up this most closed book of his psychosomatic relations. Rousseau–Haycock also construct a prosopography of medical names he attached to maladies: constipation, flatulence, vomiting, diarrhoea, gout, dysentery, cholera, an irritable bowel or irritable bladder, influenza, sciatica, rheumatism, cancer, stone or diabetes, or simply *pain*. The litany of his ailments is as long as it is varied. With his opium habits staring them in the face Rousseau–Haycock conclude that Coleridge was 'simply hypochondriacal'. But the tantalizing hypochondria diagnosis is not their final goal, accurate as they adjudge this label to be on historical grounds (naming again, if in another key). Which hypochondria is this? The Renaissance versions of melancholy or post-Restoration spleen? Narcissistic Boswellian self-pity? Or is he a harbinger of the more recent *male* hysteria and neurasthenia? An early Romantic precursor of our post-Freudian 'depression'? This vexed framing of hypochondria remains the collaborative authors' task: an arduous one given that any conclusion about a figure as notoriously multifaceted as Coleridge must always be provisional (the wars about Coleridge the plagiarist?) and in the blank stare of the European hypochondriasis that has not been studied in any detail.

The unnamable maladies of the nineteenth century could form the basis for many books about framing and imagining disease, conjuring up an exhaustive list of dramatis personae: Astolphe Custine, the aristocratic and homosexual Parisian who filled his hotel de ville with the illuminati of the day; composer-artists Chopin, Liszt, and Georges Sand; Flaubert's Mysterious Maladies; Henri Amiel (1821–81), the reclusive Genevese academic who self-consciously framed his condition to such revolting verbal proportions that by so doing he produced the longest diary in the French language, running to 17,000 manuscript pages; Charles Algernon Swinburne, the iconoclastic English poet-hill-side walker once memorialized as having the most disturbed nerves of any writer of his century; not to omit Marcel Proust, who may be the most pronounced literary valetudinarian of recent history.[67] All wrote themselves out of, or into, sickness. The 'framer' today keeps wondering (as Coleridge had already anticipated) whether it was some sort of shield in a brutal world in which one needed to take cover. If space had not been an issue for us this third section on patient's narratives would have swelled. The existence of only two chapters (one a double-header) should not indicate a lack of material or available figures for scrutiny but merely the trumpet call of the practical.

Towards a poetics and metaphorics of disease

All these figures – Coleridge, Custine, Amiel, Swinburne, Proust, along with many described in the chapters below as well – embodied (framed) their illnesses in texts of one type or another. Coleridge endlessly expressed his thoughts in letters and notebooks that survive; he composed poems on medical topics and was engaged by poetry, however second-rate when compared with his mariners, which had absorbed medical content. Custine wrote letters about (what he perceived to be his) strange sexuality to friends and especially to his male lover, the Englishman Edward Saint-Barbe. Amiel transformed his diary into mother, child, lover, all wrapped into one.[68] Proust created the vast prose canvas for an imaginary life predicated on a fiction about his health: a midnight myth in which he could invisibly move as a *malade imaginaire*. The diversity of these embodiments form a crucial part of framing: what we call in the fourth part of our book a poetics and metaphorics of disease.

Agnieszka Steczowicz notices the prevalence of paradox in Renaissance medical thought when new diseases were much discussed among doctors as a natural consequence of discovery in the era of global exploration. Many medical treatises at the time hinted at the possibility of new diseases being introduced to Europe by the men who sailed on Columbus' ships. But the conventional history of Renaissance medicine, even the syphilis and plague she foregrounds, is not her genuine topic. She starts by defining post-Ciceronian paradox as the realm of contrariety – what is contrary to common belief – and shows that by the sixteenth century paradox functioned as something of a heuristic category, a provocative tool for challenging old belief. In medicine this

literal sense of paradox as contrariety especially lent itself to the analysis of strange, or new, diseases then baffling the *eruditi*.

Steczowicz centres her discussion on sixteenth-century collections of
paradoxes devoted to illness. The concept of medical commentary as
paradox book (that is, the form of the book itself) is currently alien to
us: we could not imagine the framing of a new book about the transmission of AIDS – however strange the condition still seems to us –
through the lenses of paradox or as a compendium of paradoxes. Yet
paradox was as much an established literary genre of the Renaissance as
it was an integral mode of thinking about contradiction and incom-
mensurability.[69] The relation of medical writing – whether incorporating strange diseases or not – to literary genre is not one that has been
explored in any detail, yet Steczowicz frames her Renaissance diseases
along these lines, concluding that the paradoxical genre contributed to
new 'ontological' views of disease. Framing is presented here through an
interface of literary genre and medical history, each acting as the context for the other. If Steczowicz is correct about her two case studies –
syphilis and plague – then core historians of medicine will want to
devote more of their energy to literary genre – and, vice-versa, literary
historians to medical realism – in order to understand more fully how
these epidemics of the past were presented for the first time.

Similar vigilance to the nuance of language and literary form informs
Kirstie Blair's exhilarating discussion of heart disease in Victorian culture. Her advantage is the focus on a concrete, well-understood organ:
the heart. Blair notices that the heart had long been the perceived
anatomical seat of feeling and emotion, love and desire.[70] During the
long European Enlightenment the newly empowered nerves appeared
likely to overthrow the heart's anatomical supremacy; but a clever amal-
gam produced 'nervous hearts' by the early nineteenth century and
these anatomical types, too, always exceeded the sum of their parts to
form an organic anatomic system – also something figurative requiring
further adumbration. The more nineteenth-century British commentators worried about the declining role of feeling in society (especially
right feeling in terms of being religiously oriented), the more its physicians framed its heart disease in terms of these anxieties and fears.

The framing here is more intricate than appears at first sight. When
you have an organ as figuratively suggestive as the heart (sick hearts and
unsteady pulses were more common than diseased minds or brains) and
its pulses, every linguistic – and conceptual – turn seems ripe for interpretation. It was not, for example, chest pains they were describing but
a sentient organ exquisitely capable of responding to human beings

and social conditions: love, beauty, mortality, war, peace, all life's great revelations. Schematically the framing amounts to this approximate sequence: a society situates certain emotions in an anatomic region. These emotions, or feelings, in turn come in for criticism and doubt. Doctors, absorbing the criticism, build it into their theory of heart disease by imbuing the heart with the very attributes it lacks. This is framing conducted through lack or absence: as Blair writes, Victorian doctors 'found in the heart the qualities which its figurative uses had taught them to look for'.

How does one organ or system within the body become privileged in this way? Figuratively, the heart could denote all things irrational, mysterious, unpredictable; it is also apparent that Victorian culture was obsessed with these qualities, or affective states, especially when they led to a loss of religious faith. But it is much less apparent why a society should seek to situate its anxieties concretely in anatomic organs. Why not rest satisfied in having addressed the angst itself? If this homology of culture – doctors encoding cultural anxiety in disease theory – had really overtaken the Victorians (and there is good reason to think it had), one wonders if Blair's figurative convergencies were early strains of the scientific positivism spreading throughout western society by the end of the century. By the 1890s a wave of physiological positivism was certainly sweeping over England and Germany.

Stephan Besser's methodology in framing does not lie very far from Blair's, despite the difference in their geographies. Like Blair, he locates a metaphor – Tropenkoller, or tropical cholera – which permeates through every vein of the culture. Here it is indeed Germany rather than England, the 1890s rather than 1860s, and the heart of jungle darkness, to echo Conrad's famous novel of 1899, rather than London's late-Victorian mauve drawing rooms and plush medical societies. Claiming that Tropenkoller was coined 'on the streets' Besser proceeds to identify and situate this tropical choleric, that first appeared in the mid-1890s as the quasi-scientific designation for a bizarre form of jungle illness: nervous, inflammatory, incurable, and – most notoriously – propelling its victims to commit weird acts of sexual perversion and sadism. But what actually was tropical cholera? Was it something new? Something unique to Germans in the jungle: a new tropical illness reflecting both the German colonial experience (different insofar as Germany, in contrast to many other European powers, had relatively few colonies) and the soldier's anxieties at home?

Besser has also located novels published within the first decade of the discovery of Tropenkoller, framing its territory on two books both titled symptomatically *Tropenkoller*: Frieda von Bülow's tale of 1896 and Henry Wenden's of 1904. Von Bülow's was written at the height of concerns over the court-martial trials in Germany of those charged with colonial violence. Its genesis and plot are driven, according to Besser, by feminist concerns of the day; tensions about the sympathy all women ought to have for each other, whether at home or in remote African jungles. In contrast, Wenden's book focuses, according to Besser, on 'the sexual and pathological dimensions of colonial scandals'. The protagonist is a young, fair, blue-eyed colonial officer called Kurt Zangen who grows increasingly sadistic as he rises through the ranks of the military. His Tropenkolleric excesses are uncovered, he is apprehended, sent home, and jailed. Emerging despondent, he finally commits suicide.

Besser is astute in pinpointing the tightest frame around these works in sexual domains: 'the cultural significance', he writes, 'of Wenden's novel resides in the fact that Kurt's perversion and the obscenely detailed descriptions thereof, unite and almost pornographically expose two prime motives of contemporary debates on Tropenkoller: the idea of an out-of-control and sadistically perverted male sexuality, and the fantasy of sexual race mixing.' Each was crucial in the German *fin-de-siècle*. Perverted male sexuality had been a key facet of the German sexological debates since the 1860s; sexual miscegenation or race-blending was more recent but had also figured in much post-Darwinian biological controversy – all these against a backdrop of nervous-disease theory that was growing ever more complicated as it also became increasingly nationalized, as reflected in the idea that there actually were *German* nerves, *British* nerves, *American* nerves, *jungle* nerves.[71] Sexual life in the heart of Africa proved an exotic touchstone stimulating fantasies of excess back at home and a rationale for control in the jungle. How different would Besser's Tropenkoller appear if he *omitted* his novels. Or – to frame the matter through reversal – if he had generated a literary analysis of these intriguing, if now forgotten, fictions, no matter how intertextually adept, without also providing an adequate medico-historical context?

The persistence of figurative language in Part IV answers our rhetorical imperative in another key. Paradoxes, pulses of the heart, nervousness in the jungle: all are concepts readily grasped by the history of medicine. Yet only such a deep-layer discussion is capable of framing the points in the profundity they deserve. Otherwise each loses the cultural validity that prompted its interest in the first place. For example, Besser might have confined himself to a narrow analysis of the Tropenkoller novels but by doing so he would not have been able to explain why there is such 'a prevalence of nervous metaphors in German colonial discourse'. The nuanced analysis of discourse is an enterprise conducted on the borders of several disciplines, rarely inside the heartland of just one.

Genesis of the volume

Finally, something must be said about the genesis of this book in relation to its panel of contributors and its present organization. Our true origins lie in 1998 when a rare piece of luck brought together the principal players. A three-year institutional grant was awarded by the Leverhulme Trust (F793A) to George Rousseau, then Research Professor of the Humanities at De Montfort University in Leicester, a substantial grant permitting him to enlist the assistance of postdoctoral fellows interested in culture and disease and their layers of reciprocity. Drs David Haycock and Caroline Warman (now at Exeter College, Oxford) were a perfect pair of scholars to dovetail with George Rousseau's long-standing interest in the interfaces of literature and medicine, Haycock an Oxford-trained historian of the early-modern period, Warman a *dix-huitièmiste* focused on the literature and history of France and the Romance languages. We soon recognized that we shared a profound interest in the meeting point of different disciplines. Our main task was to compile an archive in the service of future publication. But something happened – a burst of energy and inspired thinking – which also soon gave birth to the Framing Disease Workshop.

Every year De Montfort University hosts a week-long series of cultural events in which celebrities and other speakers (artists, performers, thinkers) are brought to the campus to participate in shared programmes. We were invited to mount a symposium encompassing culture and disease. We conferred among ourselves and wondered what would happen if we assembled a dozen or so young scholars also interested in this interface. The event, we were later told, was a success: those attending had come from diverse academic corners, ranging from the arts and theatre to nursing and other healthcare professions, all agreeing that they had learned something valuable about medicine's long tentacles and literature's seduction.[72] So we repeated the experience four times – at Wolfson College Oxford, the Wellcome Trust Centre for the History of Medicine at UCL in London, the École Normale Supérieure in Paris, and New College in Oxford – on each occasion attracting a new cast of young scholars from further afield. The numbers grew so large that at the last Framing Disease Workshop in New College Oxford in

October 2002 we worried how the attendees would fit into the Salter Room. By then – Autumn 2002 – Miranda Gill and Malte Herwig had become prime movers of the group, Gill expert in eccentric modes of behaviour in nineteenth-century France, Herwig already one of the most erudite of the new generation of Thomas Mann scholars. Also active were Sophie Vasset of the University of Paris, then writing a doctoral dissertation on literature and medicine in the long eighteenth century, and Kirstie Blair of Keble College Oxford, whose chapter included in this book is guaranteed to keep the reader's pulse moving and heartbeat accelerating. Dr David Shuttleton of the University of Wales at Aberystwyth, who had been working on the interface of medicine and literature for over a decade, was eager to join and introduced us to our webmaster, Will Datsun. Sophie Vasset brought the Workshop to Paris, where many of these chapters were first heard as talks before they were reread in new versions at New College. Adam Budd of the English Department of the University of Toronto hosted our meeting at the Wellcome Trust Centre for the History of Medicine at University College London in December 2001. Budd also signed up many young scholars working in this area, even if they did not call it by any disciplinary designation proximate to 'Literature and Medicine'. And Budd, trained both as a medical doctor and professional literary historian, continued to offer us informal guidance and make suggestions for the types of symmetries we should aspire to in the sections of this book. To all these scholars, even if their own essays are not included here, we are grateful both for their degree of enthusiasm in the prospect of framing and imagining disease and their constant encouragement.

As this book goes to press, the Workshop continues to thrive and is planning for gatherings in 2003 and 2004. Our commonly articulated goal is to keep the Workshop small, and our profile low, so that we can continue to enjoy sustained and meaningful interdisciplinary dialogue without the pressures of ordinary academic life: publish, print; print, publish; run rabbit run. As our website (www.framingdisease.co.uk) states, 'we are a consortium of professional academic and independent scholars interested in the cultural understanding of illness'. Perhaps we ought to have added: united in our belief that the healing arts in dialogue are less fractured than modern disciplinary life in universities suggests.

But if a flowering of intellect and spirit among doctoral students and postdoctoral fellows as both these were continues to grow with a future life firmly in view, it does so cognizant of a past and implied genealogy of scholarship. All of us, including George Rousseau and Michael Finn (who are after all of another generation), had benefited immensely from the new history of medicine of the last generation. The works of Susan Sontag, Roy Porter, Sander Gilman, Arthur Kleinman, Oliver Sacks, Elaine Showalter, and – in Europe – Bakhtin, Augustin Cabanès, and especially such Paris intellectuals as Michel Foucault and Julia Kristeva, had paved the way in part for our views. Each of us has our own favourite list – on each a small number of names continues to reappear, the *ne plus ultra* of our heritage. Without these prior toilers in the fields of interdisciplinarity neither the Workshop and its activities nor this book would have seen the light of day.

There have also been books and articles without which our birth would have been slower. It is impossible to survey the historiography of a generation in a brief space but all of us, even if tacitly, have been enriched by such works as: the journal *Literature and Medicine* published in the USA; Marie Mulvey Roberts and Roy Porter (eds), *Literature and Medicine during the Eighteenth Century* (London: Routledge, 1993); Susan Sontag, *Illness as Metaphor* (New York: Random House, 1979); Kathryn Montgomery Hunter, *Doctors' Stories: the Narrative Structure of Medical Knowledge* (Princeton, NJ: Princeton University Press, 1991); William B. Ober, *Bottoms Up!: a Pathologist's Essay on Medicine and the Humanities* (Carbondale, IL: Southern Illinois University Press, 1989); Julia Kristeva, *Black Sun: Depression and Melancholia*, trans. Leon S. Roudiez (New York: Columbia University Press, 1989); K. C. Calman, R. S. Downie et al., 'Literature and Medicine: a short course for medical students', *Medical Education* 21: (1988): 265–9; Arthur Kleinman, *Writing at the margin: discourse between anthropology and medicine* (Berkeley: University of California Press, 1995); Marie-Hélène J. Huet, *Monstrous Imagination* (Harvard: Harvard University Press, 1993); Robert A. Erickson, *The Language of the Heart, 1600–1750* (Philadelphia: University of Pennsylvania Press, 1997); Miriam Bailin, *The Sickroom in Victorian Fiction: the Art of Being Ill* (Cambridge: Cambridge University Press, 1994); Mark Micale, *Approaching Hysteria* (Princeton, NJ: Princeton University Press, 1994); Louis A. Sass, *Madness and Modernism: Insanity in the Light of Modern Art, Literature, and Thought* (Cambridge, MA: Harvard University Press, 1994), and I would like to think that my own 'Literature and Medicine: The State of the Field', *Isis* LXXII (September 1981): 406–24, which was described at its debut as charting a field, had played a further role in the new developing field. More recently, one work has never left the tip of our collective mind: it is – of course – Charles E. Rosenberg and Janet Golden (eds), *Framing Disease: Studies in Cultural History* (New Brunswick, NJ: Rutgers University Press, 1992). It cannot be far from the mark to affirm that the present volume is both child and sequel to this distinguished predecessor. The march of knowledge is a continuum far more than a series of epistemic breaks with the past.

This book, then, reflects the recent flowering of interest in the way humans understand and decode disease in history and go about framing it. Viewed collectively, as a corporate whole, the chapters augur the type of framing we may increasingly find in the future: that is, interiors in relation to exteriors, insides and outsides, centre and periphery. They certainly demonstrate the current, continuing preoccupation with the body and the diverse methods of framing now practiced to contextualize those historical bodies. Not much lower down the scale is concern for the theoretical foundations and methodological approaches appropriate to particular problems. The chapters share the authors' concern to frame in the most suitable way possible while making a dent on the monodisciplinary status of the object, whether disease (self-starvation, smallpox, cholera, tuberculosis, madness, hysteria, etc.), author (Mann, Coleridge, the Victorian poets), or metaphorics (paradox, figures of speech, idiom, interdiscursivity, poetics).

In the follow-up second act to this volume we aim to capture malady primarily through pictorial frames. In that notion of framing there will be less transformation through verbal metaphor and a focused gaze on the pictures themselves. We hope that one offshoot of the cumulative effect will be to exert pressure on the medical profession – even medical historians – to rethink their own frames of reference. For we have collectively wondered whether their empirical view of illness based on body–mind binaries is more vulnerable, even collapsible, than they have admitted. Empirical views of illness based principally on classification and observation constitute only one dimension of a complex negotiation between patient, malady, doctor, and the vast surrounding world.

Notes

1. Jacques Derrida, 'The Parergon', *October* 9 (1979): 24–6; see the astute discussion of Derrida's essay in light of framing theories in Sneja Gunew, *Framing Marginality: Multicultural Literary Studies* (Melbourne: Melbourne University Press, 1994), especially 27–8. Also crucial for the theory of framing as it developed in the last generation is Erving Goffman, *Frame Analysis* (New York: Harper & Row, 1974) and R. C. Anderson, and Andrew Ortony, 'On putting apples into a bottle: A problem in polysemy', *Cognitive Psychology* 7 (1975): 167–80. This line

of inquiry was extended to the linguistic domain by Deborah Tannen in 'What's in a Frame? Surface Evidences for underlying expectations', in R. Freedle (ed.), *New Directions in Discourse Processing* (Norwood, NJ: Ablex, 1979), 137–81 and later in the 1990s, much more fully with examples and bibliographies, in her work *Framing in Discourse* (New York: Oxford University Press, 1993). Richard Woodfield (ed.) shows how applications are made in other fields; see his *Framing Formalism: Riegl's Work – Critical Voices in Art, Theory and Culture* (Amsterdam: G+B Arts International, 2000). Also useful are S. Cunningham, *Framing Culture* (Sydney: Allen & Unwin, 1992) and Barbara M. Benedict, *Framing Feeling: Sentiment and Style in English Prose Fiction 1745–1800* (New York: AMS, 1994). By my count more than a dozen books have appeared in the last decade with the title Framing Something – whatever it may be. But see also these works despite their lack of use of the term: Gregory Bateson, *Steps to an Ecology of Mind* (New York: Ballantine, 1972); Arthur Kleinman, *Patients and Healers in the Context of Culture: an Exploration of the Borderland Between Anthropology, Medicine, and Psychiatry* (Berkeley, CA: University of California Press, 1980).

2. D. Tannen, *Framing in Discourse*, 59.
3. Ibid., 59–60. The reference to Gregory Bateson is to his landmark *Steps to an Ecology of Mind* (n. 1).
4. Deborah Tannen and Cynthia Wallat, 'Interactive Frames and Knowledge Schemas in Interaction', in Tannen, *Framing in Discourse*, 63.
5. Extracted from Derrida's discussion of the 'violence of framing' in 'The Parergon' (n. 1).
6. Here one thinks of the vast panorama of medical history in which diseases attach to specific cultures and their internal societies, almost to the degree that centuries themselves are associated with particular maladies: the Renaissance with syphilis and plague, the seventeenth century with agues and dropsies, the eighteenth with gout and vapours, the nineteenth with consumption and cholera, and so forth. Yet every trained medical historian knows, to her peril, what false pictures of the past arise if you subscribe, even minimally, to such schemas. It is more difficult by far to explain why these disease constellations do *not* belong to particular centuries and how their rise and fall depends on other aspects of the frame (in our analogy) than the chronological one. Then there are the cultural representations of these maladies which is another matter altogether: so that the serious tone with which gout, for example, is discussed in the Renaissance differs from the astrological context it is given in the seventeenth century and the highly comic contexts that surround it in the eighteenth.
7. Something of an industry has developed in the last decade to pursue the undoing of Foucault's approaches to just the sorts of framing of disease implied by this anthology of essays. Many conferences today therefore include in their rubrics that a main goal is the exploration of how we can carry on despite Foucault, or beyond the ken of his insights. This is surely a healthy tendency in the march of analysis and scholarship provided it acknowledges that our present point was reached in no small part as a result of the totality of his contributions. We think the essays in this volume, especially those in Part II devoted to the framing and imagining of madness, demonstrate a balance between acknowledgement of the Foucaldian contribution and the desire to correct it, modify it, surmount it.

8. For the problem in painting see Norman Bryson and Mieke Bal, 'Semiotics and Art History', *Art Bulletin* 73.2 (June 1991): 174–208 who direct readers to other sources within art history and the history of aesthetics. For medicine, Friedrich Schiller anticipated some of these connections in Romantic medicine; see Kenneth Dewhurst and Nigel Reeves, *Friedrich Schiller: Medicine, Psychology and Literature* (Los Angeles: University of California Press, 1978). A generation earlier William Falconer had reached similar conclusions; see William Falconer, *A Dissertation on the Influence of the Passions upon Disorders of the Body* (London: C. Dilly, 1788).

9. For the discovery of the nostalgia diagnosis see Carolyn Anspach, 'Medical Dissertations on Nostalgia by Johannes Hofer, 1688', *Bulletin of the Institute of the History of Medicine* II (1934): 376–91.

10. Some sense of the range of these imageries in found in Richard Gordon, *An Alarming History of Famous and Difficult Patients* (New York: St Martin's Press, 1997) and Klaus Theweleit, *Male Fantasies: Volume 2, Male Bodies: Psychoanalyzing the White Terror* (Minneapolis, MN: University of Minnesota Press, 1992, 2 vols).

11. Dr Everard Maynwaring (self-styled as 'Dr in Physick and Hermetic Philosophy') explained what these wasting illnesses were in his Restoration treatise *A Treatise of Consumptions. Scorbutic Atrophies. Tabes Anglica. Hectic Fevers. Phthisicks. Spermatick and Venereous Wafting. Radically demonstrating their nature and cures from vital and morbific causes, reflecting the errours of vulgar doctrine, and Practice. Examined by Chymical Principles and the latest Practical Discoveries* (London: T. Basset, 1667). See also Hermione de Almeida, *Romantic Medicine and John Keats* (New York: Oxford University Press, 1991).

12. Here the medicalization of the imagination itself as mechanical and material organ, palpating and breathing and forever prone to disease of one kind or another, is of great interest. It has been studied in these contexts, but not within its mechanical role as imagining disease – hence a plot within the plot, as it were – wherein it is at once both passive spectator and active participant in the disease-forming activity. See John Haygarth, *Of the Imagination, as a Cause and as a Cure of Disorders of the Body, Exemplified by Fictitious Tractors, and Epidemical Convulsions* (Bath: R. Cruttwell, 1800) and, for its more monstrous shapes and forms, Marie-Hélène J. Huet, *Monstrous Imagination* (Harvard: Harvard University Press, 1993).

13. See, for example, Sarah Kay and Miri Rubin (eds), *Framing Medieval Bodies* (Manchester: Manchester University Press, 1994) and their discussion of how the Medievalist undertakes the exploration of this subject.

14. See Bateson and Tannen (n. 1 above) for applications of framing models in linguistics. In their study of medical examinations and medical interviews they evolve a classification of types of frames – frames versus schemas, interactive frames, knowledge schemas, linguistic registers – and acts undertaken by framers: fame shifting, juggling frames, interactive production of frames, conflicting frames, and so forth. We do not extend ourselves so far in this volume but we do claim – collectively – that medical contents and categories need to be situated in contexts often as challenging to construct as their companion linguistic ones.

15. Elliot G. Mishler, *The Discourse of Medicine: Dialectics of Medical Interviews* (Norwood, NJ: Ablex, 1978).

16. See Anthony J. Marsella and Geoffrey M. White (eds), *Cultural Conceptions of Mental Health and Therapy* (Dordrecht: D. Reidel Publishing Co., 1982).

17. Hence the poet Edward Young, the author of *Night Thoughts* (1742–45), assured the Duchess of Portland what his own pains were in a long medical correspondence with her. Reporting that his doctor calls 'this Rheumatic weather' worse than anything Job endured and that 'This ye Comforter Job has sent me under Pains half of which would make Him mad'. See Henry Pettit (ed.), *The Correspondence of Edward Young 1683–1765* (Oxford: Clarendon Press, 1971), p. 187, Letter 155 from Young to Duchess of Portland, 18 November 1744, Welwyn.

18. G. S. Rousseau, 'Doctors and Medicine in the Works of Doctor Tobias Smollett' (PhD. Princeton University, 1965), which demonstrates that there are well over two hundred medical practitioners – some real, others imagined – in Smollett's novels.

19. This is the point of the longest study of his works in G. S. Rousseau, *Tobias Smollett: Essays of Two Decades* (Edinburgh and New York: The Seabury Press, 1982).

20. Frank Seafield, *The literature and curiosities of dreams: a commonplace book of speculations concerning the mystery of dreams and visions, records of curious and well–authenticated dreams, and notes on the various modes of interpretation adopted in ancient and modern times* (London: Lockwood, 1869, 2nd edn. rev.).

21. These are the types of concerns Barbara M. Benedict addresses in *Framing Feeling: Sentiment and Style in English Prose Fiction* (New York: AMS Press, 1994); Miriam Bailin, *The Sickroom in Victorian Fiction: The Art of Being Ill* (Cambridge: Cambridge University Press, 1994); see also Geoffrey Sill, *Consuming Passions* (Cambridge: Cambridge University Press, 2001).

22. This conclusion seems to be the one driven home in Jadhav without his explicitly saying so; see Sushrut Jadhav in 'The cultural origins of western depression', *International Journal of Social Psychiatry* 42 (1996): 269–86.

23. Roy Porter and Andrew Wear (eds), *Problems and Methods in the History of Medicine* (London: Croom Helm, 1987) and E. Clarke (n. 25).

24. The published reviews of their book were favourable but some wondered if their contexts had been adequately drawn.

25. Edwin Clarke (ed.), *Modern Methods in the History of Medicine* (London: Athlone Press, 1971), several of whose essays are discussed below.

26. Two decades earlier, Rosenberg selected as his emphasis among the then modern (around 1970) methods of the history of medicine professional concerns as paramount; see Charles E. Rosenberg, 'The medical profession, medical practice and the history of medicine', in E. Clarke, *Modern Methods in the History of Medicine*, pp. 22–35.

27. Literature and medicine, as this subdiscipline is now known, had existed but was still in its earliest stage. The American journal by this name had just begun to appear and there were not yet the excellent studies brought out in the 1990s, for example: K. C. Calman and R. S. Downie, M. Duthie, B. Sweeney, 'Literature and Medicine: a short course for medical students', *Medical Education* 21: (1988): 265–269; R. S. Downie, 'Literature and Medicine', *Journal of Medical Ethics* 17 (1991): 93–96, 98; M. F. McLellan and A. H. Jones, 'Why literature and medicine?' *Lancet* 348 (1996): 109–11; Anne Hudson Jones, 'Literature and medicine: narrative ethics', *Lancet* 349 (1997): 1243–6;

Raymond A. Anselment, *The Realms of Apollo: Literature and Healing in Seventeenth-Century England* (Newark: London: University of Delaware Press; Associated University Presses, 1995); G. S. Rousseau, 'Bridges of Light: the Domains of Literature and Medicine', *Hysteric: Body, Medicine, Text,* Number 2: Special Issue: Sexuality in the Clinic (1996): 17–33; Michael Neve, 'Medicine and Literature', *Companion Encyclopedia of the History of Medicine,* eds W. F. Bynum and Roy Porter (London: Routledge, 1993), 1520–35.

28. Susan Sontag's *Illness as Metaphor* (New York: Random House, 1979) had appeared before 1980; *AIDS and Its Metaphors* (New York: Farrar, Straus & Giroux, 1989) would not be published until after Rosenberg's conference. It is curious that there are no references to Sontag's earlier work in Rosenberg's collection *Framing Disease* (1992).

29. In the important statement by E. Clarke and his group in 1971 (n. 25) only R. S. Roberts discussed 'The use of literary and documentary evidence in the history of medicine', 36–56.

30. It is probably the case that the jargon of literary theory had also deterred them, for by the mid-1980s literary criticism had already erected its private languages unintelligible to the uninitiated. Here it would be intriguing to read the pronouncements, ten years later, of Rosenberg's group on the matter.

31. Some of these points have been made in David B. Morris, *Illness and Culture in the Postmodern Age* (Berkeley and Los Angeles: University of California Press, 1998).

32. In just this sense a recent work such as novelist Julian Barnes' publication of Alphonse Daudet's (1840–97) extraordinary memoir about pain in chronic infectious disease is most welcome; see Julian Barnes (editor and translator), *In the Land of Pain by Alphonse Daudet* (London: Jonathan Cape, 2002). Daudet was a prolific French satirist and novelist, thought to be among the greatest writers of his age and beloved by the French reading public. During the end of his life he struggled with a fatal syphilis and described his anguish in pathetic poetic language, keeping a detailed diary of his experience of pain. Until Barnes' publication no reference to Daudet is found in the whole history of the disease; Daudet remained known only to French literary historians.

33. Aspects of these points were demonstrated for the literary structure of scientific argument in the history of science; see Peter Dear (ed.), *The Literary Structure of Scientific Argument: Historical Studies* (Philadelphia: University of Pennsylvania Press, 1991).

34. Almost two decades ago George Levine and his contributors argued for literature and science as 'one culture'; presumably the same could be claimed now for literature and medicine. See George Levine (ed.), *One Culture: Essays in Science and Literature* (Madison, WI: The University of Wisconsin Press, 1987).

35. The point is somewhat invidious and cryptic: we are eventually all patients at one time or another. The difference is some are earlier, some later, and some comment on the experience of suffering and sickness, often perceptively, before they themselves have been patients; see the brilliant account of a physician-writer who sat with his brother throughout the drawn-out course of his dying: Sherwin Nuland, *How We Die* (New York: Random House, 1993). Can anyone imagine Laurence Sterne writing *Tristram Shandy* as he did – he calls it 'a treatise 'writ against the Spleen' – if

he had not been coughing up blood and being ravished by illness all around him as he composed?

36. Joseph Collins, who went out to India, intuited Armstrong's importance in the early twentieth century. See his 'Literary leanings of eighteenth century physicians', in *The proceedings of the Charaka Club* 4 (1916), 27–44, which focuses on John Armstrong, Mark Akenside (1721–70), and Jean Astruc (1684–1766). Collins also wrote *The Way with the Nerves* (New York: Putnam's Sons, 1911); *The Doctor Looks at Literature* (New York: George H. Doran, 1923); and *The Doctor Looks at Biography: Psychological Studies of Life and Letters* (New York: George H. Doran, 1925).

37. Only the barest traces of Flemyng's life remain: whatever papers and manuscripts existed in the eighteenth century have disappeared.

38. In this literature of melancholy the writer (poet) eschews a confident iambic heroic couplet to the more insecure, if also vulnerable blank verse pentameter; see John Sitter, *Literary Loneliness in Mid-Eighteenth-Century England* (Ithaca and London: Cornell University Press, 1982).

39. *Sickness* was widely read in the eighteenth century and went into many editions. Thompson was influenced by Pope's poetry, which abounds with medical content; to what degree it made an impression on him is unknown.

40. See 'Advertisement'. Poetic framing in this mode calculatingly offers no more information than is necessary out of fear that the reader may be dislodged, and is constantly concerned as an *idée fixe* for the reader's imagination when in the act of deciding on poetic content. Here then is a salient feature of the frame: the permissible inside the border.

41. *Sickness*, I, 1.

42. Ibid. I, 391–2.

43. Ibid. II, 182–84.

44. See Marjorie Hope Nicolson and G. S. Rousseau, *'This Long Disease My Life': Alexander Pope and the Sciences* (Princeton, NJ: Princeton University Press, 1968); for Arbuthnot and the framing of disease in Augustan England, see U. C. Knoepflmacher, 'The Poet as Physician: Pope's *Epistle to Dr. Arbuthnot*', *Modern Language Quarterly* 31 (1970): 440–9.

45. *Sickness*, II. 773.

46. Ibid. I, 206–7.

47. Here I am not interested in the relative artistic merit: Thompson was a third-rank poet, Gray at least a second-, if not, front-rank writer. The matter of correlation between achievement and content requires another essay at least.

48. See G. S. Rousseau, 'Epics of Illness in the 1740s: English Poetry and the Politics of Health', forthcoming.

49. George Starr, *Defoe and Spiritual Autobiography* (Princeton: Princeton University Press, 1965) for confessions in the early-modern period.

50. Robert Mack, *Thomas Gray* (New Haven and London: Yale University Press, 2000).

51. Ross Chambers, *The Writing of Melancholy: Modes of Opposition in Early French Modernism*, trans. by Mary Seidman Trouille (Chicago: University of Chicago Press, 1993).

52. The point is also made in Allen Thiher, *Revels in Madness: Insanty in Medicine and Literature* (Ann Arbor, MI: University of Michigan Press, 1999).

53. For this tradition in the early-modern world see P. Camporesi, *The Incorruptible Flesh: Bodily Mutation and Mortification in Religion and Folklore* (Cambridge: Cambridge University Press, 1988); for its more recent French profile, S. Hesse-Biber, *Am I Thin Enough Yet?* (Oxford: Oxford University Press, 1997); P. McEachern, *Deprivation and Power: the Emergence of Anorexia Nervosa in Nineteenth-Century French Literature* (Westport, CT: Greenwood Press, 1998); and, for the corpulent reverse, Jana Evans Braziel and Kathleen LeBesco (eds), *Bodies out of Bounds: Fatness and Transgression* (Berkeley and Los Angeles: University of California Press, 2001).

54. There were many contemporary cartoons of both Seurat and Cheyne, the most recent of the former being Rowlandson's coloured caricature displayed in London's Science Museum exhibition on 'Metamorphosis 2002'.

55. Anselment, *The Realms of Apollo*, chap. 5.

56. For other approaches to this cultural profile of disfigurement see Judy Campbell, *The Invisible Invaders: Smallpox and other Diseases* (Melbourne: Melbourne University Press, 2002).

57. G. Melvyn Howe had already called attention to the importance of figurative maps in the history of medicine; see his 'The mapping of disease in history', in E. Clarke, *Modern Methods in the History of Medicine*, 335–57.

58. One of the blazing extended statements of this view is Marguerite Yourcenar's 'Humanism and Occultism in Thomas Mann', in *The Dark Brain of Piranesi and Other Essays* (New York: Farrar Straus Giroux, 1980), 199–232.

59. An example is Sir James Stonhouse (1716–95), *A friendly letter to a patient, just admitted into an infirmary. Great part of which may suit the case of any (especially of the poor) under sickness, or other affliction . . .* (London, 1795). For the general development see Allan Ingram (ed.), *Patterns of Madness in the Eighteenth Century* (Liverpool: Liverpool University Press, 1998).

60. But see also the contributions of the British physicians to the development of a coherent theory of madness: first – in the late eighteenth century – the important works of Doctors Monro and Battie and then – two generations later – its culmination in the thriving discourse found in such systematic treatises as Alexander Morison's *A Treatise of Mental Diseases . . .* (London and Edinburgh, 1826). Important here is the reassessment by Andrew Scull.

61. And in this sense he is adding to the fine work of Janet Beizer in *Ventriloquized Bodies: Narratives of Hysteria in Nineteenth-Century France* (Ithaca: Cornell University Press, 1994).

62. The anthropologists of medicine (especially the group with Professor Arthur Kleinman at its centre in America) have had a great deal to say, but much more work needs to be done in both-western and eastern traditions.

63. It may be viewed as complementary to the approach found in Mary Donaldson-Evans, *Medical Examinations: Dissecting the Doctor in French Narrative Prose 1857–1894* (Lincoln: University of Nebraska Press, 2000).

64. Rosenberg and Gordon, *Framing Disease* (1992), xiii. Naming, however, is a complex matter for all realism, not merely medical, as Ludwig Wittgenstein claimed throughout his philosophical career. For the crucial role of names and labels in the construction of meaning see Saul A. Kripke, *Naming and Necessity* (Cambridge, MA: Harvard University Press, 1972; rev. and enlarged 1980).

65. An exception is Elaine Scarry, 'How I survived my Heart Attack, Voice of the Patient', in *The Body in Pain* (New York: Oxford University Press, 1986), 123–56.

66. George Dekker, ' "*Nature's Music*",' in George Dekker (ed.), *Coleridge and the Literature of Sensibility* (London: Vision Press, 1978), 101–41. See volume one of Richard Holmes's two-volume study, *Coleridge: Early Visions* (London: Hodder & Stoughton, 1989), 'New Sensibility of Feeling', 15. On Coleridge's new sensibility and its neuroanatomical components only Jennifer Ford has recently made a persuasive case, as Rousseau and Haycock argue below.

67. Even our brilliant late contemporary novelist W. G. Sebald, whose extensive knowledge lay far afield from any of the medical domains we have been framing and commenting upon here, writes perceptively about Swinburne's nerves in *The Rings of Saturn* (London: Harvill, 1998), 162–3, especially the passage about his 'nervous crises'. The most imaginative framing of Swinburne's nervous panics and apoplexies, despite the silence about his strangely repressed sexuality – repressed to the point of complete evaporization, is found in William B. Ober, *Bottoms Up!: a Pathologist's Essay on Medicine and the Humanities* (Carbondale, IL: Southern Illinois University Press, 1989), 'Swinburne's Masochism: Neuropathology and Psychopathology', 43–88.

68. See the special issue of *Studies in Gender and Sexuality* 3:3 (2002) devoted to Amiel's framing of his maladies, especially the contributions by G. S. Rousseau and Caroline Warman and the reply by Dr Jeanne Wolff Bernstein.

69. Colie cited in Steczowicz below, chapter 12, n. 7, but see also the many important books by Ian Maclean, especially *Logic, Signs and Nature in the Renaissance: the Case of Learned Medicine* (Cambridge: Cambridge University Press, 2002).

70. The point has been made by Erickson for the period before 1800; see Robert A. Erickson, *The Language of the Heart, 1600–1750* (Philadelphia: University of Pennsylvania Press, 1997).

71. Joseph Collins, already mentioned above and writing a few years after the peak of Tropenkoller, seems blithely unaware of this nervous diaspora: see his *Way with the Nerves; Letters to a Neurologist on Various Modern Nervous Ailments, Real and Fancied, with Replies thereto Telling of Their Nature and Treatment* (New York and London: G.P. Putnam's Sons, 1911).

72. The reciprocity has been noted in different contexts: see Claudine Herzlich and Janine Pierret, *Illness and Self in Society*, trans. Elborg Forster (Baltimore, MD: Johns Hopkins University Press, 1988); G. S. Rousseau, 'Medicine and the Muses: the Idea that the Arts Heal in History', *Medicine and Literature*, eds Marie Roberts and Roy Porter (London: Routledge, 1991), 1–56.

Part I
Framing and Imagining Disease

2
Within the Frame: Self-Starvation and the Making of Culture

Caterina Albano

In an essay on the spread of anorexia nervosa, Joan Jacobs Brumberg recognizes that the shift of the condition, from a relatively obscure and isolated disorder to pre-eminence as what may be metaphorically termed a 'communicable disease', is 'a complex problem in psychiatric epidemiology warranting the attention of behavioural scientists, educators, and physicians, as well as social and cultural historians'.[1] The phrase 'communicable disease' refers to a disorder whose spread may be associated with interpersonal communication, especially among peer groups, and with the dissemination of information on anorexia. The biological, psychological, and social roots of eating disorders interact with an array of cultural factors – from the current emphasis on exercise, thinness and dieting as signs of health, to gender issues – but also with the narratives through which such disorders are constructed. As Brumberg observes, in the past decade the popularization of eating disorders through the media, the informative medical material often circulated among groups at risk, and the celebrity stories of anorexia and bulimia, have helped to transform anorexia nervosa 'from an enigmatic and rare condition into a recognisable and accessible disorder'.[2] The aetiology of anorexia and the anorectic's experience seems thus entangled in a complex reciprocity in which the medical paradigm of the disorder influences the patient's experience and description of it.[3] At the same time, the various discourses which have engaged with eating disorders, whether medical or not, are equally culturally informed with notions of the self, gender, patriarchy, forms of consumption, family relations, ideas of control and achievement, beauty and body images. As with other illnesses, this process of enculturation is so rooted in anorexia as to render it 'a metaphor for, and a manifestation of, contemporary socio-cultural concerns'.[4] These concerns may be related to gender issues as much as to the

51

cultural conflicts of a consumerist society and its glamorized image in the over-thin body of fashion icons and advertising.

Although anorexia, and more generally self-starvation, cannot be dissociated from corporeality, the disorder is nonetheless deeply encoded in a historically and culturally determined understanding of the denial of food, to the point that it is difficult to conceive self-starvation as independent from such knowledge.[5] A consideration of historical cases of self-starvation alerts us to the ways in which this cultural shaping follows well-defined modes and tends to repeat certain patterns. These patterns include the existence of competing interpretations, the popularization of fasting (often expressed in morbid curiosity), the active deployment of both food and the body as highly determined cultural signs, and the elaboration of narratives which culturally frame the denial of food. From these narratives, a tension is apparent between the private dimension of self-starvation, and its public perception and understanding. A rift emerges between the faster's denial of food and the modes in which the people who surround her respond to it. Such a rift is historically encoded in the cultural understandings of food and the body that characterize each period. In order to explore the nature of these patterns more carefully, I will use as an example the mid-seventeenth-century case of Martha Taylor, the 'Derbyshire Damosell': this case study is significant for our purposes since it stands at a moment of cultural transition in the medical understanding of the denial of food. The case survives in both medical and popular religious literature, allowing a comparison of competing interpretations, and offering an insight in the cultural perception and understanding of the denial of food in the early-modern period. In my analysis I highlight the persistence throughout this period of certain narrative tropes, especially in the description of the starving body and in the aetiology of the disorder. This may help us to shed some light upon the current cultural framing of anorexia nervosa.

A case study: the prolonged fasting of Martha Taylor, the Derbyshire Damosell

The Young Woman at Over-Haddon hath been visited by divers persons of this House. My Lord himself hunting the Hare one day, at the Towns-end, with other Gentlemen, & some of his Servants, went to see her on purpose; & they all agree, with the relation you say was made to your self. They further say on their own knowledg that part of her belly touches her Back-bone.[6]

In a letter to John Brooke, Thomas Hobbes refers to the visit that the Earl of Devonshire paid to Martha Taylor, in order to witness her prodigious fasting. Martha Taylor, aged 19, the daughter of a lead miner from Over-Hatton near Bakewell, began her prolonged fasting on St Andrew's Day in 1667. At the age of 11 Martha was hit on her hip by a miller who was her neighbour, which led to her being paralysed for two weeks. A later paralysis, with symptoms of religious melancholy and delirium, preceded the start of her abstinence. This attracted general curiosity and the concern of the Earl of Devonshire, who arranged for her to be continually watched by twenty 'maids'. The watch proved negative, for no deceit was detected. Doubts remained all the same, and in his report to the Royal Society the physician Nathalien Johnston judged Martha and her mother to be sly, untrustworthy and secretive.[7]

Martha looked emaciated in the lower part of her body, her stomach touched her spine, and she did not produce excretion and excrement. Nonetheless she was lively, accomplished, wise and well read, especially in religious matters. Hobbes observes, with a clear allusion to the social implications of the case and the family dynamics within it: 'Some of the neighbouring Ministers visit her often; others that see her for Curiosity give her Money, sixpence or a shilling, which she refuseth, & the Mother taketh. But it does not appear they gain by it so much, as to Breed a Suspition of a Cheat.'[8] Hobbes adds that 'The Woman is manifestly sick, & 'tis thought, she cannot last much longer'. For the philosopher, it is the role of the church to judge the miraculous nature of the fasting, and he prefers not to pronounce himself on the case, only commenting:

I think it were somewhat inhumane to examine these things too nearly, when it so little concerneth the Commonwealth; nor do I know of any Law that authoriseth a Justice of Peace, or other Subject to restrain the Liberty of a sick person, so farr as were needfull for a discovery of this Nature. I cannot therefor deliver any Judgement in the case.[9]

By referring to the notoriety of the case, to the basic and crucial question of the nature of the fasting and how it could be explained, Hobbes's letter highlights some of the major social, religious and medical concerns that surrounded the perception and understanding of self-starvation in the early-modern period. The aetiology of the fasting and Martha's physical condition suggest the competing readings of self-starvation; for instance, it may be viewed as deceit, as a

supernatural event, or as a natural phenomenon. More than one reading could exist simultaneously. Social, scientific and religious issues
are at stake, alluding to a cultural formulation for both the perception and understanding of the refusal of food. Hobbes significantly
restrains from pronouncing himself on the case, thus emptying it of
the social significance that is usually attributed to prolonged fasting
in the early-modern period. In so doing, Hobbes assumes an unusual
position in the debate regarding allegedly wondrous cases, whose
problematic nature is linked to the social and cultural recognition
ascribed to them.

Hobbes's belief that Martha is only ill contrasts with the account of
her fasting to be found in two other pamphlets, respectively by Thomas
Robins in his 1668 *News from Darby-shire or the Wonder of all Wonders*,
and by the author 'H. A.' in a 1669 pamphlet entitled *Mirabile Pecci*.
Both authors are among those who visited Martha and can therefore
claim to provide a firsthand reliable account of her prolonged fasting.
The details of the story coincide with those in Hobbes's letter regarding
Martha's family, the accident that caused her lameness, the development of her fasting from an early stage, and the description of her body.
H. A. also talks of convulsions, cramps, loss of speech, vomiting and
strange bleeding, all symptoms which are characteristic of the repulsion
manifested towards food in religious writing, and which coincide with
his providential reading of Martha's fasting.[10] Both authors also report
of Martha's great piety and on how she taught herself to read during her
illness. As Robins puts it: 'she hath her speech very perfect and has a
great delight to talk and discourse in the Scriptures with any Scholar'.[11]
It is in fact common to all reports of the case that all sorts of people visited Martha, especially religious men, whom she entertained discussing
religious matters. H. A., in particular, extensively describes Martha's
resilience as a sign of God's will, and suggests her piety by reporting
extracts of their conversations.[12] This is an unusual feature in early-
modern reports of prolonged fasting, in which the faster generally tends
to remain a silent presence. In accordance with the overall tone of
the account, Martha's reported speeches deploy a mystical language,
especially characteristic of women's religious writing, and are rich in
metaphors of food and feeding.

It is worth emphasizing that prolonged fasting was for many centuries
an important ascetic practice, especially for women, for whom the
denial of food functioned as a tangible manifestation of chastity, faith,
and withdrawal from the confines of their expected social roles.[13] In the
medieval period, for example, this practice became prominent for

women, who consistently adopted extreme denial of food. This, together with bodily mortification, piety, charity, the nurturing of the sick, and the distribution of food, served as overt signs of asceticism.[14] As Caroline Walker Bynum has observed, medieval mystics used bodily mortification and self-starvation as modes of altering bodily and social habits in order to gain control over their own lives.[15] Hence women tended to somatize religious experiences and ascetic practices, and turned the latter into an elevation rather than a rejection of physicality. This informed their use of metaphors of food and taste.

Early-modern 'miraculous maids' partly inherited the medieval ascetic tradition, whilst divesting it of its religious significance. Unlike medieval fasters, miraculous maids are usually presented within the confines of their domestic environment. Their denial of food is characteristically framed within the increasing interiorization of fasting that tend to coincide with contemporary forms of self-control, both in terms of diet and religious practices. Whilst early-modern regimens of health advised on proper ways of fasting as part of their dietary prescriptions, individual religious abstinence from food and drink remained an important act of faith. Equally, days of national fasting were occasionally appointed as acts of common repentance and purification, pointing to an overlapping of the individual and social dimensions of the denial of food within both the Roman Catholic and the Reformed Church.

An interesting instance of the denial of food as an ascetic practice is represented in seventeenth-century England by women prophets, such as Anna Trapnel, Elinor Channel, Martha Hatfield, and Sarah Wight.[16] Their fasting is indicative of the reformulation of religious practice, bearing similarities to medieval female asceticism, and standing alongside the more profane form of *inedia* (the refusal of food) represented by miraculous maids (as self-starving young women were usually called in the early-modern period). Most significantly for our purposes is the fact that their protracted fasting coincided with their prophetic utterances. Their speech consistently deploys images that contrast earthly food to the heavenly nourishment they claim to receive, transforming their transgressive behaviour into a divine sign. Through their fasting and prophecies, women prophets made themselves visible and audible, rendering their bodies as well as their voices a means of empowerment that allowed them to overcome the confinements of expected gender roles. Yet, as Diane Purkiss has commented, 'such somatological representation also turned women's bodies into signs which could be reread and appropriated to serve masculine agendas and discourses putting women firmly into the place assigned to them.

But such masculine co-operations were precisely what enabled women prophets to be heard'.[17]

Purkiss points to an ambiguity which is also evident in H. A.'s report of Martha Taylor and which renders Martha's voice quite problematic. She is, for example, reported as saying: 'if I was able to feed upon all good Creatures of God, where as now I cannot, yet they could none of them satisfie or solace my poor week, hungry Soul'; or, that 'I look upon my preservation without the use of creatures to be the manifestation of Infinite Power, for the benefit and advantage of them that fear God, to let them see that God can preserve life by and of himself, and for the hardening of the obstinate and impenitent; for my own awakening, and bringing into the way of holiness'.[18] Martha's words evoke the language and images in Anna Trapnel: 'I took that Scripture Neglect not the body, and went to the Lord and enquired whether I had been so, or had any self-end in it to be singular beyond what was meet; it was answered me, No, for thou shalt every way be supplied in body and spirit, and I found continuall fullness in my stomach, and a taste of diverse sweetmeats and delicious food therein, . . .'; equally Martha Hatfield claims: 'I would take food, if God would give me leave, but I cannot, I cannot'.[19] It is clear that Martha fashions herself according to both a behaviour – the denial of food – and a language which are already culturally available. Her words, as those of the women prophets and ascetics before her, signal a shift from the preservation of the body to that of the soul, thus rendering both her prolonged fasting and her starving body vehicles of God's will. Characteristically, Martha uses food images to represent God as a source of fullness and well-being, turning the starving body into both a sign and an expression of God's intervention. Yet, it is difficult to assess to what extent it is the faster, and to what extent it is the author of the reports, H. A., who translates the anxiety caused by self-starvation into a manifestation of God's agency. We may ask to what extent Martha is talking about her condition with the language which is accessible to her, and to what extent the author of the pamphlet is interfering with her discourse and having her adopt a language already culturally available. Both Martha and H. A. seem irrevocably trapped in the endorsement of a specific presentation and understanding of the denial of food.

H. A. examines Martha's starving body in search for a proof of its extraordinary condition, and wonders at it:

When you had been satisfying your Curiosity by a strict search here, you would have supposed your Hand to have been examining an half consum'd Carkass within a Grave. Here also modest Inquisition might have stood amazed to behold that colour and flesh on the Face and Armes, and yet find that vast decay in the nether Parts.[20]

H. A. turns the very improbability of Martha's body into a wondrous sign of God. The boundaries between life and death collapse, as do those between the natural and the supernatural. The problem such a description raises is not so much that of its authenticity, but rather that of its cultural significance. As in the case of Martha's voice, we are confronted by an appropriation of prolonged fasting that endorses it as much as attempting an interpretation of the denial of food. As Jacques Maître has noted in his study of religious fasting, the hagiographic claims of the complete denial of food for mystics may be considered a radicalization of fasting itself, to which both the hagiographer and the faster culturally conform. *Inedia* thus becomes a trope of feminine asceticism, as a manifestation of mysticism. Its relevance shifts from its actuality to its status as a socio-historic and psychological condition.[21]

Whilst both Robins and H. A. believe in the miraculous nature of Martha's prolonged fasting, the physician John Reynolds gives a different interpretation and tries to explain it in medical terms.[22] Though not doubting the authenticity of this protracted case of abstinence, Reynolds does not accept a supernatural explanation of the denial of food. As is often the case in medical writing on prolonged abstinence, he distinguishes between the miraculous condition of Elijah's or Moses's fasting, and that of young women like Martha. Reynolds dismisses the hypothesis of prodigious abstinence for the latter and sets himself the task of giving the phenomenon a physiological explanation. He grounds his hypothesis on Thomas Willis's theory of fermentation, as expounded in his 1659 *Of Fermentation of the Inorganical Motion of Natural Bodies*. Moving from the general to the particular, Reynolds is not concerned with Martha's case as such, but rather with the physiology of prolonged abstinence. Considering blood as the primary holder of life and its corruption the first cause of disease, he examines the mechanical fermentation of the seminal salts or mechanical spirits in the body. This fermentation is produced by 'the effect of matter and motion' in other words of the blood, or 'before it of the seed impregnated with active principles, which through their activity and heterogeneity suffer mutual collisions, or fermentations'.[23] Given the tendency for prolonged fasters to have a phlegmatic or melancholic constitution, this may result in the body using the product of fermentation instead of more proper nourishment. These ferments, moreover, tend to produce a high level of acidity, which allows the continuation of fermentation without the addiction of chyle. Reynolds also observes that 'the seminal humours in these Virgins may by a long abode in their vessels grow acid, and therefore supply the blood with a more than ordinary ferment'.[24] This proves the presence of acidity, and consequently of heat, in the body, yet if the blood produced by female seed is not purged through menstruation, this causes many disorders. As he comments:

> most of these Damosels fall to this abstinence between the age of fourteen and twenty years when the seed hath fermented the blood, that various distempers will probably ensue without due evacuations; except in our case, where through the defect of fermenting food we are enabled to bear the excess of these so much the better.[25]

Reynolds explicitly links the denial of food to femininity. His original theory of fermentation paints a pathological picture, which since the 1540s has informed the understanding of prolonged fasting, by binding it to women's physiology.

The medical debate surrounding the nature of prolonged fasting is present throughout the early-modern period. An early record concerns the case of Margaretha Weiss, as reported by Johannes Reusch in 1542, who already believed that the young woman's denial of food was due to her phlegmatic constitution.[26] Margaretha's prolonged fasting was further discussed by the philosopher Simone Portio and the physician Joseph Lange, who both tried to explain it physiologically. Portio advocates the theory, based upon classical doctrines, that fasters lived on the nutritive elements of the air.[27] Lange, instead, suggests that prolonged fasting may be interpreted as a paralysis of the stomach.[28] For Lange, appetite – the need to restore warmth and strength to the body – is proportionate to the temperature of the body, and since old people, women and animals are constitutionally colder, they require less nourishment. Such coldness of the body is increased in melancholic and phlegmatic constitutions. The body obstructed by the phlegmatic juice of concoction preserves its vital heat and does not require the support of nourishment for its survival. Lange draws his belief from the understanding of the body prevalent in his time, which viewed the implementation of the corporeal heat as vital. Though variously expressed, this theory prevailed in medical debate throughout the sixteenth and the first half of the seventeenth centuries, in an attempt to determine the natural causes of prolonged fasting.[29] Originally based on the Galenic theory of the body, these arguments gradually shifted within the changing parameters of the mechanistic conception of the body. Most significantly, it became apparent in the explanations of prolonged fasting that there was some difficulty in establishing straightforward relations between external and internal causes, and a tendency to draw similarities with other disorders, such as green-sickness, melancholy and hysteria.[30]

Characteristic of all these disorders was the intervention of physiological and psychological factors in producing a condition which foreshadowed the homology, for the female body, between the stomach and the womb, since the denial of food, uterine obstruction or amenorrhoea often occurred as related symptoms. From a 1608 dissertation in which the author describes *inedia* as a form of 'hysterical appetite' imputed to the suppression of menstruation, to Daniel Sennert's belief that prolonged fasting was due to an idiosyncratic dysfunction of the uterus, the medical reading of the disorder restated the parameters of its gendering, binding it to women's physiology.[31] Sennert's explanation of uterine obstruction produced by an excess of sulphuric salts due to the retention of seed bears similarities to Reynolds's theory. Both authors are preoccupied with re-inscribing the denial of food within a mechanistic understanding of the body, yet their theories still maintain similarities with other gendered pathologies, thus betraying a preoccupation with the socially transgressing connotation of the denial of food. The overlapping in the early modern medical understanding of prolonged fasting between the denial of food and the pathologies of melancholy, green-sickness, and hysteria, all of which foreground problems with the cultural perception of femininity and the need of monitoring sexuality, reveal a problematic cultural impasse. The denial of food subverts assumed notions of order and propriety. Through self-starvation, miraculous maids challenged the norm, by rendering themselves 'unnatural', 'super-natural', or 'pathological'.

The cultural preoccupation with the denial of food is apparent in the aetiology of the condition and in the description of the starving body, consistent in all early-modern accounts of prolonged fasting. As in the case of Martha Taylor, medical accounts present the same picture of a young woman belonging to the lower and middling classes who, as the result of a disease, refuses cooked foodstuffs, only eating small quantities of bread, fruit or broth, then denying food completely. Often bedridden, the faster may suffer from temporary paralysis, dumbness, or fits. Her body does not usually show excessive signs of emaciation, except from a collapse of the stomach that is always described as touching the spine. This is usually the most apparent sign of self-starvation, together with dryness and a melancholic or phlegmatic constitution, and the complete absence of excrement and excretion. In this medical picture, both the aetiology of self-starvation and the presentation of the starving body suggest a cultural process that produces narrative linearity in the gradual denial of food, and in the depiction of a perfectly self-contained image of the body. The accounts allude to a literal as well as symbolic impropriety of diet, yet the faster does not seem the agent of her self-starvation, but rather the passive sufferer of her condition. Beyond this coherence, we may gather the obliterated picture in which, as in the case of melancholy and hysteria, the faster makes the body into a readable sign of turmoil and inadequacy, suggesting an intertwining between external expectations and the individual's desire.

In the last part of his work, as a confirmation of his explanation, Reynolds includes a report on Martha's case. With Reynolds as well as with the other extant medical account, that of Nathalien Johnston, Martha's denial of food is reinterpreted within a rational frame which shifts the wonder of her prodigious abstinence to the physiology of the starving body. Johnston is especially concerned with the authenticity of Martha's prolonged fasting and with the fear of deceit. Yet his report adds nothing to other accounts of the case. Common to all the accounts concerning the case is the presentation of Martha's starving body as an improbable and yet wondrous vehicle of divine grace, and the tangible yet questionable proof of the truthfulness of the fasting. It is the focus of medical investigation, and most of all a spectacle that attracts curiosity and disbelief.

The case of Martha Taylor and competing readings of prolonged fasting

the palms of her hands are often moist, her countenance fresh and lively, her voice cleer and audible, in discourse she's free, her belly fla'd to her back bone, so that it may be felt through her Intestines, whenche a great cavity is admitted from the *Cartilago ensiformis* to the Navil, and though the upper parts be less emaciated (though much too) yet her lower parts are very languid, and inept for motion, and the skin thereof defiled with dry pruriginous scurf . . .[32]

By both matching the early-modern description of prolonged fasting and significantly differing from it, the case of Martha Taylor invites us to question the multiple readings of her condition and to investigate its broader cultural implications. Martha's story does not offer us any straightforward interpretations. The reasons for her prolonged fasting are carefully obliterated in the texts. Whilst it is legitimate for us to ask whether her self-starvation may be related to her alleged paralysis following a neighbour hitting her on the hip, and let us suppose that this is an encoded reference to sexual violence, this hint is no more than a supposition. Of the familial and social dynamics in Martha's story we can also draw only a vague picture, as is usually the case with early-modern reports of prolonged abstinence.

Self-starvation usually starts within the family and gradually moves outside the familial sphere. Some early-modern cases of prolonged fasting refer to the parents' preoccupation with their daughter's denial of food, and point especially to the role played by the mother, often held as the person mainly responsible in cases of deceit.[33] It is thus not an accident that both Hobbes and Johnston refer to Martha's mother when mentioning the concern with fraud surrounding the case. Because of their culturally recognized nurturing role within the family, women – and especially mothers – occupied an ambiguous position in the cultural framing of self-starvation. They appear as the closest witness to the fasting, and are the ones towards whom greater suspicion and punishment are directed in cases of deceit, as well as a metonymic referent of the fasting itself. The initial denial of cooked food and the preference for small quantities of raw foodstuffs, common to all early-modern accounts, point to a rift between the faster and her familial environment. In denying cooked food, the faster seems to jeopardize its symbolic binding value, and to withdraw from this symbolism.[34] This raises the question of whether self-starvation may be seen as an act of defiance, challenging accepted social roles for women. Although early-modern reports do not give us sufficient clues to assess the reasons of prolonged fasting for the individual, and therefore to establish to what extent self-starvation is an act of self-empowerment, nonetheless they make us aware of its social impact, and of how the denial of food functions as a form of cultural resistance.

It is evident that Martha's self-starvation aroused great curiosity. This is generally the case in all accounts of miraculous maids, to the point that one of them exhibited herself in an inn.[35] Like other human oddities in the early-modern period, prolonged fasters were perceived as wonders, attracting popular attention through the spreading of their notoriety. This curiosity crossed social classes, drawing people from all social stances to witness the prodigy of surviving without food. As for Martha, we can see how the faster acquires recognition within the boundaries of her small community, and attains a different status by becoming the focus of general attention, perhaps even gaining from

it economically. The accounts often hint at tension between the relatively humble social condition of the faster and the possible economic
advantage gained from the fasting. Such a tension is, however, treated
in various ways, especially in relation to the specific interpretation
given to prolonged abstinence. It usually plays a significant role in the
formulation of deceit. In the case of Martha, her social condition is presented as part of the general picture which allows the translation of her
condition into a wonder, and which functions as a standard narrative
pattern in the process of assessing the case. It remains marginal in the
construction of the narrative of Martha's self-starvation, and is a
contextual feature that is comparatively significant within the broad
early-modern literature of extraordinary cases, from witchcraft to supernatural wonders.

The gaining of notoriety of a case of prolonged fasting usually causes
the intervention of the civic authorities. In the case of Martha this
involved the Earl of Devonshire, who set up an investigation to ascertain the authenticity of the denial of food. The faster undergoes a careful medical examination and is put under the continuous watch of a
number of women for several days to prove that the fasting is not
fraudulent – in other words, that the faster does not eat or drink anything at all, and that her body does not produce any form of excrement
or excretion. Through such an investigation the starving body becomes
a public sign liable to interpretations, while the internal process that
has led the faster to the denial of food is overshadowed by the perception of the fasting. The authentication of prolonged fasting seems thus
to define a notion of the starving body that is already culturally
informed, and that also has various interpretations: medical, religious,
or deceptive. These interpretations almost appropriate the starving
body, shaping it according to culturally acceptable parameters. Equally,
the faster seems to fashion her own self-starvation in order to match
existing cultural expectations, and thus to turn herself into a culturally
forged wonder, open to multiple readings.

In discussing the case of Martha Taylor, Jane Shaw suggests that the
competing medical and religious readings of her fasting are the result of
a public debate prompted by the new scientific attitude which spread
throughout England in the second half of the seventeenth century,
which underlined the centrality of spirituality in the formation of the
rational self of the Enlightenment.[36] Through the case of Martha Taylor
and its competing readings, she illustrates the contamination of scientific discourse, represented by Reynolds's essay, by spirituality and the
irrational. For Shaw, 'the Martha Taylor event may also suggest, or at

least illustrate, the ways in which the rational self came to be gendered', suggesting the need to reformulate the disembodied rational male self of the Enlightenment in the light of such irrational events, and 'the miraculous bodies of women such as Martha Taylor'.[37]

Shaw's reading of Martha's case highlights the significance of manifestations of problems in the formation of the self during periods of shifting cultural parameters. The terms she considers – 'multiple interpretations' and 'gendering' – are, however, more deeply rooted in the early-modern cultural praxis than she recognizes, and may be indicative of a cultural reformulation rather than an innovative process. For, as we have observed, the coexistence of alternative or even contradictory interpretations of prolonged fasting is a common feature throughout the period, and one that persists well beyond the seventeenth century. Equally, although gender issues are apparent in cases of prolonged fasting, their relevance seems to be subordinated to the more crucial question of containing the disruption caused by the denial of food within culturally acceptable parameters. Hence Reynolds's reading of Martha's fasting conforms to an earlier tradition of medical writing, which tries to explain prolonged fasting physiologically by inscribing it within the early-modern understanding of the female body. At stake is the problematic nature of a behaviour that requires a formulation within cultural parameters. The gendering of the denial of food thus functions as a mould in which prolonged fasting can be shaped according to existing notions, such as the physiology of the female body and the social need of monitoring femininity.[38]

From the case of Martha Taylor, a number of other features that culturally shape the denial of food are also apparent. Martha reproduces, or rather is said to reproduce, behaviour and symptoms which are rooted in a tradition of prolonged fasting, thus rendering her condition recognizable. Yet, the very reproduction of culturally recognizable features also allows these parameters to be used in order to contain the problematic nature of the denial of food within culturally acceptable boundaries. In this process, the spectacle of the starving body, and the curiosity that turns it into news and makes it into a 'wonder', are important components in the shaping of prolonged fasting. In particular, the starving body becomes a cultural construct that fulfils expectations and becomes susceptible to various interpretations. These interpretations are narratives that recount the denial of food, the wonder of the starving body and how it may be understood. They acknowledge the modes in which culture appropriates and forges the denial of food by obliterating distinctions and producing a homology of details that help to support the cultural perception and therefore understanding of self-starvation. If the faster as well as those who witness the fasting are both the actor and interpreters of this process of enculturation, these narratives also testify to the unresolved fissure between the denial of food and the culture that supposedly produces and contains it. Hence in these narratives both the causes of self-starvation and the upsetting nature of such behaviour are consistently ignored.

Though the historical and cultural specificity of a case such as that of Martha Taylor is evident, the cultural patterns which we see as actively shaping the early-modern perception of self-starvation may offer us clues for detecting those which currently inform our perception and understanding of eating disorders. Historical cases, such as that of Martha, testify to instances in which an individual produces dysfunctional behaviour that violates social and cultural norms of order and acceptability. Both the difficulty and the need to find an explanation for such a phenomenon seem to cause a cultural reaction. This raises the question of whether the spread of eating disorders today is revealing not only of crucial individual, psychological, and social issues, but also of deeper dynamics which perpetrate themselves and which are expressed through the curiosity and spectacle caused by self-starvation, its formulation in narratives – from medical to biographical accounts – and the multiple interpretations of the disorder. Perhaps we may ask if, at a cultural level, we are dealing with a confused, if not ambiguous relationship between the private and the public, and a difficulty in the assimilation and channelling of information that may reach the pathology of a 'communicable disease' as proposed by Joan Brumberg. Perhaps we may question the effect of information and communication in the definition of the self in relation to our own notions of order and acceptability. As for earlier historical cases, but also in the current formation and spread of eating disorders, the public and private dimensions of the refusal of food may also be at odds. This invites us to question not only the causes that trigger eating disorders, but also the ways in which we react to them, the ways in which the denial of food interferes with the symbolic values we ascribe to food and to the body, and the modes in which we codify, define, and represent them and the manipulation enacted on both through self-starvation. As in earlier historical periods, we have elaborated a cultural picture for self-starvation that translates the denial of food into culturally acceptable terms. By dissecting the dynamics through which culture produces and endorses self-starvation, we may recognize the relationships that are established in the perception and definition of eating disorders.

Notes

1. Joan Jacobs Brumberg, 'From Psychiatric Syndrome to Communicable Disease: the Case of Anorexia Nervosa' in C. E. Rosenberg (ed.), *Framing Disease: Studies in Cultural History* (New Brunswick, NJ: Rutgers University Press, 1992) 134–54, 136.
2. Ibid., 141. See also Elaine Showalter, *Hystories: Hysterical Epidemics and Modern Culture* (London: Picador, 1997) 20–2.
3. Catherine Garrett, *Beyond Anorexia: Narrative, Spirituality and Recovery* (Cambridge: Cambridge University Press, 1998) xii.
4. Helen Malson, *The Thin Woman: Feminism, Post-structuralism and the Social Psychology of Anorexia Nervosa* (London and New York: Routledge, 1998) 94.
5. Ibid., 98.
6. Thomas Hobbes, 'Hobbes to John Brooke, from Chatworth', Letter 183, 20/30 October, in Noel Malcolm (ed.), *The Correspondence of Thomas Hobbes* (Oxford: Oxford University Press, 1994) vol. II, 701–3, 701.
7. Nathalien Johnston, 'Letter in Latin to Timothy Clarke concerning the young fasting woman in Derbyshire, named Martha Taylor, together with the apprehension of some imposture in the affair', 29 June 1669 in *The Journal Book of the Royal Society of London*, III: (1669) 389–92.
8. Hobbes, *Correspondence*, 702.
9. Ibid.
10. H. A., *Mirabile Pecci or the Non-such Wonder of the Peak of Darby-shire* (London: Printed for T. Parkhurst, 1669) 8.
11. T. Robins, *News from Darby-shire or the Wonder of all Wonders* (London: Printed for T. P, 1668) 4.
12. H. A., *Mirabile Pecci*, 28–30.
13. Peter Brown, *The Body and Society: Men, Women and the Sexual Renunciation in Early Christianity* (London and Boston: Faber & Faber, 1990) 253–40.
14. See Donald Weinstein and Rudolf Bell, *Saints and Society: Two Worlds of Western Christendom, 1000–1700* (Chicago and London: Chicago University Press, 1982) 226–33.
15. Caroline Walker Bynum, *Holy Feast and Holy Fast: the Religious Significance of Food to Medieval Women* (Berkeley and Los Angeles: University of California Press, 1987) 235–89.
16. Diane Purkiss, 'Producing the Voice, Consuming the Body', in Isobel Grudy and Susan Wiseman (eds), *Women, Writing, History 1640–1740* (London: Batsford, 1990) 139–58.
17. Ibid., 144–5.
18. H. A., *Mirabile Pecci*, 28.
19. Quoted in Purkiss, 'Producing the Voice' 146, 148.
20. H. A., *Mirabile Pecci*, 20.
21. Jacques Maître, *Anorexies religieuses, anorexie mentale, essai de psychanalyse sociohistorique: de Marie de l'Incarnation à Simon Weil* (Paris: Cerf, 2000) 82–3. For a psychoanalytical reading of religious fasting see also Rudolf Bell, *Holy Anorexia* (Chicago: University of Chicago Press, 1985).
22. John Reynolds, *A Discourse upon Prodigious Abstinence: occasioned by the Twelve Moneths Fasting of Martha Taylor, the Famed Derbyshire Damosell,*

presented at the Royal Society, 28 February 1668 (London: Printed by R.W. for Nevill Simmon, 1669).

23. Ibid., 11.
24. Ibid., 21.
25. Ibid., 21.
26. Johannes Reusch, *Propositiones aliquot de fastidiosa Spyrensis puellae inediae* (Spire, 1542). See also Geraldus Bucoldianus, *De puella, quae sine cibo & potu transigit* (Spire, 1542).
27. Simon Portius, *De puella germanica, quae fere biennium vixerat sine cibo potuque* (Florentiae, apud Laurentium Torrentinum, 1551) 14–16.
28. Josephus Langius, *Epistolarum medicalium* (Frankfurdi: apud heredes Andrae Wecheli, 1559) liber III, epistola 272, 666–79.
29. See, for instance, the debate concerning the prodigious fasting of Jane Balam between the two French physicians François Citois and Laurent Joubert. François Ciotois, *True and Admirable Historie of A Maid of Confolens in the Province of Poitiers*, translated by A. M. [Athony Munday] (London: I. Roberts, 1603); Laurent Joubert, *Des Erreures populaires* (Avignon: Guillaume Bertrand, 1578). For a contemporary comprehensive synopsis on the interpretations of prolonged fasting see Fortunius Licetus, *De his qui diu vivunt sine alimento* (Patavi, 1612).
30. On green-sickness see Langius, *Epistolarum medicalium*, liber I, epistola XXL, 100–03; Jean Varandal, *Traité des maladies des femmes* (Montpelier, 1630) 1–29; Jean Starobinski, 'Chlorosis – the Green-Sickness', in *Psychological Medicine*, 11 (981), 4459–68; S. L. Loudon, 'Chlorosis, Anemia, and Anorexia Nervosa', in *British Medical Journal*, 281 (1980), 1669–75. On melancholy see Richard Burton, *The Anatomy of Melancholy* (1621), eds. Thomas C. Faulkner, Nicholas K. Kiessling and Ronda L. Blair (Oxford: Oxford University Press, 1989); Jacques Ferrand, *A Treatise of Love-sickness* (1632), trans. and ed. by Donald Beecher and Massimo Ciavolella (Syracuse: Syracuse University Press, 1990). On hysteria see G. S. Rousseau, 'A Strange Pathology' in Sander L. Gilman et al. (eds), *Hysteria Before Freud* (Berkeley, London and Los Angeles: University of California Press, 1993) 91–141.
31. Franciscus Parcovius, *De virgineum cachexia* (Helmaestadtii: typis I. Lucij, 1608) 11. Daniel Sennert, *Practicae medicinae* (Wittembergi: Zachria Schurei 1632) liber III, chap. I, 21–40.
32. Reynolds, *A Discourse upon Prodigious Abstinence*, 34.
33. See Johannes Weyer, *De commentitiis ieiunii* (Basilaei: ex Officina Oporiana, 1577) 111, 124, 127–38.
34. Caterina Albano, 'Questioning Starvation', in *Women's Writing* 8:2 (2001), 313–26, 318–19.
35. Fabricius von Hilden, *Wund Arzney* (Frankfurt: gedruckt bey J. Aubry Hanan, 1652) observation XL, 147.
36. Jane Shaw, 'Religious Experience and the Formation of the Early Enlightenment Self', in Roy Porter (ed.), *Rewriting the Self: Histories from the Renaissance to the Present* (London and New York: Routledge, 1997) 61–71.
37. Ibid., 70–1.
38. For a discussion of the problematic ways in which self-starvation reproduces cultural assumed role of femininity see Bynum, *Holy Feast and Holy Fast*, 235–6; Susan Bordo, 'Reading the Slender Body' in M. Jacobus, E. F. Keller

and S. Shuttleworth (eds), *Body/Politics: Women and Discourses of Science* (London and New York, Routledge, 1987) 82–112; Susan Bordo, 'Anorexia Nervosa: Psychopathology of Culture', in D. Curtis and L. Helke (eds), *Cooking, Eating, Thinking: Transformative Philosophies of Food* (Bloomington, IN: Indiana University Press, 1992) 28–55; Elspeth Probyn, 'The Anorexic Body', in Arthur and Marilouise Kroker (eds), *Body Invaders: Sexuality and the Post-modern Condition* (Basingstoke: Macmillan, 1988) 201–11.

3
A Culture of Disfigurement: Imagining Smallpox in the Long Eighteenth Century

David Shuttleton

Introduction

The last reported case of naturally acquired smallpox occurred in Somalia in 1977, but the smallpox virus (*variola major*) survives under laboratory management.[1] As I write, there are newly intensified fears of smallpox being released by terrorists as a biological weapon. Smallpox still haunts the popular imagination as we share the desire of our ancestors to understand and thus control this deadly, disfiguring disease. This essay is concerned to show how the peculiarly gruesome visibility of smallpox meant that historically it was closely associated, at both a popular and scholarly level, with the psychosomatic power of the imagination. It will be argued that, for physicians and imaginative writers alike, the disfigurements of smallpox – both real and imagined – served as constant reminders of the ever-present threat of a monstrous disruption to the governable boundaries of the socialized body.

Smallpox first came to cultural prominence in England in the immediate post-Restoration period.[2] The deaths from the disease in 1660 of Prince Henry and Princess Mary, the adult brother and sister of Charles II, within months of their return from exile, alerted the whole nation to the dangers of what earlier medical texts all describe as a disease of childhood. Smallpox rapidly overtook the plague, leprosy, and syphilis as the most common pathogenic cause of premature death throughout Britain and much of Continental Europe. Modern pathology has established that the smallpox virus usually entered the body through either the nose, mouth or both (rarely through cuts in the skin surface). The primary sources of infection were from a sufferer's breath, from the corpses of victims, from handling infected clothes and bedding or by aerial infection that could cover distances of hundreds of yards. For a non-immune person, there was an incubation period of usually 12–14 days, in which time the victim was a so-called passive or non-infectious carrier. Thereafter they became highly infectious, and survivors remained so until the removal of all scabs, or, in the event of death, until decomposition or destruction of the corpse.

Smallpox followed a distinctive symptom pattern, the first sign being a high temperature, accompanied by headache, general debility and sometimes vomiting. After a few days the victim developed a characteristic rash, starting with the face, arms and upper torso, but often spreading over the whole body. This erupted into horrendous pustules that suppurated, giving off an offensive odour, polluting clothing and bedding. If pustules formed on the lips or mouth it could render eating and even drinking very difficult or, in severe cases, impossible. The severity of symptoms and survival rates depended to some extent on an individual's age and state of health at the time of exposure, but also upon the strain of smallpox contracted.[3] In fact death from smallpox could either come rapidly as a result of general toxaemia, or be protracted as a result of succumbing to secondary bacteriological infections.

Smallpox is most commonly known for leaving survivors with facial scarring (see Illustration 3.1). Apart from what most people imagine as a scattering of distinct 'pockmarks', so-called confluent smallpox could leave broad patches of scarring, resembling dark tissue-paper, covering whole areas of the epidermis. In a minority of cases, ulceration of the eyes left victims with varying degrees of blindness, or even destroyed the eyes themselves. The Scottish poet Thomas Blacklock (1721–91), who famously intrigued the literati with his ability to write 'descriptive verse' when he had no visual memory, had lost his sight to smallpox when only five months old. The disease also left Blacklock visibly scarred and a martyr to what at the time was labelled 'weak nerves'.[4] Such physical complications could be very protracted. The potter Josiah Wedgwood, who survived contracting smallpox in the Burslam epidemic of 1742 when he was 11 years old, was left with a badly scarred face, but, more seriously, with a secondary infection in his right knee which left him with a painful, immobilizing abscess, eventually requiring him to have his leg amputated in 1768 when he was 37.[5] Although victims were typically nursed in isolation, facial scarring and other long-term disfigurements amongst survivors served as permanent reminders of the threat of smallpox.

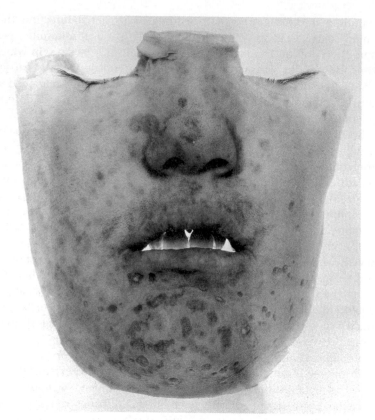

Illustration 3.1   Typical facial scars of smallpox; photograph of specimen in Hunterian Museum, Royal College of Surgeons

Smallpox and cultural framing

The apparent increase in the virulence of smallpox in the late seventeenth century may be merely a qualitative illusion as rival diseases went into relative abeyance. But epidemiologists generally agree that the greater mobility of populations and the associated expansion of cities at this time of rapid growth in trade were probably major factors in accelerating and spreading the infection to epidemic proportions. Certainly the long eighteenth century marks a concentrated period of cultural representation at a time when frequent smallpox outbreaks meant the constant threat of death or disfigurement. Apart from the evidence of material artefacts, ranging from tombstones to patent hospital ventilators, the historical role of smallpox in the cultural imaginary can be recovered from a variety of written representations in a large, underexplored archive of medical treatises, journals, and diaries alongside more imaginative literary and pictorial representations. This exploratory essay is predicated on a claim that existing accounts of smallpox, by both traditional historians and literary critics, are impoverished in so far as both have downplayed the role of the imagination in the historical framing of the disease. The former have largely constructed Whig histories in terms of progressive breakthroughs in preventive interventions: initially from the 1720s onwards, when Lady Mary Wortley Montagu played a prominent role in introducing the Turkish practice of variolation (inoculation) into English court circles, and subsequently from 1796 onwards when vaccination using serum derived from cow-pox was first promoted by Edward Jenner.[6] Traditional medical historians only examined historical medical texts for their purported accuracy in the context of subsequent paradigmatic breakthroughs. More blatantly imaginative texts such as poetry, if considered at all, have merely been used to provide illustrative 'background colour', and yet it is through such writing that we are more fully able to access the subjective, individual experiences of the disease as well as its more popular cultural meanings. Coleridge never fulfilled his plan to write a long poem celebrating Jennerian vaccination, a subject he thought worthy for a modern poet, but the topic was taken up by his humble contemporary Robert Bloomfield, whose substantial narrative poem, *Good Tidings; or News from the Farm* (1804), gains emotional force from the fact that it was prompted by the devastation reeked by smallpox amongst the labouring-class poet's own family.[7] Lady Mary Wortley Montagu's earlier canonical poem 'Satturday: After the Smallpox' registering the fears of *Flavia*, a court beauty, that her disfiguring pockmarks will mean social death, has often been considered in terms of both autobiography and genre (as mock-pastoral), but rarely placed within the wider context of other imaginative works presenting female scarring as moral retribution. An exception is Isobel Grundy's important reassessment of Lady Mary's role as pioneer inoculator, but literary scholars have yet to address the implications of Grundy's insight that '[e]ighteenth-century smallpox discourse was gendered: referring to men, it spoke of the danger to life; referring to women, of the danger to beauty.'[8] More broadly, critics have largely neglected to provide any adequate analysis of the poetics and rhetoric of smallpox; indeed in the only substantial study,

Raymond Anselment argues, unconvincingly, that smallpox resisted metaphoric meanings.[9] We need to address the many metaphoric, rhetorical and narrative meanings attached to smallpox in this rich repository of neglected literary texts; in numerous poetic elegies, in novels where smallpox serves as a punitive plot device or child inoculation provides a prompt for sentimental pathos, in the rare autobiographical writing of survivors, as well as the contrasting narratives of female and male disfigurement.[10]

But, as G. S. Rousseau has argued throughout an important essay on 'medicine and the muses', we must remain aware that the rhetoric of eighteenth-century physicians and poets (and many were both) is not so much a matter of distinct categories of knowledge, but more a continuum of explanation, in which writing and representation itself served a therapeutic role.[11] In short, we need a more interdisciplinary approach taking account of the metaphoric and cultural meanings of smallpox across medical *and* literary genres, as was done for TB, cancer and AIDS by Susan Sontag, and more recently for gout by Roy Porter and G. S. Rousseau, or the plague, leprosy and syphilis by Margaret Healy (though any such approach must always pay attention to specific textual questions of authorship, generic codes and social function).[12] This appears all the more necessary at a time when smallpox has returned to prominence in current, popular fears of disease.

Smallpox as metamorphosis: physicians, patients, and poets

Rarely were the broader symptoms of smallpox rendered with such clinical detail as in the poetic elegy on the death of Prince Henry, Duke of Gloucester in 1660, by one who attended him, the Royal Physician, Martin Lluelyn:

> The sharp disquiets of an aching brain,
> A heart in sunder torne, yet whole to pain.
> Eyes darting forth dimme fires, instead of sight;
> At once made see, and injur'd by the Light;
> Faint pulse; and tongue to thirsty cinders dry'd:
> When the reliefe of thirst must be deny'd.
> The Bowels parcht, limbs in tormenting throwes
> To coole their heat, while heat from cooling growes.
> Slumbers which wandering phansies keep awake,
> And sense not lead by objects, but mistake;[13]

Lluelyn was unusual in elaborating upon how victims remained conscious, if often delusional, even when the disease was at its most physically destructive. But if he uses a commemorative poem to provide one of the most closely observed symptomatic accounts of smallpox, we should note too that these verses also served as a defence of his own clinical methods against the charges of rival doctors and to assert his political loyalties, since he casts smallpox as the noxious legacy of Cromwell. This was also the blatantly ideological aetiology offered by Tobias Whitaker, another Royal physician, in his *Treatise on the Smallpox* (1660), which again constructs smallpox as a lingering seed of further rebellion left over from the polluted atmosphere of the usurpation.[14]

If some physicians visualized smallpox through the veil of political rhetoric, alternatively they might employ poetry as a diagnostic proof: the leading early-Georgian scholar-physician, Richard Mead, for example, in his *Discourse on the Small-Pox and Measles* (1747), argues that the horrid symptoms of 'malignant smallpox' are 'the effects of an acrid poison . . . because the same happens to those, who have been bit by the *haemorrhois*, a Lybian serpent', and by way of evidence he quotes Lucan's vivid verse description of the effects of such a bite upon Tullus.[15]

Physicians and imaginative writers habitually termed smallpox the doubly 'fierce' or 'cruel' disease because of its fearsome ability to rapidly transform the bodies of all its victims, even those lucky enough to survive. Lluelyn put it succinctly:

> Most fevers Limbecks though with these they burn,
> They leave the featur'd carcasse to the Urne,
> But thine was borne of that offensive race,
> Arm'd to destroy, she first strove to deface.[16]

With this potential to render victims unrecognizable to family, friends and indeed to sufferers themselves, poets repeatedly emphasized the trauma of social and self-alienation, perhaps none more bluntly than Thomas Shipman who, in another elegy of 1660, talks of a disease whose effects are, 'So loathsome . . . the Soul would hardly, own/The Body, at the Resurrection!'[17]

When the poet William Thompson, in his substantial poem *Sickness* (1745), a rare example of imaginative autobiographical writing by a survivor, sought to convey the subjective experience of surviving smallpox, he headed Book III 'The Progress of Sickness' with a quotation from the Book of Job: 'When I waited for Light there came Darkness./My Skin is black upon me; and my Bones are burnt with heat./My harp also is turned to Mourning'.[18] Smallpox was not infrequently associated with the 'Plague of Boils' inflicted on Job to test his faith; a biblical identification later to inform the influential Christian fundamentalist anti-inoculation arguments of the Rev. Edmund Massey.[19] But Thompson, like Mead, also turned to the classical poets, who provided powerfully mythic narratives and tropes for conveying the grotesque, transformative powers of the disease. For example, when Thompson tried to convey the experience of awakening from the delirium of a smallpox fever, he turned to Ovid's *Metamorphoses* (Book III), for a heroic analogy to covey how the 'Forehead roughens to the wonder'ing hand' as a personified 'Variola':

> Wide o'er the Human-field, the Body, spreads
> Contagious War, and lays its Beauties waste.
> As once the breathing Harvest, Cadmus, sprung,
> Sudden, a Serpent-brood? An armed Crop
> Of growing Chiefs, and fought Themselves to death.
> One black-incrusted Bark of gory Boils,
> One undistinguish'd Blister, from the Soal [sic]
> Of the sore Foot, to the Head's sorer Crown.[20]

Smallpox pictured forth the decomposition of the flesh in a grotesque anticipation of putrefaction, exposing the inherent corruption of fallen humanity. Eroding the borderline between inside and outside, nature and culture, the body of the smallpox victim was a site of conflicted desire. In this respect Anselment's observations on the representation of smallpox specifically in seventeenth-century elegiac poetry, in which he detects an ambivalent gaze oscillating between attraction and repulsion, mixing fascination with disgust, applies more generally throughout the subsequent century. It was a gaze arising out of a conflicted need to remember, and celebrate the smallpox victim for what they so recently were and horror at their monstrous transformation.[21] This is surely the 'vortex of summons and repulsion' described in Julia Kristeva's psycho-analytic 'Essay on Abjection'.[22] Suppurating pustules eroded the normally non-porous boundary between the solid – and thus definable – external surface of the body and its fluid inside, exposing what Kristeva calls 'The Horror Within'.[23] In the smallpox corpse we 'behold the breaking down of a world that has erased borders'.[24] As such smallpox marks a particularly intensified site for the disruption of the stabilizing distinction between the governable body cultural and the disruptive body natural that some sociologists argue is an essential effect of all disease.[25] We see this potential for disturbance gaining a fresh intensity in the unstable political climate of the 1790s – a time when fears of a regression to the bestial were intensified with Jenner's use of serum derived from animals (see Illustration 3.2).[26]

For survivors of smallpox, facial scarring in particular raised fundamental questions concerning the integrity and continuity of the self: does someone so visibly transformed remain the same person? What is the relationship between the damaged epidermis and inner character? By the late eighteenth century, with the emergence of materialist theories of mind–body reciprocation, smallpox disfigurement posed a problem for the fashionable adherents of physiognomy; notably in the influential theoretical expositions of Casper Lavater, who reluctantly had to concede that it is not possible to read someone's true character from a face where, as one poet phrases it at the time, smallpox had 'smeered the writing'.[27] Such metaphors of inscription are not infrequent in the literature of smallpox, as the disease is imagined as blotting out or writing over the previously legible face of its victims, leaving them open to new, and often cruel personal, social and moral

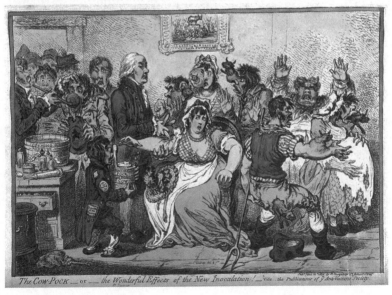

The Cow-Pock __ or __ the Wonderful Effects of the New Inoculation! __ Vide the Publications of y^e Anti-Vaccine Society

Illustration 3.2 'The Cow Pock __ or __ the Wonderful Effects of the New Inoculation!' by James Gillray, 1802

readings: the blind poet Blacklock, for example, complained of being openly mocked in the streets of Edinburgh as a walking *'memento mori'*.[28] Poets, essayists and preachers had long felt obliged to reassure the permanently disfigured that true worth lies in the angelic soul, not the corruptible flesh. When his son recovered from smallpox in the 1680s, Sir Matthew Hale addressed him in a homiletic letter: having surviving 'this spectacle of your own Mortality', the son is urged to remember his delivery – a lesson in the wages of luxurious excess – 'as often as those Spots and Marks in your Face are reflected to your view from the Glass':

> Remember by your former sickness, how pitiful an inconsiderable thing the Body of man is; how soon is the strength of it turned to faintness, and weakness, the beauty of it to ugliness and deformity, the consistency of it to putrefaction and rottenness; and then remember how foolish a thing it is, to be proud of such a Carcass. To spend all, or the greatest part of our time in trimming and adorning it, in studying new Fashions, and new Postures, and new Devices to set it out.[29]

Pockmarks served as somatic sermons against the dangers of an effeminizing narcissism; but, as already noted, it was women themselves, with their purported weakness for vanity, who were far more frequently the target of such moralizing. For women, especially young upper-class women, smallpox spelled social death.

Female disfigurement and 'menstruosity'

Lady Mary Wortley Montagu's semi-autobiographical *After the Smallpox* attests to the climate of cruel gloating in upper-class circles where female beauty was treated as a useful commodity in a marriage market. But where Montagu's *Flavia* implicitly resigns herself to this situation by retiring from court, it is the minor poet Mary Jones (1707–78), who, in her own poem 'After the Smallpox' (published 1750), offers reassurance by discrediting such crude materialism:

> What tho' some envious folks have said,
> That *Stella* now must hide her head,
> That all her stock of beauty's gone,
> And ev'n the very sign took down:
> Yet grieve not at the fatal blow;

For if you break a while, we know,
Tis bankrupt like, more rich to grow.
A fairer sign you'll soon hang up,
And with fresh credit open shop:
For nature's pencil soon shall trace,
And once more finish off your face,
Which all your neighbours shall out-shine,
And to your Mind remain a Sign.[30]

More broadly, smallpox was overdetermined in association with femininity as poets and moralists inherited established classical and biblical tropes already laden with moral meanings. The disfiguring power of smallpox (see Illustration 3.3) exemplified that all disease is evidence of the Fall which, according to Genesis, stemmed from specifically female transgression. This moralistic interpretation of smallpox as Eve's punitive inheritance to vain women is made explicit in *Inoculation; or Beauty's Triumph* (1768) when the poet Henry Jones supplicates the second-generation inoculator Daniel Sutton:

Oh! Hadst thou power to purge the darker Passions
From the human Breast, with moral medicine,
And inoculate the Soul; couldst thou, SUTTON,
Quick kill the Seeds of each Distemper there,
Of each irruptive fever, that deforms
The maker's Image in th'immortal Mind,
And blots bright beauty in the outward Frame,
With marking, deep degrading Spots, those banners
Of frail Defect, those legacies of EVE,
That give th'angelic Face the Lye,
And bring the fatal Apple to our View.[31]

This Old Testament notion of inherited sin was often overlaid onto an older Aristotelian discourse linking the generative female body with disease as related types of monstrosity. Indeed the leaky porosity of the smallpoxed body was implicitly feminine, in as much as the disruption of the classical bounded and sealed male body resembled the grotesque female body, as described by Bakhtin, which is 'unfinished, outgrows itself [and] transgresses its limits'.[32] Such sinful and monstrous associations are implicit in Thompson's Miltonic personification of smallpox as the female fury 'Variola', and his Ovidian description of his own transformation in her malign hands:

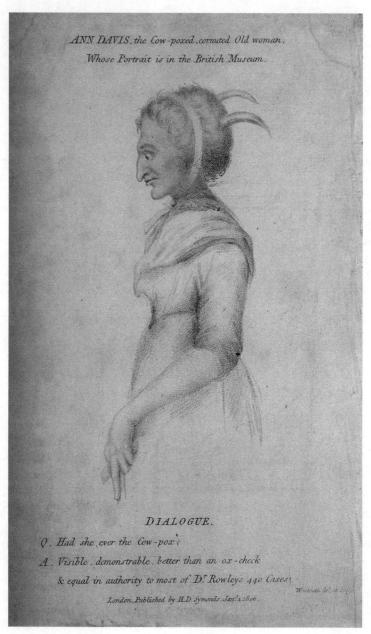

Illustration 3.3 'Ann Davis, the Cow-poxed, cornuted Old Woman', stipple engraving by T. Wolnoth, 1806

> But am I awake? Or in Ovidian Realms,
> And Circè holds the Glass? What odious Change,
> What Metamorphose strikes the dubious Eye?
> Ah, wither is retir'd the scarlet Wave,
> Mantling with Health, which floated through the Cheek
> From the strong Summer-beam imbib'd? . . .[33]

Thompson alludes here to Ovid's story of how, when asked by Polyphemus for a love potion that would make Scylla reciprocate his affections, instead, acting out of sexual jealousy Circè uses her magic skills – learnt from Hecate – to cast a spell over the pool where Scylla bathes: when she enters the pool she watches her own body transforming into that of a monster. While the image of self-alienation, as the victim catches sight of themselves in a mirror, was a more common, implicitly narcissistic trope in poems concerned with the loss of female beauty, Thompson offsets any risk of unmanliness by suggesting that it might be the witch Circè who actually holds his mirror. Thus smallpox is confirmed as the product of a monstrously threatening femininity, for, according to Ovid, Circè was Goddess of the Sun whose palace 'thronged with victims she had transformed into beasts' (*Metamorphoses*, Bk IX). This linkage between smallpox and the monstrous feminine was in fact implicit to the Galenic aetiology of the disease inherited by Restoration and Georgian scholar-physicians and poets in which Aristotelian notions of the porous generative female body were reinforced by Old Testament taboos regarding female blood as a source of pollution.[34]

It was traditionally claimed that smallpox grew from a so-called seed, 'seminaria' or ovum implanted in the blood of the foetus by the stagnated menstrual blood of the mother during gestation. Eruption of this seed of corruption was subsequently triggered by certain external conditions, such as bad air or miasmas, and treatment involved the purging of bad, coagulated blood and a return to humoural balance. Writing on smallpox in 1660 Tobias Whitaker employed the telling neologism 'Menstruosity' to describe this phenomena, concretizing in one word an established false etymological linkage between *menstrua* and *monstrum*.[35]

Closely allied to this 'innate seed' theory was the popular belief that smallpox might be triggered by the sight of someone bearing the outward marks of the disease or, indeed, simply by having their 'Fancy' overtaken by fearful images of the threat of smallpox. From the sixteenth century onwards the 'innate seed' theory was often posited

alongside a more modern model of specific particle contagion, as first
formally proposed in an influential treatise of 1546 by Girolomo
Frascatoro of Verona (1478–1553), that talked in terms of external physical transmission (through direct contact with victims, their bedding, or
by breathing in particles floating in the air of sick-chambers).
Nonetheless learned physicians continued to endorse the popular belief
that the disease could be triggered by so-called 'conceit' even into the
age of inoculation.

This persistent traditional association of smallpox with the power of
the imagination provides a context for an anxiety detectable in much
eighteenth-century writing on smallpox over the possible dangers of
representing, indeed even mentioning the disease in the first place.
Medical texts and imaginative literature alike tended to assume the
reader's familiarity with the disfiguring effects of smallpox, while deliberately avoiding any panic-inducing details. We have seen how the poet
Thompson sought to express his own personal experience of the disease, but in his own preface and annotations he betrays a self-conscious
anxiety over his theme:

> Sickness being a subject so disagreeable, in itself, to human Nature,
> it was thought necessary, as Fable is the soul of Poetry, to relieve the
> imagination with the following, and some other Episodes. For to
> describe the anguish of a distemper without a mixture of some more
> pleasing incidents, would, no doubt, disgust every good natur'd and
> tender reader.

> It cannot be suppos'd that I should treat upon sickness in a medi-
> cinal, but only in a descriptive, a moral, and a religious manner . . .
> I have just taken notice of the progress of the Small-pox, as may give
> the reader some small idea of it, without offending his imagination.[36]

Thompson's anxiety over 'offending the imagination' was not just a
matter of personal distaste: such disquiet needs to be read within the
wider context of a contemporary culture of smallpox in which a belief
in the contagious power of the imagination remained active.

Contagion by conceit

The role of fear in the likelihood of contracting or surviving smallpox
certainly formed part of popular knowledge at this time. In 1711
Jonathan Swift reports to Stella that Lady Betty Germaine's companion,

one 'Poor Biddy Floyd', a noted beauty, has lost her looks to smallpox: Lady Cartaret later explained that a cousin of hers had taken ill with smallpox at the house of a mutual friend and since died: 'it was near Lady Betty's and I fancy Biddy took fright'.[37] Similarly, in 1763 when the elderly James, Earl Waldegrave contracted smallpox he immediately made out his will and, as reported by his anxious friend Horace Walpole, observed that

> the great difference between having the smallpox young, or more advanced in years, consisted in the fears of the latter, but that as I had so often heard him say, and now saw, that he had none of those fears, the danger of age was considerably lessened. Dr Wilmot says, that if anything saves him, it will be this tranquillity.[38]

It was indeed common for physicians to caution their colleagues against frightening patients, and smallpox patients in particular (it was common practice to hide any mirrors in the sufferer's house).[39] Dr John Woodward (1665–1728), writing on the management of smallpox in 1718, suggests that the physician's 'Masterpiece, and chief Care is to raise the Fancy, steer and rightly rule the Passions, and continually keep up the Hopes of the Patient'.[40] He explains this in essentially humoural terms, based on the pyrolic spasms of nausea:

> This is a great Art: and so necessary that the best Medicines, directed with the utmost Wisdom, in the Small-Pox . . . will prove generally ineffectual and fruitless without it. The reason of which will be evident to those who are rightly inform'd of the Contrivance of the Body of Man: and know that the Stomach, which is the Fountain of those Principles that supply, form, and raise the Small-Pox, is likewise the Seat of the Passions. Now every unseasonable Rouseing of them must needs disturb the Oeconomy, and regular Egress of those Principles; upon which Oeconomy, and Regulation, the Event of the Disease depends. I am the more particular in this, because 'tis certain there are greater Numbers hurryed out of Life by the Disorders brought on by fright, Surprize, Apprehension, the bustle and indiscreet Shew of Concern by Relations, Friends, and those about the patient, than by the Malignity of the Disease.[41]

As this implies, the role of 'the Passions', essential to Galenic understandings of disease and a key term in eighteenth-century psychology, was crucial to contemporary understandings of how the disease acted.[42] Indeed carefully recorded case histories of contagion by 'conceit' are common in medical treatises published throughout the early part of this period.

In *A Particular Treatise of the Smallpox and Measles* (1689), by the Utrecht professor of physick and anatomy, Isbrand de Diemerbroeck (1609–74), often reprinted as part of his popular 'Anatomy', we find several such cases with the authorial commentaries.[43] A brief summary suggests that in these short narrative examples we are being invited to consider several means by which the disease might be triggered by mental association. Diemerbroeck's 'History V' recounts the story of how two young sisters encounter a young lad . . . newly cured of the Small Pox' who 'was got abroad, and coming along in the street, at least thirty paces distant from them, having his face all spotted with red spots, the remainders of the footsteps of the disease; with which sight they were so scared that they thought themselves infected already.'[44] Diemenbroek then recalls how he 'endeavour'd by many arguments to dispel these idle fears', by prescribing a purge and ordering them 'to walk abroad, visit Friends, and by pleasant Discourse and Conversation, and all other ways imaginable to drive those vain conceits out of their Minds'. But 'all that I could do signified nothing, so deeply had this conceit rooted itself in their Imagination' until 'at length, without occasion of Infection, they were both seized' (the history ends with his reassurance that by 'observing my prescription exactly, without scratching off the Pox with their Nails, [they] were both cured with very little or no prejudice to their beauty').

In his 'Annotations' Diemerbroek observes: 'How wonderful the Strength of Imagination is, we have experienced in many Persons, for that by the Motions of the Mind it frequently works Miracles' and 'thus in these two Gentlewomen through the continual and constant Cogitation caused by the Preceding Fear, that Idea of the Small Pox, so strongly Imprinted in their Minds, and thence in their Spirits and Humours, begat therein a disposition and Aptitude to receive the Small Pox'. He also reports visiting a 'Noble *German*, who Dreamt that he was drawn against his Will to visit one that was Sick of the Small Pox, and was very much disfigur'd'; being 'unable to drive the dream out of his thoughts', after three weeks this nobleman fell 'into a fever and was pepper'd with the Small Pox'.[45]

Such cases continued to be published throughout the eighteenth century.[46] In Thomas Fuller's *Exanthematologia, or an Attempt to Give a Rational Account of eruptive fevers, especially of the measles and smallpox*

(1730) – one of the most substantial early-Georgian medical studies – he observes that there 'have been very numerous Instances of people that have got the Small Pox (but not the Measles, or any other Sorts that I have heard of) by mere Fancy and Fear'. Fuller discusses several examples of his own, one of 'the most unaccountable' being that of a young man, 'who being scared with seeing one that lately had it, was taken ill upon the spot . . . and had them come out upon the very next day'. Alluding to the usual, essentially humoural explanations, Fuller thought this case 'beyond all Rule and Precedent; for there was no Time for Assimilation or Concoction of the matter before Expulsion'.

A distinct subset of Fuller's cases involve the mediation of objects bearing fearful associations: a young woman is sent a gold chain 'which another had worn in the Small-Pox, to keep them . . . out of their Throat' but it 'chanced to bring Terror, and caused her Fancy to work her up into a kindly Small-Pox; out of which she recover'd'. She in turn tells Fuller how a gentleman who once 'lay sick of the Small-pox, order'd his servant to send a key; which he had not lately touch'd and lay in a chamber far distant from him to his Mother' who 'conceited it brought Infection' and soon fell fatally ill with the disease. In each such case it is emphasized that the object had never been in direct contact with a victim: rather, they trigger the disease at a distance purely by prompting mental associations.

In a related case Fuller describes that of a gentlewoman who, being accidentally brushed by some soil when passing a Sexton digging a grave, went home

> most terribly frighten'd, fancying some Corps that had dy'd of the Small-Pox had broke out upon her; upon which she fell in Travail, brought forth a Child full of them; both Mother and Child dy'd. So the Distemper bred upon both from nothing at all but a mistaken Conceit.[47]

Fuller adds three whole quarto pages of citations to further reports of pregnant women bearing children infected with smallpox in the womb.[48] He remarks that as 'strange a Thing as breeding of the Small-Pox by the force of fear and Fancy' is no more to be wondered at than the common knowledge that 'longing-women' can 'by the pure workings of the Imagination, form the Spirits into such Ideas, figures, and Species, as to Imprint marks upon their Foetus in the Womb'.[49]

While it cannot be stated categorically that the majority of smallpox case histories concerned women, and in particular mothers, the role of the purportedly vulnerable and unruly female imagination was prover-bial. In William Wycherley's stage-comedy *The Country Wife* (1674), a play riddled with metaphors of disease, the misogynist fop Sparkish quips that 'we men of wit have amongst us a saying that cuckolding, like smallpox, comes with a fear, and you may keep your wife as much as you will out of danger of infection, but if her constitution incline her to't, she'll have it sooner or later, by the world . . .' (IV, iv). To make full sense of such assertions, we must turn to contemporary physicians like Fuller, who offers a brief explanation of the psychosomatic reciproca-tion at work:[50]

> Now when a Person is taken with a through pannic and Fright, and thinks of nothing but Infection, that extraordinary Perturbation and Terror may form the Spirits into such Species, and create such an Alteration of the Particles of the Body, as will directly and pecu-liarly act upon the latent ovula as effectively as an actual Contagion might do.[51]

Conventional medical historians either ignore or dismiss these early-modern psychosomatic accounts of contagion, which disrupt their own categorization models. For example, in his 1992 essay 'Explaining Epidemics', Charles E. Rosenberg provides terms for distinguishing between two alternative early-modern ways of understanding epidemic disease.[52] The first is a 'configuration' model, predating the knowledge of specific infectious agents, which attributed an epidemic to 'a unique configuration of circumstances, a disturbance in the "normal" health-maintaining and health-constituting – arrangement of climate, en-vironment, and communal life'. Alternatively there is, what Rosenberg terms, a 'contamination' model that often 'reduced itself down to person-to-person contagion, of the transmission of some morbid mate-rial from one individual to another'. But as Rosenberg describes 'con-tamination' as 'logically alternative' to 'configuration', crucially he also concedes that 'historically the two have often been found in relatively peaceful, if not logical co-existence'.[53] While this certainly chimes with my own reading of eighteenth-century accounts of smallpox in which several models are often offered together, Rosenberg adds the following footnote to his account of *configuration*:

> Smallpox constituted something of an exception. Although eighteenth-century physicians did not understand the nature of the 'virus' that was passed from individual to individual during

inoculation . . . it was clear that the epidemics of this great killer were caused by a specific, reproducible 'matter'.[54]

Rosenberg's two models remain indispensable for discussion purposes, but his claim for the exceptional nature of smallpox requires some qualification. Although the development of inoculation did gradually lead to the dominance of a theory of external contagion from 'reproducible matter', it is also evident that, however illogical, configuration explanations persisted long into the age of inoculation; moreover these persisted alongside the belief, clearly dependent upon a continued adherence to the 'innate seed' theory, that smallpox could be triggered by the imagination.

Writing as late as 1779, in a pamphlet supporting the inoculator John Coakley Lettsom, the pseudonymous 'Uninterested Spectator' argues for the advantages of inoculation by comparing the progress of the mild form of the disease amongst the inoculated – who may only bear a few pustules – with the victims of the natural, confluent form, whose 'miserable body . . . is covered with indistinguishable millions'.[55] Though it might be argued that the confluent patient is 'confined to his chamber' while the 'inoculated one is abroad in the street, obvious to the approach of every passenger', the latter case is preferable because if the confluent patient dies, 'his chamber must be thrown open releasing a stream of malignant particles, in their highest state of energy, dispersed at once among the neighbourhood'. Moreover, if the confluent patient lives, he must come abroad at some stage,

and in general he [the confluent patient] will come out much too soon, and object of disgust and terror, deformed by the violence of the distemper, and loaded with contagion. The inoculated patient is almost perpetually in the air, the action of which will gradually dissipate the effluvia exhaling from his body, and prevent their accumulating in his garments; . . . A confluent patient, I apprehend, might communicate the disease by the most instantaneous interview; the inoculated patient, I should suppose, could communicate it only by an approximation of some considerable duration.

ADMITTING what has often been asserted, that fear, by acting on the nervous system, sometimes produces the smallpox, the natural disease must be infinitely more mischievous than inoculation; the confluent subject walks the streets, as before hinted, imprinted with alarming tokens of his dangerous condition, so visible and peculiar as not to be mistaken; the inoculated subject has at most only a few pustules not to be distinguished from common pimples but by close examination, and often has none.[56]

Note here how the theory of contamination by conceit has accrued a fashionable explanation in terms of delicate nerves while, in keeping with Rosenberg's 'illogical' juxtapositioning, the account as a whole moves comfortably between an explanation in terms of airborne 'reproducible matter' and one in terms of contagion by fear.[57] It is also telling that all this is offered in defence of what the writer terms the 'modern regimen' of inoculation, especially when we consider Rosenberg's own comment on how the equilibrium model of health active in the eighteenth century, in which 'the idea of specific disease entities played a relatively small role', continued to dominate 'even when a disease seemed not only to have a characteristic course but (as in the case of smallpox), a specific causative "virus", the hypothetical pathology and indicated therapeutics were seen within the same explanatory framework'.[58] Indeed many eighteenth-century inoculators devised regimens to be adopted in preparation for the operation. By the late eighteenth century, fashionable inoculators were establishing isolation houses in the countryside where, for those who could afford it, individual fears were

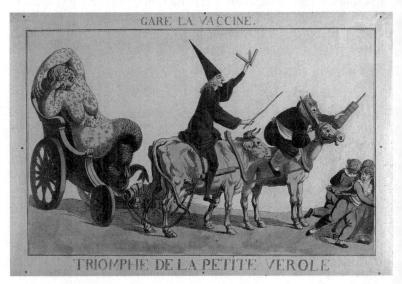

Illustration 3.4 'Gare La Vaccine: Triomphe de la Petite Verole', etching with watercolour, *c.* 1800

quelled by regulated sociability with fellow risk-takers as part of the pre-inoculation regimen.[59]

As I have begun to illustrate, attention to both medical and imaginative texts reveals how smallpox was rhetorically framed within inherited conceptions of disease as punishment for sin, as seed of inherited corruption and within specific gender ideologies. In particular it was fearfully imagined and framed within an accepted model of psychosomatic interaction. Conventional disease histories often begin by outlining the current state of 'objective scientific' knowledge, against which the type of older, imaginative models I have just been recovering are measured and found wanting, if not absurd. Although I have prefaced my own discussion of early-modern smallpox culture with a summary of modern pathological knowledge, I want to conclude by drawing attention to the cautionary words of a contemporary social historian J. R. Smith, who, in opening his own summary of the 'Classification and Pathogenesis of Smallpox', remarks that 'it must be pointed out, however, that medical opinion, even as late as the 1960s, was by no means unanimous on the subject'.[60] While this serves to remind us that even our current knowledge of a given disease is socially and culturally constructed within contested discourses, to make this claim does not automatically require a collapse into postmodern solipsism: smallpox was not just a linguistic construct, and to imply so would be an insult to those many generations who suffered the pain of illness and loss.[61] To suggest the importance of the imagination in the historical framing of smallpox is not to claim that smallpox was merely *imagined* (though this does not preclude the possibility that fear might eventually be proven to directly impact on the immune system). But Smith's aside does nevertheless alert us to the historical contingency of the epistemic frames – be they scientific, religious, psychological, pictorial or poetic – within which we imagine a given disease.

Notes

1. The last-known death occurred in Birmingham, England in 1978 when a photographer's assistant was infected after the virus accidentally leaked from a research laboratory.
2. The standard histories are James Moore, *The History of the Smallpox* (London, 1815), Charles Creighton *A History of Epidemics in Britain*, 2 vols [1891, 1894] reprinted 1963 (London: Frank Cass and Co.), C. W. Dixon, *Smallpox* (London: J. and A. Churchill, 1962), Donald R. Hopkins, *Princes and Peasants:*

Smallpox in History (Chicago and London: The University of Chicago Press, 1983) and J. R. Smith, *The Speckled Monster: Smallpox in England, 1670–1970, with particular reference to Essex* (Chelmsford: Essex Record Office, 1987).

3. By 1977, the World Health Organization recognized ten viral strains. Of the prevalent types of *variola major* identifiable in eighteenth-century accounts, the two most severe strains were that now known as malignant, confluent or black smallpox (Type 2), with a mortality rate of about 75 per cent, and malignant semi-confluent smallpox (Type 3), with a 25 per cent mortality rate: Smith, *The Speckled Monster*, 179–182.

4. Henry Mackenzie, 'Life of the Author' prefacing *The Poems of Thomas Blacklock* (London, 1791).

5. Smith, *Speckled Monster*, 19.

6. Isobel Grundy, 'Medical Advance and Female Fame: Inoculation and its After-Effects', in *Lumen* XIII (1994), 13–42, is an important riposte to the standard histories: Genevieve Miller, *The Adoption of Inoculation for Smallpox in England and France* (Philadelphia: University of Pennsylvania Press, 1957) and Peter Razzell, *The Conquest of Smallpox* (Firle: Caliban Books, 1977) (as well as Creighton, Razzell, Smith and Hopkins above); for vaccination see John Baron, *The Life of Edward Jenner*, 2 vols (London, 1827, 1838), E. M. Crookshank, *History and Pathology of Vaccination* (Philadelphia, 1889), Edward J. Edwardes, *A Concise History of Small-pox and Vaccination in Europe* (London, 1902), F. D. Drewitt, *The Life of Edward Jenner* (London, 1931); Peter Razell, *Edward Jenner's Cowpox Vaccine: The History of a Medical Myth* (Firle: Caliban Books, 1980); Derrick Baxby, *Jenner's Smallpox Vaccine: The Riddle of Vaccinia Virus and its Origins* (London: Heinemann, 1981), Paul Saunders, *Edward Jenner: the Cheltenham Years 1795–1823* (Hanover, USA and London: University Press of New England, 1982) and W. Le Fanu, *A Bio-bibliography of Edward Jenner* (London: Harvey and Blythe, 1951); see also James Johnston Abraham, *Lettsome 1744–1815: His Life, Times, Friends and Descendents* (London: Heinemann, 1933).

7. Creighton, *A History of Epidemics*, 588 (Coleridge to Jenner).

8. Grundy 'Medical Advance', 15; another exception is Jill Campbell, 'Lady Mary Wortley Montagu and the "Glass Revers'd" of Female Old Age' in Helen Deutsch and Felicity Nussbaum (eds), *'Defects': Engendering the Modern Body* (Ann Arbor, MI: The University of Michigan Press, 2000) 213–51 (though the emphasis here is on the discourse of female aging).

9. Raymond Anselment, *The Realms of Apollo: Literature and Healing in Seventeenth-Century England* (Newark: University of Delaware Press, 1995) 196.

10. This essay, part of a book-length project, mainly refers to poetry. I shall be discussing the specific discourse of male smallpox disfigurement, including its visibility in portraiture, elsewhere.

11. G. S. Rousseau, 'Medicine and the Muses: an Approach to Literature and Medicine' in Marie Mulvey Robert and Roy Porter (eds), *Literature and Medicine During the Eighteenth Century* (London: Routledge, 1993) 23–57, passim.

12. Susan Sontag, *Illness as Metaphor* [1978] *and Aids and its Metaphors* [1989] (Harmondsworth: Penguin, 1991); Roy Porter and G. S. Rousseau, *Gout: the Patrician Malady* (New Haven and London: Yale University Press, 1998); Margaret Healy, *Fictions of Disease in Early Modern England: Bodies, Plagues and Politics* (Basingstoke: Palgrave, 2001).

13. Martin Lleulyn, 'An Elegie on the Death of the Most Illustrious Prince Henry, Duke of Gloucester' (Oxford, 1660) (quoted in Anselment, *Realms*, 194).
14. Details in my paper 'The Seeds of Further Rebellion: The Rhetoric of Smallpox at the Restoration', *Controlling Bodies*, Glamorgan University, July, 2002 (forthcoming).
15. Richard Mead, 'Discourse on Smallpox and Measles' in *The Medical Works of Richard Mead* (London, 1762) 154.
16. As quoted in Anselment, *Realms*, 194.
17. Ibid, p 197.
18. William Thompson, *Sickness: a Poem* (Oxford, 1745) 243.
19. Grundy, 'Medical Advance', 24.
20. Thompson, *Sickness*, 246.
21. Anselment, *Realms*, 197.
22. Julia Kristeva, *Powers of Horror: an Essay on Abjection* (New York: Columbia University Press, 1982) 1.
23. Ibid
24. Ibid. 53, 3–4.
25. Bryan S. Turner, *The Body and Society* (London: Sage, revised edn 1996) 213–14, 222–4.
26. See James Gillray's satirical engraving 'The Cow-Pock - or - the Wonderful Effects of the New Inoculation' (1802) in which the bodies of the vaccinated sprout cows.
27. Johann Casper Lavater, *Essays on Physiognomy; designed to promote the knowledge and love of mankind*, 3 volumes in 5 (London, 1789–98) I, 100; and II, Chapter iii; Temple Luttrell, 'Physiognomy, if Always an Index of the Mind?', *The Edinburgh Magazine or Literary Amusement*, Thursday 14 March 1782, 306.
28. Blacklock, *Poems*, 87.
29. *A Letter from Sr Matthew Hale, Kt, sometime Lord Chief Justice of England, To one of his Sons; After his recovery from the Small-Pox* (London, 1684) 3, 5 and 15.
30. Mary Jones, *Miscellanies in Prose and Verse* (Oxford, 1750) 79–80.
31. Henry Jones, *Inoculation; or Beauty's Triumph,: a Poem in Two Cantos* (Bath, 1768) 7–8.
32. Michel Bakhtin, *Rabelais and his World*, trans. H. Iswolsky (Cambridge, MA: MIT Press, 1968) 27.
33. Thomson, *Sickness* (1745) 246 (see also p. 229 ff).
34. Kristeva, *Powers of Horror,* 71ff.
35. Whittaker, *Treatise*, 6.
36. Thompson, *Sickness*, 41 and 'Advertisement to the Reader', v–vi.
37. Jonathan Swift, *Journal to Stella*, edited by Harold Williams, 2 vols (Oxford: Clarendon Press, 1963) II, 217.
38. *Horace Walpole's Correspondence with George Montagu*, 2 vols, edited by W. S. Lewis and Ralph S. Brown, Jr (London and New Haven: Oxford University Press and Yale University Press, 1941) II, 56.
39. Antoine Luyendijk-Elshout, 'Of Masks and Mills: the Enlightenment Doctor and his Frightened Patient' in G. S. Rousseau (ed.), *The Languages of Psyche: Mind and Body in Enlightenment Thought* (Berkeley and Oxford: University of California Press, 1990). A key text was Thomas Cadogan, *De Animi Pathematum, vi et modo agendi in inucendis vel curandis morbis* (Leiden, 1767).

40. Thomas Woodward, *The State of Physick: and of diseases; with an inquiry into the causes of the late increase of them; but more particularly of the small-pox* (London, 1718) 69.
41. Ibid., 69–70.
42. *Galen on the Passions and Errors of the Soul*, trans. Paul W. Harkins, introduction by Walter Riese (Columbus: Ohio State University Press, 1963). A substantial literature on 'The Passions' in eighteenth-century medico-philosophy can be usefully accessed through the introduction to Geoffrey Sill, *The Cure of the Passions and the Origins of the Novel* (Cambridge: Cambridge University Press, 2001).
43. Isbrand van Diemerbroeck, *The Anatomy of Human Bodies ... To which is added a particular treatise of the small-pox and measles ... Translated* [from Latin] *by William Salmon ...* (London, 1689; reprinted 1694).
44. Ibid., 29.
45. Ibid.
46. For example, 'The Case of a Lady, Who Was delivered of a Child, Which had the Smallpox pox Appeared in a day or Two after its Birth', dating from 1700 was later written-up by Dr Cromwell Mortimer for the *Transactions of The Royal Society*, Volume 46 (1749–50), 23–4.
47. Diemerbroek, *Anatomy*, 189–90.
48. Thomas Fuller, *Exanthematalogia, or, An Attempt to give a rational account of eruptive fevers, especially of the measles and small pox* (London, 1730) 190–3.
49. Ibid., 189.
50. For the medico-philosophical background see G. S. Rousseau, 'Pineapples, Pregnancy, Pica, and Peregrine Pickle' in *Tobias Smollett: Bicentennial Essays Presented to Lewis M. Knapp*, ed. G. S. Rousseau and P.-G. Boucé (Oxford University Press, 1971) 79–109; P.-G. Boucé, 'Imagination, pregnant women, and monsters, in eighteenth-century England and France', in G. S. Rousseau and R. Porter (eds), *Sexual Underworlds of the Enlightenment* (Manchester: Manchester University Press, 1987) 86–100; M.-H. Huet, *Monstrous Imagination* (Cambridge, MA: Harvard University Press, 1993); Dennis Todd, *Imagining Monsters: Miscreations of the Self in Eighteenth-Century England* (Chicago and London: University of Chicago Press, 1995) and citations to further studies p. 283, note 26). Todd analyses the notorious case of Mary Toft, the 'Rabbit Woman of Godalming' who, in 1726, claimed to have given birth to 17 rabbits.
51. Fuller, *Exanthematalogia*, 149.
52. Charles E. Rosenberg, *Explaining Epidemics and Other Studies in the History of Medicine* (Cambridge University Press: 1992) 295.
53. Ibid.
54. Ibid., footnote 4, 295.
55. Anon, *A letter to J. V. Lettsom M.D. occasioned by Baron Dimsdale's remarks ...* (London, 1779) 22–3.
56. Ibid.
57. Faced with the synchronic coexistence of multiple explanations of smallpox, we might refine Rosenberg's somewhat bifurcated schema by borrowing the model of dominant, residual and emergent discourses or 'structures of feeling' as proposed by the cultural historian Raymond Williams in *Marxism and Literature* (Oxford University Press, 1977) chapter 8. In this respect the 'con-

tagion by fear' theory survives, as in my last quoted example, as a perhaps residual, but powerful structure of feeling articulated alongside what were to become the more dominant, emergent external contagion models, even in the same text. Rather than push for a coherent, purely progressive explanatory narrative of smallpox, we should seek to extend our methodological frameworks, to embrace and explore the wide and complex range of meanings generated by the disease during this crucial period.

58. Rosenberg, *Explaining Epidemics*, 13.
59. Smith, *Speckled Monster*, 98 (illustrations).
60. Ibid. 179.
61. For summary accounts of the theoretical ontology of illness and disease as social constructs see Turner, *The Body and Society* (London: Sage, revised 1996) passim and Healy, *Fictions of Disease*, 5–10.

4

'This Pestilence Which Walketh in Darkness': Reconceptualizing the 1832 New York Cholera Epidemic

Jane Weiss

On Tuesday 2 July 1832, Susan Warner, a 12-year-old in Brooklyn, wrote in her journal, 'The Cholera is in New York; Father told us so last night. I do not feel much afraid.'[1] Her offhand comment underplays the epidemic's impact, both for New Yorkers of her time and for twentieth-century historiography. The city's newspapers did not share her sanguinity: as the menace moved south from Quebec, the headlines read like montages in horror films as a monster crept toward the metropolis.[2] In the fast-growing city, the threat of Asiatic cholera provided a flashpoint for every sort of social anxiety, producing discourses involving class and industrialization, religion and secularism, immigration and political unrest, physicality and sexuality, and not least the power of language in an already media-conscious city.

The explosive energy of this discourse, as much as the catastrophic mortality rates, may be what has attracted the attention of postmodern cultural scholars. Charles E. Rosenberg's *The Cholera Years: the United States in 1832, 1849, and 1866* effectively invented contemporary medical historiography upon its publication in 1962. Although Rosenberg acknowledged the range of philosophical stances available in 1832, the chronological arrangement of *The Cholera Years* served to reinforce the trajectory of linear narrative, not the heterogeneity of the contemporary responses to the epidemic; Rosenberg's thoughtful documentation of competing ideological factions made a far smaller impression on subsequent historians than his narrative of evolution from 'then' until 'now', as Rosenberg recognized in a conclusion added in 1987.[3] 'Cholera,' the narrative asserted, 'a scourge of the sinful to many Americans in 1832, had, by 1866, become the consequence of remediable faults in sanitation.'[4] Subsequent studies, including R. J. Morris's *Cholera 1832: the Social Response to an Epidemic* and David T. Z.

Mindich's *Just the Facts: How 'Objectivity' Came to Define American Journalism*, have built on Rosenberg's chronology, contrasting representations of and responses to recurrent cholera epidemics as indices of sensibility, from moralistic theology toward the secularized pragmatism of the *fin de siècle*. Mindich's examination of the *Morning Courier and New-York Enquirer*'s cholera reporting in 1832, that of the *New York Herald* in 1849, and the *New York Times* in 1866, reinscribes Rosenberg's linear narrative, tracing the evolution of journalistic paradigms from sentimental moralizing to scientific detachment.[5] Valuable though these studies are, diachronic narratives drawn from a limited number of sources offer little resistance to the pull of teleology, constructing the past as a direct route to an inevitable destination: our own values and priorities.[6] Yet Warner's affectless note hints that the summer of 1832 comprised myriad micro-events experienced differently by various communities, most of which are inevitably suppressed in current historians' accounts. The counterpoint between these marginalized positions and the received chronicle may be a reminder that our own readings of the past are contingent on present ideological frames.

Identity and rhetoric

Cholera's arrival in the United States had a dramatic impact on discourses surrounding national identity, not least the rhetorics taking form in nascent American literary culture. Rosenberg's account encapsulated the American public's association of Asiatic cholera with Europe, prompting panic and revulsion as it swept westward in 1831, arriving at Warsaw in April, Berlin in August, England and Wales in October, and then Paris in March 1832.[7] Its spread wrought havoc with civic arrangements and attempts at prevention. Quarantines and barricades – even when enforced by troops – were useless in checking its inexorable westward march. Many Americans nonetheless took satisfaction not only in their geographical distance from the catastrophe, but also in the immunity they assumed would follow from their superior virtue and manner of life. In December 1831, the front page of the *New-York American* assured readers that the disease 'originated at Hamburg in a miserable resort called the Deep Cellar, frequented by beggars, vagrants, and other abandoned objects of both sexes; and to this profligate class of people it has hitherto been confined.'[8] In January 1832, the Paris correspondent of the *New-York Whig*, a newspaper serving the city's liberal elite, reported that 'at St. Petersburg the lower order are ignorant, brutal, and superstitious, and would not consent to be cured, but when seized with the complaint, abandoned themselves to despair and death' and, moreover, 'the medical knowledge possessed in Russia is very small.'[9] The *New-York Daily Advertiser* warned censoriously that cholera 'first appeared in England immediately after Christmas, – a festival strangely and impiously perverted into a period of revelry and intemperance.'[10]

The rhetoric of the *New York Mirror*, a weekly miscellany of poetry, fiction, and sketches addressing upper-middle-class readers, was more colourful. In a series titled 'First Impressions from Europe', the *Mirror*'s correspondent, Nathaniel Parker Willis, reassured readers that feckless French decadence exacerbated the scourge, while regaling New Yorkers with piquant descriptions of victims' disgusting torments. Borrowing from Heinrich Heine's widely circulated letter from Paris, Willis adorned the report with fashionably lurid Gothic touches, but underlaid his recounting of doomed Parisian frivolity with distinctly American censure:

> If you observed the people only, and frequented only the places of amusement and the public promenades, you might never suspect its existence. The weather is June-like, deliciously warm and bright; the trees are just in the tender green of the new buds, and the public gardens are thronged all day with thousands of the gay and idle, sitting under the trees in groups, laughing and amusing themselves, as if there was no plague in the air, though hundreds die every day ...
> I was at a masque ball at the Theatre des Varietes, at the celebration of the Mi Careme, or half lent. There were some two thousand people, I should think, in fancy dresses, most of them grotesque and satirical, and the ball was kept up till seven in the morning, with all the extravagant gaiety, noise and fun with which the French people manage such matters. There was a cholera waltz, and a cholera galopade, and one man, immensely tall, dressed as a personification of the cholera itself, with skeleton armor, and other horrible appurtenances of a walking pestilence. It was the burden of all the jokes, and all the cries of the hawkers, and all the conversation; and yet, probably, nineteen out of twenty lived in the quarters most ravaged by the disease, and many of them had seen it face to face, and knew perfectly well its deadly character![11]

Like Heine, Willis found pathos in such death-defying gaiety, but, unlike Heine, he registered consternation at the un-American blend of festivity and tragedy.

Of course, New Yorkers also proved themselves capable of mingling frivolity with horror. Foreignness and ethnicity were the premises for most examples of cholera humour, a genre that emerged with the first forebodings of the epidemic. The English, the Irish, the affectedly aristocratic or sordidly poor were the protagonists of comic anecdotes, along with young 'men-about-town' and the merely absent-minded. The *Truth Teller*, serving Roman Catholic readers in the city, led the way, amusing its readers with grotesque squibs, such as this anecdote reprinted from an unspecified London paper:

> *Who's got the Cholera Morbus?* – The excitement which is now so general throughout the metropolis occasioned by the fear and alarm which pervade the minds of every class of society, at the expected visit of this dreadful scourge, was considerably heightened by the following circumstance, which lately occurred at a newspaper office in Fleet-street. The editor had sent down to the printer, to be composed, a long article on 'the cholera morbus.' From its extreme length, it was divided into six parts, and given to as many compositors to 'set up.' Just after a timid gentleman, who had been for many weeks past adopting every precaution to prevent an attack of this fatal complaint seizing him, came into the office to chat away half an hour with the 'Reader.' He had not been there five minutes before the 'reading boy' entered in great haste, and inquired, 'who's got the cholera morbus?' 'I have' – 'I have.' – 'I've got it,' loudly responded the aforesaid half-a-dozen compositors. 'The d—l you have!' shrieked out the timid gentleman in question, more dead than alive with fear and agitation, 'then I'm off' – and, 'suiting the action to the word,' he jumped down the first flight of stairs, and was clear off the premises in a twinkling.[12]

Rival papers predictably retaliated with jokes mocking the Irish, and ethnic humour rapidly became a staple of the genre, reflecting widespread anxiety about the connection between immigrant communities and immigrant disease. The *New-York Whig*, meanwhile, appropriated cholera humour to the Whig party's signature cause, antimasonry:

> TOASTED ON BOTH SIDES. – An Antimason, sound to the core, was invited into a shop in Waltham, which he was passing by, on the 4th, to hear a toast which one of the cable-tow gentry proposed to give for his special edification. It was a second hand concern, said to have

originated, at one of the St. John festivals, from the worthy edition of Boston Transcript, and ran thus–
  'Antimasonry: like the Cholera, it only takes the lower classes.'
The hit was received with great applause, but the tables were soon turned by the Antimason proposing to acknowledge the compliment, which he did in the following manner:
  'Masonry: like the *gallows*, it takes only those who are *hoodwinked* and *haltered!*'[13]

Flashpoints: foreignness, elimination, intemperance

The exotic origin of the epidemic, and its inevitable association with foreignness, meshed seamlessly with cholera's other unsavoury connotations. The undeniably disgusting corporeal symptoms of diarrhoea and vomiting which the infection produced exacerbated Calvinist aversions to physicality; although cholera's bacterial causes would not be fully understood until 1883, the disease's connection with bodily waste necessitated elaborate code languages.[14] Moral and ritual terms were inseparable from practical measures. Controversy swirled about the causes of the disease; authorities were divided over whether cholera was contagious or caused by atmospheric influences – a term which could denote the weather, or connote mysterious spiritual influences.

  The elevated mortality rate among the impoverished and immigrants further complicated popular comprehension of cholera. An association of physicians cautiously noted that 'wherever large bodies of men have been congregated, as in camps and caravans, or crowded into a narrow space, as on shipboard, the proportion of persons attacked has been greatest, and the fatality the most appalling . . . The disease is most apt to attack the poor, the filthy, and the intemperate.'[15] An advertisement for the fashionable resort of Lebanon Springs headlined 'A Retreat from the Cholera' promised that the spa was 'situated among the mountains, inland from any water course, and entirely out of the way of emigration'.[16] As the advertisement's chosen phrase implied, many American citizens were apt to associate the spread of cholera less with travel from place to place than with the arrival of immigrants, whose lingering foreign taint was cast as a threat to the body politic of the United States. On 19 June, the *New-York Daily Advertiser* excerpted a 'letter written from Montreal' whose unnamed author asserted that 'the Asiatic Cholera had not attacked any but emigrants . . . Between 27,000 & 30,000 emigrants had arrived at Montreal this season, and so great a multitude, long deprived of many comforts, would hardly fail ... to bring into active operation the seeds of disease'.[17] Even newspapers whose editors rejected the theory that Asiatic cholera was contagious nonetheless attributed infection to the incursion of foreigners. On 27 June the *Morning Courier and New-York Enquirer* scolded,

> We are informed that yesterday morning a considerable number of emigrants arrived in the village of Brooklyn, who had been landed during the night at New Utrect, on Long Island. They were very properly immediately sent back by the authorities of Brooklyn. If some measure is not taken to prevent the landing of emigrants in this manner on our coast, the quarantine laws will become perfectly useless.[18]

At the same time the *New-York American* emphasized that the New York State Board of Health had named 'freedom of intercourse' as a factor 'increasing the prevalance of cholera'.[19] The spread of cholera through American cities thus seemed to index the penetration of immigrants into the New World, despoiling its innocence and its sense of difference.

New York journalists also identified cholera with the epicurean pleasures and social promiscuity afforded by the burgeoning hospitality industry. The *New-York Daily Advertiser* suggested that bars and restaurants be shuttered, warning that 'these receptacles of vice and intoxication, are the resort of that description of people, who are considered as the most exposed to the attacks, and to the fatal consequences of this pestilential disease'.[20] Yet xenophobia and asceticism were not the only contemporary responses to the epidemic, even though observation of cholera's spread and its effects tended to reinforce this aetiological theory. Crowding, poor sanitation, malnutrition, and alcoholism did elevate the risk of contracting and dying from Asiatic cholera, but New York's different communities processed these facts in diverging ways.

The unusually blunt 'Report of the Cholera Committee', widely reprinted in the city's commercial press, interlaced sensible recommendations for street-cleaning with language redolent of Puritan sermons. The introductory remarks warned that 'the season has already arrived when various causes, combined with the prevalence of great heat, produce in this city nauseous effluvia, a visiated [*sic*] state of the atmosphere, a kind of Malazia [*sic*], in which the destroying angel, should he visit our city, would walk unseen in the midst of us, enveloped in a pestilential vapour.' This Gothic imagery is followed by straightforward directives that heaps of waste be treated with quicklime, and that 'hydrants [be] opened several times each week, and to allow the water from the reservoir in 13th street to have issue for several hours at a time. During this process, the sweepers employed by the Corporation should use their brooms in washing out the gutters.' Individuals, the committee warned, should avoid intemperance, which the report defined as indulgence not only in liquor but in 'seasonable and unripe fruits', lest 'the new enemy in our neighborhood should . . . find us predisposed to be operated upon by his malignant influence'. At the same time, the committee urged vigilant monitoring of one's emotional state: 'Exciting causes should not be produced by anxiety or fear. The exercise of equanimity would tend to ward off the evil, and render the affliction mild.'[21] The equivocal terms of the report, like the conditions of the disease itself, could render cholera a spiritual malaise to be fought off through industry, temperance, and purifying rituals – or into a forum for the exercise of reason and common sense, or an urgent arena for humanitarian aid and social justice. Ideologies framed cholera's most anarchic and terrifying manifestations; while the chaos inflicted on individual lives or families could not be contained, the course taken by the disease reified communal values rather than shaking them.

Denial, emotion and evangelism: the *Morning Courier and New-York Enquirer*

The cultural response to the 1832 cholera epidemic foregrounded by current historiography is represented by the *Morning Courier and New-York Enquirer*. No New York newspaper embraced the epidemic with more zest than James Watson Webb's publication, which aimed at a wider readership than its fellow broadsheets, anticipating the techniques of the 'Penny Press' tabloids by several years. Although the *Courier* sold for six cents for a copy – too expensive for most New Yorkers – its colourful prose and aggressive editorials drew unprecedented circulations.[22] The epidemic was ideal matter for the *Courier's* 'take-no-prisoners' approach. Nominally Jacksonian politics were subordinate to Webb's propensity for sensationalism, trends, and random potshots.

Initially, the *Courier* denied the inevitability of the epidemic. As late as 27 June, the paper offered a disparaging review of the official Cholera Committee's statement ('consisting of course of the most wise, judicious, and learned, of the New York Medical Profession', the reporter chortled), beginning with 'This report is an oddity.' The critic continued:

> The committee say they are appointed to consider the means of prevention and treatment of the Cholera Morbus. Let us see how they have acquitted themselves. They say that they 'do not pretend to a knowledge of the means that will present a *recurrence* of an epidemic pestilence, such as is dreaded and apprehended in the Asiatic Cholera.' In this, I admit the correctness of the views of the learned Committee: for, of a disease that has never yet *occurred* here, it would be difficult to conceive a *recurrence*.

The reporter scoffed at the committee's high-flown personification of the disease, saying that the precautions should have been employed against other diseases, 'and then their unkind and *"destroying Angel, should he visit our city, and walk unseen in the midst of us, enveloped in a pestilential vapour"!* would have passed by us, unseen, unfelt, and unsmelt, on the balmy wings of northern zephyrs.' Excoriating the committee's warnings against raw fruits, he credited 'good strawberries and Boston's particular Seidlitz water' for his own robust health.[23] On 4 July, after the first cases were recorded, the *Courier* doggedly insisted:

> We hear from every quarter, on the highest medical authority, that it is at least questionable if the Asiatic Pestilence exists at all in New-York. There have been a few, isolated cases of highly malignant cholera morbus, resembling the Canadian, but certainly nothing that can bear the name of an epidemic . . . we are now in a singular situation. If it shall be found that alarm, or fear, or *terror*, added to the common cholera morbus, constitutes the disease an epidemic, and spreads it by sympathy in every direction, what feelings of indignation ought not to be aroused against those daring triflers with the public health, who endeavor to create that terror – who stimulate that fear – who excite that alarm? . . . there can be no excuse, no apology for those who wilfully endeavor on the appearance of a few sporadic cases to assert pertinaciously that the pestilence is among us.[24]

On 7 July, the *Courier*'s lead editorial snidely commented, 'We are disappointed. Yesterday we expected *fifty* new cases at least; the Board of Health only report *thirty-seven*. This is one of the best proofs we have seen of the mildness of the disorder.' An article headlined 'Fashionable Society' lampooned the cowardice of socialites fleeing their usual summer haunts:

> The shocking audacity with which the 'Cholera Panic' marched into the saloons and boudoirs of fashionable society has never been exceeded, from the call of Abraham down to the present day . . . This derangement of fashionable society was about to be melancholy in the extreme . . . Only think of it – the Cholera had the impudence to threaten Saratoga, Balston, Lake George, the Green Mountains, and every fashionable avenue – every fashionable resort.[25]

But when mortality rates soared, the *Courier* came into its own. Webb launched an unprecedented Sunday 'Cholera Edition', selling some 10,000 extra copies. The 'Cholera Edition' compiled a bewildering variety of medical recommendations, moral fulminations, political accusations, and invocations to prayer. 'This pestilence, which walketh in darkness, continues its ravages among us', thundered the lead editorial on 25 July, 'and is daily sacrificing hundreds of victims to its unmitigated fury, as if in derision of the authorities and presses which have set it at defiance, and attempted to deceive the people into the belief that it does not exist, or if it does, that it is neither to be dreaded nor regarded.' The editorialist unblushingly castigated the stolid *New-York Evening Post* for having 'the hardihood to attempt to disseminate the belief that the Cholera does not exist among us!' and charged that 'hundreds of deaths have and will occur from the manner in which the exercise of a sound discretion in leaving the city has been prevented by our authorities and one or two of our daily papers.'[26]

Once its presence was admitted, Asiatic cholera was a spectacular opportunity for sensation and moralizing. The *Courier's* columnists treated the disease as an act of God, presaging the emergent Second Great Awakening which would reach its acme at the mid-century. The 25 July issue featured a cholera-themed sermon:

> If you leave the city for your own sake or your families, do not flee like *cowards*, caring not for those of your fellow creatures left behind, but extend the hand of charity to the needy, aye, and even to the *dissolute*, if they are in need. By charity, I mean no *paltry* pittance – if you fall, fall like Christians, or at least like men. Above all, confide in the most High. 'Surely he shall deliver thee from the noisome

pestilence; he shall cover thee with his feathers, and under his wings shalt thou trust.'[27]

Federalist rationalism: the *New-York Whig*

The *Morning Courier and New-York Enquirer*'s combination of sermonizing and purple prose offered a frame for the epidemic that attracted an unprecedented number of readers, and the ideology it represented has dominated recent narratives contrasting American social responses to successive cholera epidemics. But the paradigm reflected in the *Courier* was not the only frame available to New Yorkers in 1832. One alternative was represented by the dignified *New-York Whig*, the organ of the conservative neo-Federalist faction. Beginning in January 1832, the *Whig* scrupulously reported Asiatic cholera's progress through Europe, often printing correspondence from medical academicians or military surgeons. Articles debating the merits of various cures and the mode of causation uniformly employed a moderate, empirical tone. A lengthy column appearing on 11 January, its author identified as the 'Surgeon Major, &c. of the late Polish Army', ended with the sober reflection, 'Do I think the Asiatic European Epidemic cholera morbus will arrive in America? I answer candidly, I *think* it will, inasmuch as other epidemics have generally made the tour of the world, and this one follows, as has been observed, the general laws of all epidemics.'[28] A front-page editorial on 27 June read,

> No doubt the disease will reach from the lakes to the Atlantic. We recommend to all to prepare their hearts for it, to prepare their lives for it, that they may receive it with the greatest coolness, when it does come, and be in the best frame, successfully to combat it, or cheerfully to yield to it, as the Allwise Providence may direct.

The term 'Allwise Providence' suggested the impersonal Deism of eighteenth-century Federalists; the recommendations, moreover, took the form not of prayer or repentance, but dietary regimens and chemical disinfectants. Another article on the same page explicated the properties of chloride of lime:

> The disinfecting properties of this cheap substance render them interesting at all times, and especially so when the noonday pestilence sweeps over the North. We fancy many of our readers ask,

What is chloride? Whence comes its great cleansing, purifying, sweetening power? How can it disinfect a sick room, or foul ship, or filthy sink? How is it able to destroy the fatal breath of the cholera?

We answer, in our humble way, a *chloride* is a compound of two substances, of which one is always *chlorine*, and the other may be lime, soda, water, &c. a great variety. It is *chlorine* that possesses this great power, and that is united with lime and soda, solely for the convenience of using it, and not because they change its native properties and powers of disinfection . . . In its pure, airy form, shut up in white bottles, it has a greenish color. From this color, it takes its name, chlorine, *chloros* being the Greek for green.[29]

The evocative vocabulary of the first paragraph is followed by a dispassionate, neutral report on the chemical substance, consistent with the *Whig's* rationalist stance. While the *Whig* attributed the spread of the disease to 'atmospheric conditions' rather than contagion and urged temperance and serenity as mitigating factors, the editors avoided moral pronouncements that would attribute infection to vicious or dissolute behavior; disease, in the rationalist paradigm, was a result of physical imbalance, not a Divine punishment for sin. Indeed, on 4 July, the *Whig* prominently positioned the whole text of a letter by Governor E. P. Throop, refusing to proclaim an official 'day of fasting, humiliation, and prayer' in New York State. Like President Andrew Jackson, Throop rejected such a declaration on the grounds that it would violate the separation of church and state. Jackson's political coalition, the Republican party, was noted for its anti-intellectual ethos, laissez-faire economic policies, and racy rhetoric, and although Jackson himself had little enthusiasm for organized religion, his constituency participated enthusiastically in the revival meetings and fervent, spontaneous prayers of the nascent Second Great Awakening, while the fading Whig party perpetuated the rationalism of eighteenth-century humanist philosophers.[30] Throop and Jackson's twin pronouncements therefore confounded existing political allegiances: the Jacksonian *Courier and Enquirer* roundly condemned the president's irreverence, while the *Whig's* editorialists were uncomfortably obliged to commend Jackson's loyalty to the Constitution. Throop wrote:

While the duty of individuals and religious communities, to humble themselves before God and in times of public calamity by pestilence or otherwise, is clearly pointed out and exemplified in the Scriptures,

I feel bound, as a civil officer, to look for the rule of my duty in the powers conferred upon the Executive by the institution, and the laws enacted under its authority ... The repugnance of the people of this state to the mingling of civil and ecclesiastical authorities is not left to inference alone; it is strongly expressed in the constitution of 1777.[31]

On 18 July, the *Whig*'s lead editorial underscored the Enlightenment creed that the known was less alarming than the unknown: 'This alarming disease', the essay read, 'has now been in the city a fortnight. It has lost much of its terror on acquaintance.' The editorial counterbalanced praise for wholesome behaviour with acknowledgment of the disease's amorality:

Its victims are generally of the looser sort of our population; yet many are tried with the cholera, whose temperance is above impeachment, even when forced to shrink at the attack of this touch-stone. The most abstemious, frugal, and temperate are brought sometimes under the dominion of its influence; but such have a manifest advantage in the conflict over those of an opposite character.[32]

Another editorial in the same issue declared that 'Truth is better than error, *the precise truth.* We always desire to know it for ourselves; we are willing to state it for others. When truth frightens, it is time to be alarmed.'[33]

The *Whig*'s editorial stance did not preclude moral reflections or emotion, but these were likely to take aestheticized forms, often in verse. On 18 July, the *Whig* printed a poem that counterbalanced conventional piety with recognition of social pleasures:

> When Pestilence invades our streets,
>   And frights our friends away,
> How calm, but solemn, seem the hours
>   To us who lonely stay!
>
> Our wonted places now no more
>   Their wonted faces shew;
> And silence seldom yields to sounds
>   Of voices which we know.
>
> But, oh what hours are these for pray'r,
>   When scarce the world intrudes?

> For now we feel that God is near,
>> The more in solitudes.

> We pray for those who're absent far;
>> And ah! how blest we'll feel,
> When wakes again the social pray'r,
>> Where lonely now we kneel.[34]

Another verse, 'Thoughts on the Cholera', which appeared on 25 July, incorporated neoclassical rhetorical strategy. The anonymous author complained that in the face of imminent death 'The crowded city has no heart/No soul to feel the woes/That circle round the stranger's head/and his existence close', and opted instead for the countryside:

> There 'neath the shades where budding life
> Its dearest pleasures found,
> And my native stream goes sparkling by
> With a lulling silver sound,
> 'T would be a privilege when dead
> To find my last and dreamless bed.[35]

The poem neither pleads for intercession by a personalized God, nor asks for deliverance. Rather, refuge from disease is located in the tropes of Virgil's and Horace's bucolic poetry, the staples of European neoclassical education; death itself is envisioned as a natural phenomenon rather than a moral or spiritual ordeal. The Elysian Fields, not a Christian heaven, was the *Whig*'s anticipated end.

Social justice: the *Truth Teller*

A third set of responses to the epidemic, framed by a third paradigm of human interaction with disease, is exemplified by the *Truth Teller*, which served the burgeoning Roman Catholic population. Occupying the far end of the continuum from the *Courier*, the *Truth Teller* stressed the social reverberations of the epidemic, and proposed civil and medical measures to limit its casualties. Reflecting the European roots of its audience, the *Truth Teller* began reporting the epidemic's spread as early as January 1832. An editorial began with the sombre warning:

We allude to that dreadful disease which has been ravaging the kingdoms of the Continent during the last twelve months – which is now within twenty-four hours' sail of this country, and whose entrance into the country, we fear, that it is beyond the power of human skill to prevent. The next object of consideration therefore, with all who are anxious for the public safety, must be to endeavour to confine the ravages of the disease within as small a compass as possible – to diminish the number of those who might otherwise suffer from it, by diffusing as universally as possible, both among the medical world and the people generally, such information as seems calculated to contribute to these ends.

A lengthy excerpt from 'that able periodical, the *Foreign Quarterly Review*' followed, offering technical descriptions of symptoms and typical progress, and recommended treatments, including vigorous liniment massages and doses of turpentine, olive oil, magnesia, and mint water. Finally, the article urges fumigation of houses and public places.[36] On 11 February, the paper featured a tract by the British naval physician Sir Gilbert Blane, which strenuously asserted that Asiatic cholera was contagious, contradicting the dominant medical hypothesis of the period.[37] As the epidemic progressed, the *Truth Teller* continued to provide the most authoritative medical advice, however unavailing the cures and preventative measures proved.

The *Truth Teller*'s editorial signature was its insistence on organized social reform. Absent from its pages were denunciations of suspicious foreigners and unwashed slum-dwellers, or references to divine judgments. Like the *Whig*, the *Truth Teller* approved of the president's and the governor's refusal to declare an official day of prayer, commenting, 'No apprehensions need be entertained of the success of the "Church and State" party, so long as the people have the good sense to elect such men to the head of the Government and State.'[38] Instead, the epidemic provided the impetus to lobby for improved housing, drains, and water supplies for the poor. A satirist speaking for cholera claimed, 'I prefer lodgings always in narrow courts, and in cellars under ground; in chambers where no windows will open; and in the neighborhood of gasometers, ponds, or the purlieus of public-houses.'[39] By June, the *Truth Teller* lamented, 'It is truly inexplicable why there should be such indifference in the minds of the Corporation' to improvements in street-cleaning and endowed public hospitals. The following week, a review of François Gabriel Boisseau's *Traite du Cholera Morbus* ended with the plea, 'what must now be the feelings of our Citizens when they reflect on the awful condition of the city–loaded with filth, and emitting the most insupportable stench! If it be not too late, we implore the Corporation to set to work, and endeavor by proper measures to arrest the threatening calamity.'[40] The editors praised the 'active spirit of benevolence' of immigrant communities welcoming refugees from their homelands, and commended the public-spiritedness of 'our Reverend Clergy' who tended parishioners at their own peril.[41] As the epidemic waned, the *Truth Teller* continued to denounce the living conditions endured by the city's poor. An editorial on 3 August analysed the reduced incidence in the Sixth Ward, the setting for the notorious Five Corners slum, as a triumph of urban renewal:

> The quantity of filth and dirt removed out of the neighborhood of Five Points cannot be conceived, and it is only a matter of astonishment to us, who afterwards examined the place, that the persons employed could possibly escape the infection . . . Every house, every alley, was visited, the free use of the chloride was pursued, and the Street Inspector, with a perseverance which will not be soon forgotten, was himself present at the purification of the filthy rookeries.[42]

'Purification' implies ritual, but the *Truth Teller* frames the performance as a civic, communal ritual, collectively redeeming the neighbourhood's residents without reference to their individual moral merits. Maintaining close connections to European institutions, the readers of the *Truth Teller* were, perhaps, less heavily invested in the myth of American exceptionalism. Instead of presenting the immigrants and indigents who peopled Five Points as the cause of infection, the editorialist presciently offered governmental investment in sanitation as the single most powerful form of action against cholera.

Conclusion

By December 1832, the cholera epidemic had killed 3,515 New Yorkers.[43] Few of Manhattan's approximately 200,000 residents remained untouched by grief or fear, even if not by the disease itself.[44] But the epidemic did not affect all residents equally, or elicit unified responses within what was already one of the most heterogeneous urban centres in America. In retrospect, the *Courier*'s emotive religiosity and accusatory politics may appear most representative of the era's emergent consciousness, anticipating both the cresting of the Second Great Awakening in the mid-century and the appearance of the Penny Press in 1833. The rationalism voiced by the *Whig*'s journalists might retrospectively be dismissed as harking back to the humanism of the late colonial and Federalist eras, recalling a fading eighteenth-century faith in an orderly, enlightened natural world; in fact, the *Whig* ceased publication the following year. The *Truth Teller*'s advocacy of sanitation and acknowledgment of contagion seem prescient today, although they had scant impact on the city's policies; Roman Catholics were a minority population with little influence until their numbers swelled in the 1840s. But in 1832, these three positions existed simultaneously, in constant dialogue; differences among the populations of the rapidly-growing city defined New Yorkers' daily experiences more sharply than the potentially unifying fact of Asiatic cholera could.

More importantly, the three paradigms reflected by the editorial stances of the *Courier*, the *Whig*, and the *Truth Teller* do not exhaust the positions that were available to New Yorkers in 1832; rather they represent a past framed by the critical methods, beliefs, and materials available to a scholar 170 years later. At the close of *Culture and Society*, in his interrogation of the impact that canonical literary historiography has on the mythic narratives that form a society's sense of cultural identity, Raymond Williams warned, 'What we receive from the tradition is a set of meanings, but not all of these will hold their significance if, as we must, we return them to immediate experience.'[45] Whilst Williams validated the conscious appreciation of complex, ever-changing relationships among multiple, coexistent structures of thought and feeling that would eventually define postmodernism, the 'inherited tradition' of the literary canon, he cautioned, would necessarily circumscribe readers' conceptions of their cultural legacy.[46] Even more than literary critics, historians attempt to wrest meaning from the past through the power of narrative, stories that forge disparate data into legend; but, unlike literary critics, historians do not have recourse to Williams's touchstone of 'immediate experience', or applicability to the present without the grave risk of distortion of their subject, the past.

This falsifying touchstone nonetheless remains as seductive for historians as for literary critics. The textual and archaeological materials remaining from the past – the minutiae from which meaningful narratives may be drawn – may be scanty or unrepresentative, forcing historians to make inferences based not on what was, but on what was left. When plentiful remains do survive, their very abundance may demand that evidence deemed expendable will be discarded. To extrapolate an intelligible account from the surviving evidence inevitably involves selectivity, and principles of selection follow from the values and priorities of the time in which the account is composed, on the unexamined assumption that these values and priorities apply as well to the time being reconstructed. Yet the past is not a mirror of the present, or a road leading to the present; rather, it is a foreign country, whose large and diverse populations hurry about on their own errands, oblivious of the nature or existence of would-be visitors from the future. Indeed, the appeal of teleology – the examination of phenomena in the faith that they inevitably lead to a specific goal – may be irresistible; we are attracted by those who resemble us, or who lead to or explain ourselves. The problem with conceiving the past as an explanation or mirror of ourselves is that such a conception presupposes that we are the destined, inevitable terminus of the process. Of course, our beliefs and assumptions are as dynamic and contingent as those consigned to 'history'; the premises and values that seem obvious to us now will inevitably become outmoded, even embarrassing, under pressure from circumstances we cannot now anticipate.

As we look at the events of the summer of 1832, the ideological frames of our own times or communities shape the picture in our minds, foregrounding some threads of history and consigning others to the background, while sheer distance reduces some details to invisibility. Although Rosenberg's *The Cholera Years* made an admirable attempt to reflect the range and complexity of New Yorkers' responses to the 1832 epidemic, critical discourse in the generations following its publication has reduced the nuances of Rosenberg's portrait to the first snapshot in a 'before-and-after' sequence illustrating the progression from theologically grounded moral judgment to the self-conscious 'objectivity' of the era following the Civil War. Such metonymic substitution of the rhetoric of the *Courier* for the sensibility of 1832 may satisfy the historian's craving for linearity but it obscures the reality that there was no single sensibility of that era or any other, and that the majority of the voices of 1832 remain unheard. Federalist humanists sparred with increasingly fervent Protestant theologies; cholera as divine judgement on the intemperate warred with cholera as a public sanitation problem; antipathy to an infection widely perceived by Americans as a foreign invasion jostled against the perceptions of the immigrants themselves. The texts and artifacts on which are inscribed the responses of still more of New York's subcultures – those of African-Americans, Jews, immigrants from Germany and Holland – demand further study. Perhaps consciousness of the multiple frames through which New Yorkers of 1832 gazed at their present may enlarge the frames which contain our picture of the past.

Notes

1. Susan Warner, journals, Constitution Island Association Archives, West Point, New York.
2. *Morning Courier and New-York Enquirer*, 27 June 1832: 2; *New-York Whig*, 27 June 1832: 1; *Truth-Teller*, 23 June 1832: 206.
3. Charles E. Rosenberg, *The Cholera Years: the United States in 1832, 1849, and 1866* (Chicago: University of Chicago Press, 1962 and 1987) 55–64.
4. Ibid., 5.
5. David T. Z. Mindich, *Just the Facts: How 'Objectivity' Came to Define American Journalism* (New York: New York University Press, 1998), 95–112. See also Norman Longmate, *King Cholera: the Biography of a Disease* (London: Hanish Hamilton, 1966), R. J. Morris, *Cholera 1832: the Social Response to an Epidemic* (London: Croom Helm, 1976), Margaret Pelling, *Cholera, Fever, and English Medicine* (New York and Oxford: Oxford University Press, 1978), and Geoffrey Bilson, *A Darkened House: Cholera in Nineteenth-Century Canada* (Toronto: University of Toronto Press, 1980). On the reception of cholera in London, and the troubles invovled in distinguishing between 'imported' Asiatic cholera and 'domestic' cholera morbus, see George S. Rousseau and David Boyd Haycock, 'Coleridge's Choleras: Cholera Morbus, Asiatic Cholera and Dysentery in Nineteenth-Century England', *The Bulletin of the History of Medicine* 77 (2003): 298–331.
6. The limitations of a teleological approach are apparent in G. William Beardslee's 'The 1832 Cholera Epidemic in New York State: Nineteenth-Century Responses to *Cholerae Vibrio*', *Early America Review* (Fall 2000): 4–12.
7. Rosenberg, *The Cholera Years*, 15–16. *Asiatic Cholera Pandemic.* University of California at Los Angeles Department of Epidemiology. Accessed at http://www.ph.ucla.edu/epi/snow/pandemic1826-37.html.
8. 'Fatality of Cholera', *New-York American for the Country*, 30 December 1831: 1.
9. 'O. P. Q. on the Cholera', *New-York Whig*, 11 January 1832: 2.
10. *New-York Daily Advertiser*, 19 June 1832: 2.
11. [Nathaniel Willis], 'First Impressions of Europe', from the *New York Mirror*. *New-York Whig*, 13 June 1832: 3.
12. 'Who's Got the Cholera Morbus?', *Truth Teller*, 4 February 1832: 45.
13. 'Toasted on Both Sides', *New-York Whig*, 25 July 1832: 2.
14. John Duffy, *A History of Public Health in New York City* (New York: Russell Sage Foundation, 1974).
15. 'Board of Health', *New-York American for the Country*, 29 June 1832: 2.
16. 'A Retreat from the Cholera', advertisement, *Morning Courier and New-York Enquirer*, 26 June 1832: 4.
17. *New-York Daily Advertiser*, 19 June 1832: 2.
18. 'Emigrants', *The Morning Courier and New-York Enquirer*, 27 June 1832: 2.
19. *New-York American for the Country*, 29 June 1832: 2.
20. *New-York Daily Advertiser*, 19 June 1832: 2.
21. 'Report of the Committee on Cholera', *New-York Daily Advertiser*, 20 June 1832: 2.
22. James L. Crouthamel, *Bennett's* New York Herald *and the Rise of the Popular Press* (Syracuse: Syracuse University Press, 1989) 11.

23. Hyder Ally [*sic*], 'Report of the Committee on Cholera', *Morning Courier and New-York Enquirer*, 27 June 1832: 2.
24. 'Health of the City', *Morning Courier and New-York Enquirer*, 4 July 1832: 2.
25. 'The Cholera', *Morning Courier and New-York Enquirer*, 7 July 1832: 2; 'Fashionable Society', *Morning Courier and New-York Enquirer*, 7 July 1832: 3.
26. 'The Cholera', *Morning Courier and New-York Enquirer*, 25 July 1832: 2.
27. Howard, 'Thoughts on the Cholera', *Morning Courier and New-York Enquirer*, 25 July 1832: 2.
28. Paul F. Eve, *New-York Whig*, 11 January 1832: 2.
29. 'Chloride of Lime', *New-York Whig*, 27 June 1832: 1.
30. Nathan O. Hatch, *The Democratization of American Christianity* (New Haven: Yale University Press, 1989), 133–41.
31. E. P. Throop, 'Correspondence', *New-York Whig*, 4 July 1832: 3.
32. 'The Cholera', *New-York Whig*, 18 July 1832: 3.
33. 'The Health of the City', *New-York Whig*, 18 July 1832: 5.
34. 'Thoughts amid the Cholera', *New-York Whig*, 18 July 1832: 6.
35. Ibid., 2.
36. 'The Cholera', *Truth Teller*, 14 January 1832: 20. Though based in London, the *Foreign Quarterly Review* also published a New York edition.
37. Gilbert Blane, 'Warning to the British Public against the Alarming Approach of the Indian Cholera', *Truth Teller*, 11 February 1832: 51.
38. 'The Fast Day', *Truth Teller*, 30 June 1832: 214.
39. 'Warning from the Cholera', *Truth Teller*, 11 February 1832: 53.
40. 'Cholera', *Truth Teller*, 2 June 1832: 182; 'A Treatise on the Cholera Morbus', *Truth Teller*, 16 June 1832: 199. Boisseau's *Traite* had first been published in Paris, but was now translated into English and made available in a New York edition as *A Treatise on Cholera Morbusor, Researches on the Symptoms, Nature, and Treatment of the Disease; and on the Different Means of Avoiding It* (1832).
41. 'Public Meetings', *Truth Teller*, 30 June 1832: 215; 'Cholera', *Truth Teller*, 21 July 1832: 239.
42. 'The Cholera', *Truth Teller*, 3 August 1832: 54.
43. Howard Markel, 'Cholera', in *The Encyclopedia of New York City*, ed. Kenneth T. Jackson (New Haven: Yale University Press, 1995), 219.
44. Nathan Kantrowitz, 'Population', in ibid., 923.
45. Raymond Williams, *Culture and Society 1780–1850* (1958; Harmondsworth: Penguin, 1963) 287.
46. Ibid., p 309.

5
Mapping Colonial Disease: Victorian Medical Cartography in British India

Pamela K. Gilbert

In the early nineteenth century, new techniques in cartography and printing made maps far more widely available in Europe than had previously been possible. From the late 1820s on, social, sanitary and medical experts began to combine statistics and cartography in thematic maps that enabled medics, sanitarians and urban dwellers alike to understand their environment in new ways. The cholera pandemic of the late 1820s and early 1830s sparked a host of medical maps, which were used both as epidemiological tools and as arguments for developments in social policy. As such, they also became powerful representations of and arguments for certain models of the social body, as well as revolutionary tools for envisioning both diseases and diseased populations. Such maps became crucial in defining community and the boundaries of place, at the levels both of social imaginary and of policy.

British metropolitan sanitary mapping sought to modernize the city, to create a utopian and fully 'civilized' metropolis. Within that project, areas of poverty and disease (often, though not always, coterminous) were coded as dark, barbaric places to be brought into the light of the nineteenth century. At the same time, especially in the decade following 1857, India increasingly came to be seen as permanently barbaric, the 'other' against which Britain would define itself. This vision of progress, related as it was to a developmental narrative of increasing metropolitan civilization and health, invoked its opposite, the unhealthy and barbaric colony. Because cholera was considered a disease endemic to Bengal, we find British medics in India struggling to manage – or exculpate themselves from their failure to manage – the spread of disease. The land of India itself came to represent the opposite of progress and civilization as it was identified with a disease that seemed to the British to be an essential characteristic of the area. In part, this was accomplished through maps that represented this conceived space of India to viewers in the British Isles.

Although early mappings of cholera in India showed clear continuities with British domestic theories of disease, it began to diverge significantly by the mid-century. In these later maps, the projection of barbarism onto the 'other' could be confirmed through the construction of both the land and the people as essentially unhealthy and not susceptible to the remediation of which metropolitan public health programmes were exemplary. Cholera, an 'Indian' disease emerging from the Gangitic delta which also struck hard at the urban working and underclasses at home, became a symbol not only of geographic connection between periphery and metropole, but also of a barbarism connected with a heterogenous and problematic geography. By 1867, after the International Sanitary Conference had laid the responsibility for cholera pandemics at the British doorstep,[1] the pressure on British officials in India to 'modernize' and sanitize led to two clearly marked trends – one, a continuing effort to address sanitary problems in India, using similar methods to those used in Britain, and the other, denial of the current scientific knowledge of cholera in Europe as inapplicable to the disease-producing, static landscape of India.

In this essay, I would like to focus on the British mapping of cholera in India, and especially the differences in representations of the land and disease between metropolitan and colonial mappings. After some brief remarks offering an overview of mapping in the period, I will examine in some detail a squabble between medical officers of India that is illuminative of the political and representational issues surrounding the mapping of cholera in late 1860s British India: the exchanges of Cornish, contagionist medic of Madras, whose territory suffered successive 'invasions' of cholera from Bengal, and Bryden, surgeon and statistical officer of the Sanitary Commission in Bengal. The battle was fought with multiple maps, drawing both on earlier medical maps of the same areas and on contemporary maps. In these maps it is possible to trace the different traditions in spatial representation of India which illustrate dominant British attitudes regarding metropolitan versus colonial land and disease.

By the 1860s epidemic, more than three and a half decades after the first cholera maps of England were drawn up, substantial changes in mapping had occurred. Probably the most well-known is that derived from Snow's meticulous epidemiological mappings of water contamination and its responsibility for the devastating St James's epidemic of the mid-1850s, which transformed medical mapping from a model of surface sanitary contamination (visible filth) to depth (invisible circulating contamination).[2] However, another major change during this period was a continuing attention to history – both that of the particular land under investigation and its development and of epidemic activity in the area.

By the mid-nineteenth century, cholera mapping in Britain was characterized by an attention to history – that of prior epidemics and death rates of a given area, and, following Snow's argument that cholera was spread by water contaminated with sewage, increasing attention to drainage and other underground features of the landscape. This spatialization of epidemiological research in Britain was not restricted to the surface topography of land and built environment, but had already assumed a palimpsestic historical organization of space. A quick example here will have to do – a map of the St James's epidemic most famously mapped by John Snow. (This map, however, is not Snow's; it was created by the General Board of Health; Illustration 5.1).[3] Seeking an explanation in history and the historical uses of space, residents of St James used a geological model which assumes that strata of the ground under their feet contain both evidence and potentially active residue of past uses of the environment – here we see that the map responds to their concerns, including the site of a sixteenth-century plague pit, the disturbance of which by modernizing public works projects was believed by some to have been responsible for the outbreak. (This hypothesis was rejected by the Board.) The Appendix to the St James Vestry report on the same epidemic also has recourse to a model of a palimpsest of microspaces within macrospaces, containing a street-by-street and house-by-house 'mapping' of the micro-organisms found in the water of every place where cholera occurred (with hand-coloured pictures) and narratives (by Hassall, Illustration 5.2).[4] Attentive to Snow's theory, the report also summarizes micro-organic content by water company. The enclosed map of the St James's epidemic is accompanied by charts which 'map' the houses in order, so that the report maps space at the level of the community, the historical use of the land during an earlier epidemic (the plague), the micro-level, and the structural level of individual houses – a mapping which mediates between several conceptions of meaningful space – from that of legal units of property and historical use of terrain, to that of water source and content.

The rhetoric of civilization and barbarism, culture and anarchy pervades the sanitary project as it does liberal discourse in general in this period. If a lack of sanitation reveals a lingering barbarism in the heart

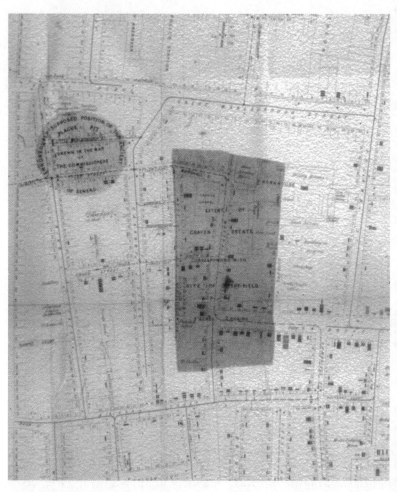

Illustration 5.1   'Corrected Map' by the General Board, showing suppressed and actual location of plague pit: detail

of the civilized social body, wherein dirt = viciousness = 'Otherness', insular maps increasingly refine their search for this barbarism in micro-mapping, seeking it in that which was hidden, below ground, and therefore from the past history of the city. On the one hand, this displaces authority over the social body's condition from the general community to a designated group of professionals who can surgically intervene in the environment (engineers, doctors). On the other, it displaces barbarism onto an inadequate past, a failing infrastructure that

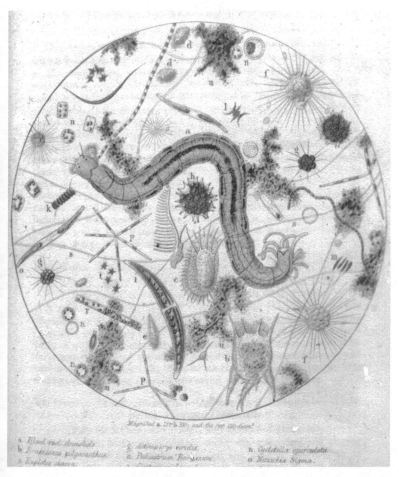

Illustration 5.2 Water Content Mapping: example from General Board Report: detail

can be redeemed in the interests of modernization, which becomes equal to civilization.

Barbarism, backwardness – antimodernity, really – is thus figured as a feature of landscape, often below the surface in its sewage, its cesspools and wells, its soil quality and the level of the water table; it is a history which can be fixed, purged. Matching landscape, both natural and built, to properly socialized bodies engaging in properly socialized behaviours is a matter of eliminating these layers of dissonance and reinscribing all within a single layer of time – modernity – and type of space – abstract, transparent. However, in order to do this, all those layers must be mapped to identify the points of incongruity. Thus the city and its maps function as palimpsests, showing levels of space and discrepancies between times – the time of modernity and the barbaric relics of the past which infect the modern body (largely through the bodies of the backwards, barbaric working classes and Irish underclass). Maps are both a means of achieving a more perfectly modern space and its ideal representation.

The result of this emphasis (if not also its cause) was that medical mapping developed an image of London consonant with other images of its modernity, in which filth was coded as barbarism, and modernity associated with a malleable landscape in which filth and circulation could be contained and managed, and in which openness, light, and freedom of circulation was associated with modernity and civilization. The goal, as Lynda Nead points out, was to restructure London by mapping its dark spaces and transforming them, through urban planning and restructuring, into their clean modern opposite.[5] Thus, by the 1860s, these mappings posited a multilayered urban surface that could be manipulated and brought into a historical narrative of progress. As David Pike points out of the building of the Underground railways,

> The fantasy of the empty city reflects the emptying out of both its literal and its metaphorical undergrounds, its sources of disease as well as of difference. The Underground replaced one type of underground space – the space of poverty, slums, crime – with another – a space increasingly sanitized and middle-class ... The Underground displaced the lower depths from representational space just as it did from the physical space they occupied in the city.[6]

Mid-nineteenth-century Britons distrusted the underground (both metaphorical and real) layers of difference which had, they thought, produced disease and were redolent of earlier historical periods of cultural – and perhaps biological – evolution.

Anglo-Indian medicine, however, takes a rather different trajectory. Although disease mapping in England was increasingly preoccupied with charting the historical geography of epidemics preparatory to transforming the environment (for example, by embanking the Thames and laying new sewage infrastructure), no historical disease maps were made in India until the early 1870s, and even then they were initially invoked in the service of an ahistorical vision of an unchanging

geography of endemic disease. First, the vastness of the land under survey was not conducive to the kind of detail needed for a detailed
palimpsestic mapping. Furthermore those carrying out medical mapping in India were often completing these projects as part of required
reports, and had little research interest in medical topography per se.
But, perhaps just as importantly, India was not presumed to be
meliorable in the way the English (and especially English urban) landscape was. Despite the presence of detailed early cholera maps from the
1820s and early 1830s, British medics in India did not refer to these earlier documents in their mapmaking, mapping each year of outbreak as
a singular event until the late 1860s.

The 1860s found British medics within a wider global context, in
which England and India were not wholly separate problems, but were
located in a global continuum. Discussions of attempts to reinstitute
modified *cordons sanitaires*, in particular targeting Muslim pilgrims
crossing the Red Sea, made international collaboration and British
responsibility for communication between areas under their own
administration and the larger world a necessary, if unpleasant object of
contemplation. The enormous increase of British troops, and thus, also,
medics, in India following the Rebellion or Mutiny of 1857 also did
much to bring the two medical literatures (insular and British-Indian)
together by increasing contact between the two professional groups.
Indian maps of the 1860s tend to assume some kind of human activity
as the cholera vector – usually religious pilgrimage – and map this
movement, as sanitary questions across larger India are less remediable
than those of particular camps and fair locations. By contrast, at this
time maps in Britain are more concerned with specific sites and water
supplies, which are seen as demanding identification and remediation.

Finally, the later maps of India are preoccupied less with epidemiological questions than with administrative issues – such as how
disease got out of hand in a particular camp. This is in part because its
aetiology was more clearly understood, but also, I suspect, in large part
because responsibility for sanitary 'failures' were laid squarely on
colonial administrators' shoulders. Further, the system of local sanitary
authorities accompanying their reports with sanitary maps meant that
there was a thorough and reasonably accurate, if stylistically inconsis-
tent mapping of data in Britain on a detailed scale which enabled central government to turn their attention to larger issues. A large map
literature not only fostered its own continuance, it also provided a firm
basis for the burgeoning of the study of epidemiological topography.
Only later did colonial disease mapping catch up. The birth of tropical

medicine as a specialty with claims to both professionalism and respectability is part of this outward-looking movement and British mapping of itself into a larger and radically interconnected world.

In the late 1860s, the need to exculpate themselves from responsibility for poor sanitation is quite evident in reports written by British sanitary authorities in India. One report begins by referring to the issue with entertaining candour:

> With reference to paragraph 7 of Goverment Resolution No 398 of 1867, dated 25th February, 1867 . . . I have the honour to submit the following report on the measures . . . necessary to prevent *Bombay being regarded by European nations as* a base whence Cholera habitually spreads westward by the sea;[7]

Perhaps in part also for this reason, a small flurry of counterarguments did appear from insular medics clinging to meteorological and other explanations, and sometimes by refuting the claim that cholera had come from India. D. K. Whittaker, reporting for the *London Quarterly Review* on the Cholera Conference and recent cholera research, goes through an impressive number of historical documents in order to conclude that although cholera may be endemic to India, it does not, necessarily, emerge primarily from the Ganges valley. He remarks of the cholera conference's conclusions that,

> It has been a favorite French notion to throw the onus of the production of cholera in India on English domination, and to attribute it to the neglect on the part of the English Government of the great canals and works of the Mohamedan emperors. This idea was broached before the Conference, but was entirely dissipated by our able English representatives. We need not inquire where those great works were situated, or at what period they fell into decay, It seems sufficient to remark, that cholera is first known to us in districts in which there never were such works, and that its great centre in India at present is in a part of India where none such ever existed.[8]

Although Whittaker makes some reference to the importance of sanitation and drainage in the Ganges, he immediately turns to religious pilgrimage, both in India and to Mecca, as the real target of concern, thereby shifting the blame onto the recalcitrant Indians rather than focusing on the land, which was a British responsibility.

Despite the fact that English physicians had almost universally accepted the efficacy of sanitary measures, in particular the provision of clean water, whatever their reservations about the exact nature of cholera and its spread, a substantial minority of Indian medics – including, crucially, in Bengal, the acknowledged endemic centre of cholera outbreaks – reverted to a climatic theory of cholera which, amazingly, was not only anti-contagionist, but also anti-sanitarian. W. R. Cornish complains that, 'even in the present day so unsettled are the views of the profession that the old battle between the "contagionists" and "non-contagionists" bids fair to be fought over again with all its original fierceness'.[9] This debate is best exemplified by the exchanges of this same Cornish, the contagionist medic of Madras, whose territory suffered successive invasions of cholera from Bengal, and Bryden, of Bengal, surgeon and statistical officer of the Sanitary Commission. Bryden first published his views in the late 1860s. He concluded that cholera was born out of the endemic region into the epidemic ones on the monsoon winds, that it was non-contagious. Furthermore, because it was native to part of Bengal, and it was not related to sanitary conditions, sanitary measures would have no effect on it – in fact, it was a natural disaster beyond human control. As might be imagined, this conclusion, running counter to all conventional wisdom in Europe, most in India, and the findings of the International Conference, raised eyebrows. In response, Bryden writes loftily:

> Those who can know little of the harmonies of epidemiology and of the rigid laws which govern these harmonies, who would accuse me of sitting down with this vast collection of facts before me and ambitiously distorting each into a place in a system, which as a system has no real existence. Different observers will interpret the same facts differently. An uneducated man has no difficulty in satisfying himself that the ice-groovings on a boulder are the work of the stone-mason. In science, there is a recognizable limit to diversity of interpretation, and he whose education is the more complete can go further in advance of the man who has no intimate knowledge of the subject he professes to treat.[10]

He refers to the conference directly, and refutes their findings. In 1874 he published an expanded version of his argument, claiming that Indian authorities have never ascribed to the contagionist views of the conference, quoting Jameson and his followers at length, but failing to mention Scot or his own contemporaries in Madras, with whom, by then, he had had long and acrimonious disputes centred precisely around Scot's map.[11] In this same 1874 document, he refers to the attraction which plans to quarantine Bengal have for many people, but asserts that such a step would make no difference to the spread of disease.[12] In short, the demands of the International Sanitary Conference split British medics into two camps – one which basically agreed with the general consensus in Europe, and one which was decidedly reactionary. The disagreement between these two groups would propel British medical mapping in India into a new phase.

Surgeon W. R. Cornish of Madras was appalled and infuriated by Bryden's argument, the more so since 'his' region was regularly invaded. Countering Bryden and his use of Jameson, Cornish draws upon the mapping of his own area by Scot, who had been as in favour of the contagionist thesis as Jameson was opposed to it. Cornish is clear that the cholera is Bryden's problem:

> malignant or epidemic cholera is not a natural product of Southern India – instead it invades from the North ... we have been in the habit of supposing that the disease was a true endemic of the soil [in some of Southern India where it lingered for three or four years]; but, although the conditions of the soil and climate in such districts probably approach very nearly to the conditions of the natural habitat of cholera in Lower Bengal, yet there are probably some points of difference as yet unascertained.[13]

And again, he stresses that in his district, 'Cholera is like a foreign plant in them, that has found a fairly congenial, but not wholly natural soil, so that after a certain definite time the plant dies.'[14] He then quotes Scot's 1820s work on cholera in India verbatim and at length, concluding that subsequent epidemics have all followed the same route, and pointedly asserting that Scot's work is 'all the more valuable at the present time, because it was compiled not to illustrate any "theory" of invasion, but to record, in a connected form, the testimony of officers of the Medical Department, who had personally witnessed the outbreak.'[15] He explains that he has 'redrawn' Scot's map (work in fact carried out by V. Vardaraja Moodely), and has added several arrows to show the direction of the monsoon winds, both from the Southwest and the Northeast. (Unfortunately, he has also removed the marked roads, which in Scot so clearly showed human transmission; the topographic detail of mountains is also missing.)

Cornish then launches into an indignant refutation of Bryden, whose maps, he states, are 'wholly misleading':

if we are to trust to Dr. Bryden's figures and maps, the invading cholera of that year stopped short in what he calls the 'eastern division of the epidemic area,' viz, the districts eastward of Gwalior, Saugor, and Jubbulpore . . . It is somewhat strange that a cholera map should have been drawn for 1859 so as to show a complete exemption of the western and southern tracts, the more especially as it is evident from the report that Dr. Bryden was acquainted with the fact of the invasion of Bombay in that year.[16]

He repeats his version of Bryden's maps (seven times, each showing a different time period) and extends them to show the South and the geography and temporality of epidemic invasion there – incidentally, by repeating them, he reiterates the endemicity of the Northeast (see Illustration 5.3). Cornish's long-held argument is for human transmission; as is customary in this group, religious pilgrims and coolies are seen as responsible for the spread of cholera. (In this way, the importance of the government's responsibility for sanitary improvements, expensive to make and difficult to maintain in India, is downplayed.) Cornish finds Bryden's casual dismissal of Hurdwar pilgrims as vectors monstrous. The keynote of his argument, however, is his reproduction of Scot's map, with the addition of arrows showing wind direction during the monsoons, which, he argues, shows clearly that the monsoons do not spread cholera.[17] He insists that every epidemic since Scot charted the first one has followed the same path.

Cornish is basically happy with the condition of Madras, reiterating that it is pilgrims who spread disease:

> simple sanitary precautions should be enforced, at all times, with the class of people who constitute the bulk of pilgrim visitors to celebrated shrines, but it does not help forward the progress of sanitary science to credit attempts at enforcement of cleanliness and decency, with the power of averting an advancing wave of cholera . . . The intensity of cholera, and the prolongation of its epidemic visitations, are, I am convinced, largely due to the habits of the people in gadding about to divers places where festivals are held, and their unnatural modes of living during such seasons.[18]

However, he argues, against Bryden's total dismissal of sanitary improvement, that such improvement does make a material difference, observing dryly that if Bengal cannot be improved vis-à-vis sanitation, it must be a very different place than it was a few years earlier,

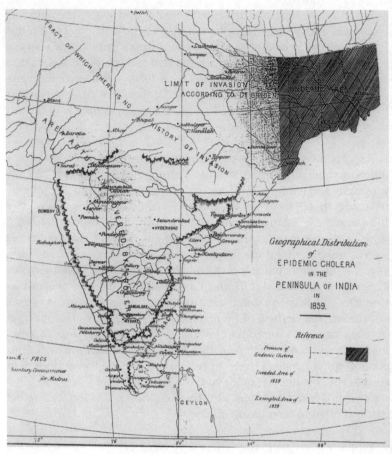

Illustration 5.3   Cornish's reprint of Bryden's map with added material: detail

when the 1861 Cholera Commission found its sanitary conditions
wanting.[19] He concludes, pointedly, that he trusts that soon, 'a systematic effort to attack and defeat cholera in its endemic home, shall
be made with every prospect of modifying those periodical invasions
of epidemics which now carry terror and dismay, and destruction of
life, over nine-tenths of the habitable globe'[20] – including his own
innocent corner of it.

Cornish is not the most eloquent defender of the faith, and his waf-
fling on the topic of sanitary improvements – Madras doesn't need
them, but Bengal does – contribute little to his argument. Bryden rose,

exultant, to the challenge, reproducing Cornish's reproduction of Scot's map and, adding several lines denoting areas of successive epidemic invasion, managing through a rather spectacular manipulation of data to adduce Scot's map as evidence for his own theory: 'In the map [Scot's], I have inserted in the North, stations where Jameson's record tells us were first invaded in May 1818 . . . This cholera, had a definite boundary line in the South, which I have dotted in on Scot's map. . . . demarcations shown between May and July 1818'[21] and likewise between July and August, and August and October, which, according to Bryden, showed cholera's advance 'per saltum' – that is., in leaps covering simultaneously an entire region affected by monsoon winds. He exults in the happiness of having more data to fill out his theory and chides his predecessors,

> Records of the epidemic intervening are made up of fragmentary data which were never placed in order to form a consistent history, probably because it was deemed impossible that a connected history of cholera could be written for any year or any epidemic, although the simple narration of Scot and Jameson now show us that all through these fifty years an accurate and connected record might have been kept up.[22]

Future splutterings by Cornish and others were grandly ignored. It is hard, from the vantage point of the present, not to indict Bryden for a callous, cynical and self-serving misuse of evidence in the interest of exculpating the Bengal authorities from responsibility, both for past epidemics and for any sanitary improvement. His arrogant dismissal of his critics as 'uneducated' makes him no more likeable. However, it is also important to keep in mind the fact that medics living in the endemic area may have had a very different experience to those living outside those regions. Bryden, the regional heir of Jameson, shares his views, and that may be because their experiences were similar. In fact, recent research suggests that weather patterns do contribute to the epidemic spread of cholera. However, it is difficult not to hold Bryden, with the experience of other medics all over the world to draw on, to a higher standard of the openness he so ostentatiously claims. In answering critics who wondered why measures which had worked in Europe wouldn't be useful in India, he responded, simply, 'on the ground of homology, I am prepared to believe that the aspect of cholera in Europe may be very different from that presented to our study in India. As I remarked in my original report – "The relative value of the primary and secondary truths probably differs much in different countries and among different races".'[23]

What must interest us about this spat, in addition to its illustration of the tendencies of medical theories to follow local political interests, is that it sparked the first detailed historical analyses of cholera epidemics and use of multiple maps to reinvest the epidemics with a sense of historical narrative. Bryden uses few maps, preferring charts, and all his care is directed to a story of a timeless cycle – a homogenous land visited by an annual cycle of monsoons which must always have the same result – his narrative is one of inevitable repetition, a land caught in time. He is thus in direct opposition to his contemporaries in Britain in his portrayal of disease and geography. His maps tend to strip the land of its features, including mountains, rivers, roads, etc., since those are extraneous to his argument (and also suggest other possible theses). However, in giving the disease a history and a narrative extending backward in time and space, he opens the door for Cornish, however blunderingly, to use his maps to show several *different* trajectories of the epidemic in successive years. Despite his claim that the cholera always follows generally the same path (that is, invading his territory from Bengal), his maps tell us that there are many variations in the path of the disease, just as his narrative focuses on the possibility of melioration through sanitation (and possibly quarantine of pilgrims, a notion dear to Cornish's heart).

Despite Bryden's call for a continuous narrative, then, it is Cornish who actually gives us a narrative – that is, a sequence of events defined by change. Townsend, who appears to have teamed up with Cornish in order to question Bryden's results, of course, had long been interested in a vision of an India subject to progress through drainage.[24] It is in the 1860s, then, that we begin to see a concerted drift among some medics and other mappers toward a layered, historically more nuanced vision of India's land.[25] This, of course, may be partially related to the rise of Orientalist study which was related to political management, and I don't want simply to glamorize it as anti-racist or anti-imperialist. However, the emergence of this trend did enable a vision of Indian land to emerge in the British imaginary which could be emplaced in a narrative of progress and change – and, perhaps, a vision of India which suggested the possibility of a history which extended beyond the boundaries of British occupation – both backwards and forwards in time.

Finally, though his motives must remain obscure, it is certainly clear that the intended effect of Bryden's fatalistic arguments was to excuse the British government in Bengal from making any efforts towards melioration of conditions. Cornish and Townsend repeatedly demanded inquiries into Bryden's investigations, but Bryden did not budge an inch, was promoted to surgeon major, and, four years after the initial publication of his thesis, brought out the definitive and greatly expanded version of the same argument, analysing several years of data, to arrive at exactly the same conclusion. Of course, his voice was one among many, and was not definitive in policy-making.

Abstract space in India, then, is not at this time, as in London, the space of the palimpsest. Unlike England, where the landscape had layers which were defective, but meliorable, India did not. The land of India itself was seen as guilty of disease production. Whereas low-lying, damp areas in England were seen as unhealthy and vulnerable to colonization by disease until drained, India, and the people and behaviours that were mapped onto the land, were considered to constitute an ecological entity productive of evil. David Arnold has also observed the increasing tendency in the first half of the nineteenth century for Britons to imagine the entire diverse geography of India as homogenously tropical,[26] and the tropics themselves represented a sullied Eden, a condition of humanity simultaneously childlike and degenerate.[27] (In fact, about half of India sits above the tropic of Cancer.) William Sanderson writes in 1866, 'Cholera is known to have originated in India, which has long been well-populated, even in the prehistoric period . . . Cholera could originate only in dense masses of population depositing excreta and other animalized matter over surfaces, from which it is carried by the percolation of the rainfall to the sources of the water supply . . .' (10).[28] Although medics speak of the sedimentation of a very old culture being the very source of cholera in India, that sedimentation was not in the mid-century seen as layers of change in a country moving towards modernity, as it is in England. Instead, it is simply the sedimentation of a stagnant culture caught endlessly in a single moment of past time. When India is seen as having degenerated from a past glory, at some point in the distant past, this progression or regression is presented as having stopped. Micromapping is not necessary because there are no distinctions in the layers – the level of the graticule is the appropriate level of abstraction for the imposition of a British logic and British settlements – at an appropriate distance – from the monstrous and monumental barbarism of India. Although this was undoubtedly often not the intention, or even the perception, of the mapmakers, other factors – often economic and political – contributed to a representation of India that depended on and perpetuated this perception. Those Britons who objected to this view – and there were many – were largely ignored, as were the natives who lobbied for such assistance. While English visions of space became increasingly layered, susceptible of what we might call a 'realist' narration of progress and the structural equivalence of bodies, representations of Indian space tended to become ever more solidly 'mythic' – tending towards narrative embedded in static or cyclical time and embodying fixed characteristics.

This 'denial of coevalness', as Johannes Fabian puts it[29] – the distancing of another in space and time which simultaneously legitimates the scientific gaze and neutralizes difference by casting it in the distant developmental past in relation to the observer – obviously has its appeal, from a simply economic and administrative standpoint. Sanitizing India would have been expensive; if India was, however, by its essential nature unsanitary, then it was impossible to expect that British administration should have much impact on it. This attitude made it possible for a time to leave Indians in the Augean stables which imperialism had helped create, but which, in the perception of many British, was simply an unalterable part of the Indian landscape.[30] But at last, in the late 1860, British medics in India begin to be able to map it as a land with a medical history – and, perhaps, a future.

Notes

1. Samuel Abot, translator, *Report to the International Sanitary Conference of a Commission from that Body on the Origin, Endemicity, Transmissibility and Propagation of Asiatic Cholera* (Boston: Alfred Mudge and Son, Printers, 1867).
2. John Snow, *Snow on Cholera. Being a reprint of two papers: On the mode of communication of cholera; On continuous molecular changes* (New York: Commonwealth Fund, 1936).
3. *Report of the General Board of Health on the Epidemic Cholera 1848 and 1849* (London: W. Clowes and Sons, 1850).
4. *Report of the Cholera Outbreak in the Parish of St. James, Westminster during the Autumn of 1854. Presented to the Vestry by the Cholera Inquiry Committee, July 1855* (London: Parish of Saint James, Westminster, 1855).
5. Lynda Nead, *Victorian Babylon: People, Streets and Images in Nineteenth-Century London* (New Haven: Yale University Press, 2000).
6. David L. Pike, 'The Underground Railway in Victorian London'. n.d. Accessed 8 November 2002. http://www.iath.virginia.edu/london/Archive/On_line_pubs/Underground%20Railway/Underground%20Railway.html
7. T. G. Hewlett, *Report of Measures Recommended in Bombay to Prevent Cholera Spreading Westward by the Sea towards European Nations* (Bombay: The Education Society's Press, Byculla, 1867) 1 (my emphasis).

8. D. K. Whittaker, 'The Cholera Conference', *The London Quarterly Review* 27 (Jan. 1867): 16–29, 22.
9. W. R. Cornish, *Cholera in Southern India: A record of the progress of cholera in 1870, and resume of the records of former epidemic invasions of the Madras Presidency* (Madras: H. Morgan, 1871) 1.
10. James L. Bryden, *Epidemic Cholera in the Bengal Presidency: Report on the General Aspects of Epidemic Cholera in 1869: a Sequel to 'A report on the cholera of 1866–68'* (Calcutta: Office of the Superintendent of Government Printing, 1870) 2–3.
11. James L. Bryden, *Cholera Epidemics of Recent Years viewed in relation to Former Epidemics: A Record of Cholera in the Bengal Presidency from 1817–1872* (Calcutta: Office of the Superintendent of Government Printing, 1874) 243–4. He is using James Jameson, *Report on the Epidemick Cholera Morbus, as it Visited the Territories subject to the Presidency of Bengal in the Years 1817, 1818, and 1819* (Calcutta: Printed at the Government Gazette Press, by A. G. Balfour, No. 1 Mission Row, 1820). He ignores William Scot, *Report on the Epidemic Cholera as it has appeared in the territories subject to The Presidency of Fort St. George* (Madras, 1824).
12. Bryden, *Cholera Epidemics*, 2.
13. Cornish, *Cholera in Southern India*, 2.
14. Ibid., 3.
15. Ibid., 14.
16. Ibid., 15.
17. Ibid., 78.
18. Ibid., 149–50.
19. Ibid., 151.
20. Ibid., 160.
21. Bryden, *Cholera Epidemics*, note, 6.
22. Ibid., note, 2.
23. Ibid., 40.
24. Dr. S. C. Townsend, Sanitary Commissioner, Central Provinces and Berars, *Report on the Cholera Epidemic of 1868* ([no pub. data on titlepage] 1869).
25. A good example of such a study (which rehistoricizes the land) is that by Captain J. Forsyth, Bengal Staff Corps. *Report on the Land Revenue Settlement of British Nimar: District of the Central Provinces. 1868–1869* (Nagpore: Printed at the Chief Commissioner's Office Press, 1870). This document gives a full historical background before and after British government, and relies in part on older Hindu land descriptions. It argues for improvement, in this case land irrigation, and in addition to a detailed analysis both historical and geological, it contains a map, which shows 'ancient and modern divisions' of the territory and includes 'Old Pergunna' and 'Old Tuppa' placenames. This is one of the emerging trend of studies, not yet a dominant one, which begins to reinsert India into a historical tradition, and acknowledges that the land has changed over time and can be changed again.
26. David Arnold, *The Problem of Nature: Environment, Culture, and European Expansion* (London: Blackwell, 1996).
27. See, for example, much of the work by Charles Kingsley or Tennyson.
28. William Sanderson, *Suggestions in Reference to The Present Cholera Epidemic, for the Purification of the Water Supply and the Reclamation of East London, with*

Remarks on the Origin of the Cholera Poison (London: William Macintosh, 1866) 10.

29. Johannes Fabian, *Time and the Other: How Anthropology Makes its Object* (New York and Guildford: Columbia University Press, 1983).

30. It also made it possible to ignore that in fact India had changed a good deal in the nineteenth century, what with massive British public works projects, which, recent scholarship suggests, had a role in causing endemic cholera to get out of hand. See, for example, Ira Klein, 'Imperialism, Ecology and Disease: Cholera in India, 1850–1950', *Indian Economic and Social History Review* 31.4 (1994): 491–518.

6
Framing the 'Magic Mountain Malady': the Reception of Thomas Mann's *The Magic Mountain* in the Medical Community, 1924–2000

Malte Herwig

Ever since its publication in 1924, Thomas Mann's novel about disease and degeneration, *The Magic Mountain*, has exercised the imagination of general readers and physicians alike. Probably no other novel in the history of literature has attracted such attention in medical circles. In 1925 alone, around a dozen medical journals in the German-speaking world published reviews of Mann's highly controversial satire on sanatorium life. Though by no means all of these reviews were negative, Mann felt obliged to answer the attacks of some medical critics in an open letter to the *Deutsche Medizinische Wochenschrift*, the main organ of the medical profession in Germany, in which he defended the novel's aim as genuinely 'medical' ('ärztlich').

It is this claim by a writer who counted medicine among the 'neighbouring spheres of his art'[1] which I would like to investigate here on several levels. Within the broader scope of this volume – identifying ways of framing and imagining disease – I am specifically interested in the way in which Mann's novelistic account of disease was received in the medical community. Its members scrutinized the novel's image of disease in the light of their own medical schooling, clinical experience, and professional interests. From this interaction between the author, his novel and its medical readers a new frame for tuberculosis emerged: the 'Magic Mountain Malady' ('Zauberberg-Krankheit').

While much has been written about the thematic significance of disease for Mann's work, his confident self-portrayal as a kind of literary doctor ('Among my inner possibilities there has always been that of a medical existence'[2]) has never been tested against whatever use medical practitioners felt his writings might have for their work. Thus my approach is in the widest sense *rezeptionsgeschichtlich* and I shall consider actual responses from physicians in order to show how definitions of disease were negotiated between the medical establishment and those who offered alternative interpretations. Did physicians challenge the writer's authority in treating disease as a literary topic? Did they find that lessons could be learned from the image of disease presented in *The Magic Mountain* – lessons for understanding a disease's significance in an individual or social context, for the institutional set-up and therapeutic practices that had been built up around the treatment of tuberculosis, or for reforming healthcare policy? In general terms, this case study may help to illuminate the relation between medical accounts, the personal experiences of suffering individuals, and the image of a disease as it exists in the public mind. The central question thus is whether fictional narratives can usefully enhance our understanding of disease and thereby fulfil the 'medical aim' that was envisaged by Mann.

The medical reviews I survey in this short essay[3] give evidence of the complex process in which definitions of tuberculosis not only as a biological but also as a social and psychosomatic disease were negotiated in the Germany of the 1920s and 1930s. From the debate between Mann and his medical critics, the framing of disease definition in imaginative literature emerges as a powerful tool of cultural diagnosis ('Kurkritik' as 'Kulturkritik' as Mann quipped) and social control, which competed with the authority of institutionalized medicine, not least because of *The Magic Mountain*'s widespread popularity. However, I also hope to show that there is more to physicians' sustained interest in Mann's novel than a concern to legitimize status relationships and assert authority over a medicalized society. Over the past two decades, it has become common currency among social historians of medicine to understand disease as being shaped by social, historical and linguistic antecedents and to view medical science as an interpretive practice. As Sander Gilman writes in *Disease and Representation*: 'Like any complex text, the signs of illness are read within the conventions of an interpretive community that comprehends them in the light of earlier, powerful readings of what are understood to be similar or parallel texts.'[4] The secure place *The Magic Mountain* has on curricula in the Medical Humanities, its role in reading therapy and as a frequent point of medical reference ensure the novel's status as such a powerful text about disease.[5] Health geographers appreciate the novel because it allows them to form more embedded accounts of illness and health, as Wil Gesler wrote recently in *Health & Place*: 'One of the most important ideas that can be carried away from *The Magic Mountain*, I believe, is that knowledge about disease and death, health and life, can be gained in ways that depart from traditional positivist studies'.[6]

One result of what we might call the humanistic turn in medicine is the importance given to narratives for framing disease and investing it with meaning. In Howard Brody's words, 'the primary human mechanism for attaching meaning to particular experiences is to tell stories about them'.[7] Literature situates and contextualizes disease and invests the experience of disease with meaning. These interpretations not only help patients to 'make sense' of their condition, but they can also serve as critical correctives to prevailing medical thought and practice. As Peter Conrad has pointed out, 'new disease designations are not solely the product of medical discovery or knowledge, but often . . . emerge from a complex interaction with sufferers and interested publics'.[8] In this negotiation of disease between individual patients, the medical profession and the general public, imaginative literature like Thomas Mann's *The Magic Mountain* has played and continues to play an important role, as I will show below.

Negotiating disease: the German sanatorium of Dr Mann

During the years that he was writing *The Magic Mountain*, Thomas Mann – sometimes dressing up as a doctor – visited hospitals, surgical theatres, and X-ray laboratories. He also observed operations, read a considerable amount of medical literature that he had either acquired himself or had received from physician friends, and consulted with doctors about his novel at every opportunity. Having gone to such lengths in his attempt to render a faithful and accurate description of medical matters, Mann could be forgiven for initially having high hopes for the novel's reception: 'All doctors and former patients who hear about the enterprise are thirsting for the satire' he wrote to his friend Ernst Bertram on 16 March 1920.[9] However, when *The Magic Mountain* was published in 1924 it was precisely the elements of scathing satire in Mann's description of life in a Swiss mountain sanatorium that met with fierce opposition from medical critics, who saw their profession as being undermined by what they considered a deeply negative portrayal of the sanatorium's chief surgeon and staff.

Before we consider the justifiability of such criticism it is worth asking why doctors deemed it necessary at all to review a work of literary fiction in medical journals and on what basis they felt able to offer their views on the novel. From the reviews that appeared within five years of the novel's publication it quickly becomes apparent that the medical community saw the need to assert its authority in the public debate that was generated by Mann's descriptions of disease. *The Magic Mountain* had soon reached a wide audience and many doctors felt they had to correct what they believed was a misleading and biased account of tuberculosis and its treatment. Alexander Prüssian writes in the *Münchner Medizinische Wochenschrift*:

> In the whole of world fiction there is probably no parallel for a two-volume novel treating largely one specific disease and its course with such an abundance of technical terms. This is done in such an obvious and biased manner that, in view of the extremely wide readership and the author's distinguished artistic reputation, the medical community is required to take a stand.[10]

Similarly, Hermann Schelenz points out that even those physicians who are not usually interested in literature – and particularly those involved in the fight against tuberculosis – ought to take note of the book because it contained a great deal of substance worthy of medical consideration ('ärztlich Nachdenkliches').[11] In the *Zentralblatt für innere Medizin*, G. Zickgraf writes that Mann's book is of great importance for doctors because its literary treatment of medical problems and institutions is vastly superior to ordinary descriptions of disease and medical issues.[12] Like Mann, Loewy-Hattendorf sees literature and medicine as neighbouring areas, and he alerts his colleagues in the *Zeitschrift für ärztliche Fortbildung*, a journal devoted to further education in the medical profession, to the fact that many medical and scientific problems discussed in specialist periodicals are also treated 'in poetic disguise' in great works of literature, among them Mann's *The Magic Mountain*, which he comments upon at length.[13]

Most reviewers draw a distinction between the artistic qualities of the novel and its medical subject-matter, terminology and specific descriptions of disease. It is only the second aspect which the majority purport to judge competently. Consequently, nearly all physician reviewers disregard the novel's symbolic meaning and instead focus on the painfully realistic and accurate portrayal of the sorry state of Swiss sanatoria. While the majority concede that Mann's description of the symptoms, course and treatment of tuberculosis is realistic and accurate, many reviewers take particular issue with the medical characters in the book: Hofrat Behrens, the sanatorium's medical director, his assistant Dr Krokowski and the nursing staff are frequently criticized as improbable, exaggerated, cynical, cold, and odious. Writing in *Die Therapie der*

Gegenwart, Felix Klemperer concludes that the disagreeable and some-times brutal Behrens is, as a doctor, a very distasteful colleague ('als Arzt ... ein sehr wenig erfreulicher Standesgenosse').[14] Prüssian criticizes Mann's 'downright devastating characterization' of the medical person-nel and his emphasis on the repulsive and disgusting aspects of the dis-ease on which, to Prüssian's taste, the author dwells too extensively at the expense of ethical values ('ethisches Pathos'): 'Reading his book the layman will think that almost everybody suffering from tuberculosis of the lung is bound to degenerate spiritually as well as morally.'[15] Schelenz, one of Mann's most vociferous critics, goes even further and warns of the 'considerable damage' that the book may well cause:

> To be precise I consider the main damage that non-medical readers will form a completely wrong picture of sanatoria and their work-ings. We have nothing to hide about the way our sanatoria work, yet we will never think it desirable that unqualified amateurs venture criticism of us or our patients.[16]

In *Die Tuberkulose*, Dehoff takes a similar 'us and them' stance and con-demns the 'improper description and criticism of medical measures and personalities by non-physicians even in the form of a novel'.[17] Unlike more moderate reviewers such as Loewy-Hattendorf, she denies Mann the right to comment upon something which he 'cannot judge objectively' and even accuses him of inciting hostility to the medical profession ('Anfeindung der Medizin'). From these remarks it becomes clear that the medical establishment – especially, of course, those who specialized in tuberculosis like Schelenz and Dehoff – felt threatened by what they read as a highly critical (if fictional) account of the shortcomings of sanator-ium care. Thus we have an interesting example here of what Charles Rosenberg called the process of 'negotiating disease'. According to Rosenberg, 'disease definitions and hypothetical etiologies can serve as tools of social control', which structure and legitimize social relations.[18] Public debates about specific diseases are such acts of social negotiation, 'in which interested participants interact to produce logically arbitrary but socially viable, if often provisional, solutions to a dispute'.[19]

It comes as no surprise that the strongest criticism of Mann's novel came from those who were themselves working in tuberculosis care and felt immediately affected by the depiction offered in *The Magic Mountain*. Before the discovery of streptomycin by Schatz and Waksman in 1943, the treatment of tuberculosis consisted mainly in (often long-term) sanatorium care, rest cure and occasional surgical interventions such as an artificial pneumothorax[20] or thoracoplastic surgery. The sanatoria were dependent on a steady stream of wealthy European patients willing to spend considerable money and time in these often luxurious institutions. In *The Magic Mountain*, Mann makes much of the elaborate meals served in the 'Berghof' sanatorium and he also satirizes the frivolous games and entertainments which the patients indulge in to pass the time. He was, in fact, not the first one to highlight the serious institutional shortcomings to be found in spas like Arosa and Davos: In 1920 Alexander Prüssian had published a report in the *Münchner Medizinische Wochenschrift*, in which he relates his impressions of a trip to Arosa and Davos.[21] Prüssian's criticism of the conditions in these spas – especially the many distractions and entertainments which the patients were allowed to indulge in – foreshadows much of what Mann describes. However, it was only four years later with the publication of *The Magic Mountain* that (in this case) Davos felt exposed before a European public and local doctors and administrators saw their business threatened by what they regarded as a defamatory caricature. Although a Davos doctor like Dehoff rejects Mann's medical views, she nevertheless fears that less discerning ('minder urteilsfähige') people may be misled by them,[22] and Schelenz brings out what Dehoff only implies: reading *The Magic Mountain* may deter potential patients from seeking a cure in Davos. Their outright rejection of Mann's framing of tuberculosis therefore has to be seen in the context of social and professional control which I mentioned above: It is an attempt to assert the medical establishment's authority over the definition of disease against alternative definitions such as those offered in imaginative literature.

Thomas Mann's self-confessed lifelong obsession with disease and degeneration certainly make him, in Rosenberg's terminology, an 'interested participant' in the negotiation of disease definitions, and he did not shy away from publicly asserting his own authority in an open letter entitled 'Vom Geist der Medizin' to the very journal on whose pages Schelenz had challenged it. In this brief text, Mann rebuts criticisms by invoking a number of medical authorities who had commented favourably on the novel, and he closes with the prediction that it would only be a matter of time before he received an honorary medical doctorate. Mann's self-confident stance was not so much a sign of imperious arrogance but, as I have already suggested, resulted from a genuine feeling that his aims in *The Magic Mountain* were akin to those of medicine. Thus, he rejects the importance his critics gave to the medical surface narrative and emphasizes instead its pedagogical aim: 'its service is service to life, its commitment is to health, its aim is the future. That means it is medical.'[23] How much the public image of tuberculosis was indeed influenced by Mann's portrayal of the disease in the *Magic Mountain* is illustrated by an anecdote which the delighted author related to his translator Helen Lowe-Porter in a letter of 15 January 1927: 'An Englishman arrives at Davos and his first question is: "Where is the German Sanatorium of Dr. Mann?" Isn't that heartening?'

Blaming disease: the doctor's or the patient's fault?

Whether the anecdote about Dr Mann's sanatorium is true or not, there is enough evidence to suggest that Mann's depiction of tuberculosis was widely influential. Moreover, despite the scandal that the novel's publication had caused in large parts of the medical community, some physicians quickly jumped to Mann's defence and drew attention to the possible benefits that the 'Tuberkuloseroman' could have for medicine. Klemperer assures his colleagues: 'It obviously is of use to us physicians. It is the source of much stimulus',[24] and Zickgraf cautions against dismissing criticism simply because it comes from outside the medical community: 'Anybody, I think, is entitled to criticize, and if it is done in such a subtle manner we should rather think about the causes of this criticism and whether we cannot remove them.'[25] Those who welcome Mann's commentary all agree that his description of the deplorable shortcomings of sanatorium care may be exaggerated for literary effect, but nonetheless concede that it has a grain of truth in it. On a more profound level, there is a consensus among the novel's medical advocates that its most interesting achievement lies in showing how an illness like tuberculosis affects the psyche and how, conversely, the course of the disease is influenced by psychological and social constraints and the harmful milieu the patients live in. Far from seeing it as an attack on the medical profession, Margarete Levy appreciates the book as 'a very serious appeal to the conscience of doctors to protect their patients from the psychologically damaging influence of this milieu'.[26] Instead of dismissing the autocratic Hofrat Behrens and his dubious assistant Krokowski as defamatory caricatures of their profession, Helmut Ulrici, himself the director of a clinic, places the blame for the deteriorating state of the Berghof sanatorium and its inhabitants firmly on the medical characters rather than their author:

Instead of giving a supportive example through his rounded character, the Hofrat's cynical wit increases moral disorientation, and he completely fails to see the intellectual ruin of his charges, and even the objectionable activities of his assistant, who exploits the patients' apparently heightened sense of last things in order to draw them into erotic discussions and highly questionable psychoanalytical experiments. This too is just another example of the psychological decline of those patients.[27]

Unlike Schelenz and Dehoff, Ulrici and Levy appreciate the fundamental difference between narrator and author in a work of literary fiction; their judgement is not clouded by professional misgivings and they allow themselves to be drawn into the novel's argument about disease. This is all the more important since *The Magic Mountain* was published at a time when the psychological side-effects of tuberculosis in general – and sanatorium care in particular – were only just about to become conceptualized in medical discourse (see my remarks below on Amrein and Stern). All positive reviews of Mann's novel draw attention to this desideratum and make a point that fictional literature has been ahead of clinical medicine in this regard. Where scientific knowledge was lacking, useful insights into the psychological effects of diseases might therefore be drawn from fictional accounts, especially of course from the genre of the psychological novel which had been developed and fine-tuned in the nineteenth century. Levy consequently argues in the *Deutsche Medizinische Wochenschrift*:

> There is very little medical literature so far about the relation between tuberculosis of the lungs and psychological phenomena, whereas laymen have for a long time shown great interest in this problem . . . This is where the doctors' work, a sensible psychotherapy alongside and together with the actual medical therapy, ought to start. Thomas Mann's novel is a downright challenge to do just that, and that is why doctors should not see it as an attack on them, but as a stimulus to reflection and understanding.[28]

Indeed, *The Magic Mountain* is a classic example of 'disease as social diagnosis' impacting on discussions of health policy and social environment: 'Disease thus became both the occasion and the agenda for an ongoing discourse concerning the interrelationship of state policy, medical responsibility, and individual culpability.'[29] Insightful medical reviewers came to realize that there was a more profound conception behind the panorama of physical and spiritual degeneration Mann had drawn. Thus, Ulrici draws attention to the inner lives of the patients described in the novel: 'the poet requires a social context in order to show the powerful influence of physical suffering on psychological development and the corrupting effects of futile resistance against spiritual degeneration and loss of personal values'.[30] *The Magic Mountain* also puts much of the blame on the patients themselves, whose egocentricity and wilful seeking of pleasure and distraction or, alternatively, indifference and fatalistic self-abandon contribute much to their own decline. Medical responsibility and individual culpability are criticized in equal measures in the novel, and both are framed within the wider context of the sanatorium's social milieu. Mann tried to encourage this reading in his open letter and also in his private correspondence with doctors. In a letter of 15 November 1927 to Willy Hellpach, he praises the illuminating manner in which Hellpach's review treats the medical aspects of *The Magic Mountain*, but concludes that by only considering this aspect, the doctor's literary diagnosis has missed an important point. Mann quips: 'he quite sees the criticism of the cure, but not the cultural criticism' ('Das Kurkritische ist durch und durch gesehen, nicht aber das Kulturkritische').

By combining medical and cultural frames of reference, Mann's description of tuberculosis drew attention to the psychosomatic, social and environmental factors that influenced the course and eventual outcome of the disease. The ensuing debate shows how much the diagnosis and treatment of this chronic illness was conceptualized along the lines of firmly held social values – in particular, notions of character, sexuality and work. While Klemperer finds Mann's description of the sanatorium as a 'place of depravity and licentiousness' ('Stätte der Liederlichkeit und Zuchtlosigkeit') exaggerated and often disgusting, he acknowledges: 'Tuberculosis and its institutional treatment pose a psychological danger for the patient, they lead to emotional confusion and dissolution, as a consequence of which the desire to get better is lost and the "young people go to the dogs".'[31] One of the pioneers in this area of research was Otto Amrein, the director of the Altein sanatorium in Arosa. In 1919 Amrein published a pamphlet, *Die Tuberkulose in ihrer Wirkung auf Psyche und Charakter*,[32] in which he outlines the negative influence that tuberculosis can have on the psyche of patients. Although he mentions somatic causes (the effect of toxins generated by the disease), he devotes most attention to the environmental and institutional aspects and the side-effects of tuberculosis treatment in sanatoria. In particular, children and adolescents suffer when they are forced to live for months and even years in an institution far away from home, the family and school. According to Amrein, one of the greatest dangers to the patients' psyche is idleness and a lack of meaningful occupation. Thus, they carelessly seek thrills and entertainments that seriously endanger their prospect of being cured. Alternatively, they may become indifferent and lose any interest in work and a productive life. The corresponding states of mind – irritability or apathy – recur literally in some chapter titles in *The Magic Mountain* ('Die große Gereiztheit'; 'Der große Stumpfsinn'). Amrein's advice is that patients should receive ethical guidance and that doctors need to impose a strict discipline and regimen of work in their institutions, for 'work is one of the best educators of character'.[33] He also views it as very important to educate patients about the proper attitude to adopt towards their disease and the experience of suffering: 'nor should one forget (toxin or no toxin) that the patients' mind can also be influenced by wrong *ideas of and a wrong attitude* toward suffering'.[34] In 1920, Prüssian confirmed Amrein's statements in his travel report from Davos and Arosa (cited above). Many of the incidents that Amrein and Prüssian mention (including increased libido due to high temperature, and psychological afflictions like *Thermometromanie* – the patients' urge to constantly check their temperature) are described vividly in *The Magic Mountain* and it is conceivable that Mann had read both accounts.

Naming disease: the 'Magic Mountain Malady'

What is interesting is that *The Magic Mountain* served to reinforce this medical debate, which thereby came full circle. In his review, Klemperer identifies as the central idea in Mann's novel a 'psychoanalysis of tuberculosis and its treatment'[35] – an idea which he commends as medically incisive, useful and important:

> Finally, I find brilliant confirmation and justification of the psychologist Thomas Mann in a book on 'The Psyche of the Tuberculosis Patient' by Professor Erich Stern (Gießen), which has only recently been published – months after Mann's *Magic Mountain*; whether and how far it is influenced by the novel I cannot say. In his chapters 'The Psychology of the Chronic Tuberculosis Patient' and 'The Influence of Sanatorium Life on the Patient' Stern completely mirrors Mann's views and reaches the same conclusions.[36]

Even if he cannot confirm it, it is interesting to note that Klemperer at least considers the possibility that Stern's medical text[37] may have been influenced by the novel. Like Loewy-Hattendorf, Ulrici, Zickgraf and Levy, he finds Mann's book immensely useful in its description of the patients' attitudes towards their disease. This emphasis on individual experience ('Erleben') is, according to Klemperer, one of the most important lessons for doctors to take away from reading the novel. He asks rhetorically whether current therapeutic measures – rest cure, long-term institutional treatment – may not have become too schematic and one-sided by focusing too much on disease instead of health. By using *The Magic Mountain* as an occasion to strike a blow for the patient: 'we ought to treat the patient, not the disease'[38] Klemperer negotiates between what Arthur Kleinman distinguished as illness experienced by the patient and disease as defined by the medical profession.[39]

The manifest impact of Mann's psychological and social framing of tuberculosis in the medical community is demonstrated by the term 'Zauberberg-Krankheit' (Magic Mountain Malady), which came into use within a few years after *The Magic Mountain*'s publication to describe the psychological side-effects of tuberculosis care that Mann had drawn out so vividly in his novel. At the '9. Internationaler Ärztlicher Fortbildungskursus' in 1927, Willy Hellpach delivered a lecture which was reprinted under the title 'Die Zauberberg-Krankheit' (The Magic Mountain Malady) in *Die Medizinische Welt*. Hellpach had obtained his qualification as a university professor with a study of social pathology, which he defined as the influence of the social environment ('mitmensch-liche Umwelt') on the occurrence, manifestation and development – in qualitative as well as quantitative terms – of a pathological disposition or disease in an individual. In his article, he presents *The Magic Mountain* as a socio-pathological panorama of the detrimental effects that a milieu like the traditional sanatorium can have on the patients' attitude toward their sickness. This is how Hellpach characterizes Mann's framing of the 'Zauberberg-Krankheit':

It is not the physical aspects of tuberculosis of the lungs alone, it is that psychological component which, perhaps in conjunction with every tubercular disposition or primary infection, is fostered by the hothouse atmosphere of the sanatorium and now itself becomes a silent but constant psychosomatic source of continued, indeed exacer-bated physical illness, and eventually presents an insuperable barrier to recovery. The sanatorium milieu systematically paralyses the anti-tubercular will to get well again, and it generates a pathological sloth-fulness: this is the Magic Mountain Malady.[40]

Whether this disease really exists as pictured by Mann or not, Hellpach hesitates to judge in the absence of proper scientific knowledge about the psychology of tuberculosis. Like Levy in 1925, he declares that the psychosomatic effects of tuberculosis have not been sufficiently concep-tualized by clinical medicine, which means that the doctor's judgement is based to a large degree simply on the ability to judge human nature ('Menschenkenntnis'). What Hellpach does affirm is Mann's unique ability to describe the causes, symptoms and characteristics of the 'Zauberberg-Krankheit' – that is, the geopathological effect of the Alpine setting and the psychopathological social environment of the sanatorium, both of which contribute to ensnare patients in the psychological trap their disease has become.[41] In 1930, Hellpach elaborated these psychosomatic ideas in a lecture on the 'healing power of the mind' ('Heilkraft des Geistes'), in which he emphasizes the importance of the patient's will to become well again. To foster this will, he continues, the doctor cannot rely on biomedical science alone because 'the patient must never be merely a scientific case, he must be cured by the physician with or without science, with a lot of or a little science'.[42] Hellpach does not shy away either from criticizing the economics of institutional care (Mann was frequently attacked for caricaturing the profit motive that also played a role in luxury sanatoria) and stresses that an important part on the road to recovery was for the patient to eventually emancipate himself from his doctor again and turn his mind to normal, healthy life.[43] Thus, Hellpach takes the central message of *The Magic Mountain* – 'Lebensdienst' (service to life) – as a call for institutional reform and changes in health policy: by forcing patients to contribute to the cost of their treatment, one could not only protect the system more effectively from unnecessary claims, but would also encourage them to stay in a sanatorium only as long as absolutely necessary and thereby minimize the psychological side-effects caused by long-term care.

Hellpach's stance clearly marks a point in the public debate about tuberculosis, at which, inspired partly by imaginative literature like the *Magic Mountain* or Klabund's story *Die Krankheit*,[44] medical thinking about tuberculosis turned towards broader conceptualizations of the disease, which included social and moral values. If, as Randall McGowen writes, medicine emerged during the nineteenth century 'as one of the dominant paradigms used to think about the nature and destiny of humanity',[45] this process has to be seen as a multilateral negotiation between the various strands of cultural knowledge to which imaginative literature and medical thought both contributed.

Showcasing disease: Thomas Mann and the canon of the Medical Humanities

Thomas Mann once remarked about Gerhart Hauptmann that one of the most humane characteristics of his art was its penchant for the pathological, his inclination to view the human condition in terms of illness – be it social, psychological or physical.[46] In his novels, stories and essays, Mann himself adopted this 'medical paradigm' of the human condition, and as his texts became canonical among a wide audience, so did the philosophy of disease and health they espoused. In a eulogy on the occasion of Mann's eightieth birthday in 1955, a writer in the *Pharmazeutische Zeitung* celebrates Mann as the 'nosographer of our epoch'.[47] Inspired perhaps by Mann's remark about music and medicine as neighbouring spheres, Fromm describes the author's medical narratives as a four-movement 'Symphonia pathologica': curiously omitting *Buddenbrooks*, he includes *The Magic Mountain* ('Tuberculosis Pulmonum'), *Doktor Faustus* ('Lues Venera' and 'Meningitis Cerebrospinalis') and, finally, *The Black Swan* ('Carcinoma Uteri') and describes the medical paradigm of the human condition as the tenor ('Grundakkord') of Mann's oeuvre.

Since Mann's death in 1955, *The Magic Mountain* and its author have become regular objects of celebration in the medical community. One incidence of this is the frequent reference (verging on the reverential) that is made to Mann in medical training and further education. To give just two examples, in 1965 the *Zeitschrift für ärztliche Fortbildung* printed an anniversary article on Mann and the 'spirit of medicine',[48] and 1974 saw the reprint of Mann's 'Vom Geist der Medizin' of 1925 together with a commemorative article by Heinz Saueressig in the *Deutsche Medizinische Wochenschrift*.[49] These articles continue along those favourable lines of argument that some of the early reviewers developed, particularly the medical paradigm of the human condition. Saueressig writes that tuberculosis 'is, after all, a kind of illness particularly suited to making clear the relation of man and society to illness as such'.[50] The articles also emphasize the relevance of Mann's novel for current debates in medicine and health policy. On the occasion of a congress on 'Prevention, Therapy and Rehabilitation' in Davos, Schretzenmayr declares, in the *Deutsches Ärzteblatt*, that it is 'the symptomatology and psychology of the Magic Mountain Malady, which we doctors are nowadays more interested in than ever before'.[51] Schretzenmayr diagnoses a contemporary revival of the disease which Mann had framed 'with such narrative skill and eloquence' in the form of what he calls 'Sozialkur-Krankheit': the social phenomenon that, thanks to the opportunities offered by national health insurance schemes, normal patients take regular cures for granted even if these are not medically indicated. Like Hellpach in 1927, Schretzenmayr uses *The Magic Mountain* as ammunition[52] to argue for a reform of medical welfare and more excess payments on the part of the patient:

> Thomas Mann is right! Doctors and makers of social policy ought to read the novel a second time, especially today – on the eve of decisive health-insurance and welfare reforms. A reading could open the reformers' eyes: encouraging individual responsibility for their own health on the part of those who are well and those who are sick is the antibiotic against the modern contamination with Magic Mountain Malady.[53]

What Schretzenmayr, unlike Hellpach, fails to mention is that in Mann's novel part of the blame is also laid squarely on the profit motive of the medical institutions and practitioners. Had Mann written his book in the 1970s, Hofrat Behrens and Co. would surely have been all too happy to welcome a great number of over-insured, middle-class patients in their health farms.

It is telling that an author whose novel had once been regarded by many doctors as a slur on their profession is nowadays used to achieve just the opposite: He now serves the medical community as a means of cultural legitimation and representation, a guarantor of social status and humanistic *Bildung*. By this I do not mean to diminish the insights (discussed above) which Mann's writings offer into disease and health. But it is a curious and telling reversal of fortunes in an author's reception that illustrates the vicissitudes in the social negotiation of disease. As with any process of canonization, the 'classic' status of an author, a work of art, or a theory does not necessarily indicate some universal truth contained therein, but has to be understood in terms of cultural significance and its relation to other discourses in a given society and period.

To illustrate the extent to which Mann has become idolized and instrumentalized by parts of the medical community, one need only look at some of the most recent articles published in medical journals. In 1970 Schretzenmayr had already used a drawing of the author and colourful reproductions of paintings by Ernst Ludwig Kirchner to illustrate his article, which bore the technicolour title 'Der Zauberberg in Farbe' ('The Magic Mountain in Colour'). This ornamental showcasing of the author is taken even further in Richard Carter's 'The Mask of Thomas Mann (1875–1955): Medical Insights and Last Illness', which was published in a section 'Our Surgical Heritage' in the *Annals of Thoracic Surgery*.[54] In his richly illustrated piece, Carter certainly offers an accurate, if limited summary of Mann's life and work – and above all his death – and its relevance for medicine, calling the author 'one of the most medically perceptive writers of the century'.[55] Drawing on an interview with Professor Christoph Hedinger, who had performed the autopsy on Thomas Mann at the Zürich Cantonal Hospital, and on Hedinger's autopsy report of August 1955,[56] Carter concludes that Mann's death was 'due to a spontaneous rupture of the left common iliac artery about a centimetre beyond the aortic bifurcation' and relates with clinical detail how a 'massive exsanguinating internal hemorrhage'

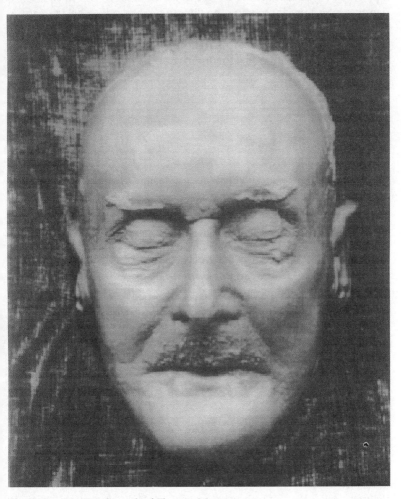

Illustration 6.1 Death mask of Thomas Mann

occurred just before 'the literary giant quietly dropped off to his final rest at 10 minutes to 8:00 on the evening of August 12, 1955'.[57] For good measure, Carter also throws in the anecdote that the hospital's chief surgeon, Professor Wilhelm Löffler, 'attended two Nobel laureates during their final illnesses – James Joyce and Thomas Mann'.[58] We have read Mann's diaries, but only now have we literally been allowed a voyeuristic glance into 'the guts of the great man'.[59] This, presumably, is not how Roland Barthes imagined the death of the author (Carter actually prints a photo of Mann's death mask – see Illustration 6.1). On the contrary it demonstrates how, by treating the 'literary giant' and 'Nobel laureate' as a patient, the medical profession constituted him as their subject and appropriated him as 'one of us'. The medical profession's former *bête noire* has become lionized in the interest of institutional self-representation, and the 'mask of Thomas Mann' has become a fetish of medicine.[60]

Appendix A

Chronology of selected medical responses to Mann's *The Magic Mountain* (published 1924):
First reactions
1925
Dehoff. 'Der Zauberberg (Kritisches Referat)'. *Die Tuberkulose* 4 (1925): 42–5.
Klemperer, Felix. 'Ärztlicher Kommentar zu Thomas Manns "Zauberberg". Ein Beitrag zur Psychologie der Lungentuberkulose'. *Die Therapie der Gegenwart* (1925): 601–6.
Levy, Margarete. 'Bemerkungen zum "Zauberberg" von Thomas Mann'. *Deutsche Medizinische Wochenschrift* 51 (1925): 1166.
Loewy-Hattendorf, Erwin. 'Ärztliche Probleme in der modernen Dichtkunst'. *Zeitschrift für ärztliche Fortbildung* 22.19 (1925): 603–6.
Prüssian, Alexander. 'Der Zauberberg'. *Münchner Medizinische Wochenschrift* (1925): 696–7.
Schelenz, Hermann. 'Thomas Mann: "Der Zauberberg" vom Standpunkt des Tuberkulosearztes aus gesehen'. *Deutsche Medizinische Wochenschrift* 51 (1925): 831–2.
Ulrici, Hellmuth. 'Thomas Manns "Zauberberg" '. *Klinische Wochenschrift* 4.32 (1925): 1575.
Zickgraf, G. 'Noch eine ärztliche Kritik über den Zauberberg'. *Zentralblatt für innere Medizin* 46 (1925): 869–76.
Mann's defence
Mann, Thomas. 'Vom Geist der Medizin'. *Deutsche Medizinische Wochenschrift* 51.29 (1925): 1205–6.
Revisions
Hellpach, Willy. 'Die "Zauberberg"-Krankheit'. *Die Medizinische Welt* 1.38 (1927): 1425–9.

—— 'Die Heilkraft des Geistes'. *Schweizerische Medizinische Wochenschrift* 60.25 (1930): 573–9.

The Path to Glory

1950s

Fromm. 'Symphonia Pathologica. Zum 80. Geburtstag von Thomas Mann, dem Nosographen unserer Epoche, am 6. Juni 1955'. *Pharmazeutische Zeitung* 100 (1955): 597–9.

1960s

Stein, R. 'Vom Geist der Medizin – und vom Geist der Literatur. Vier Jahrzehnte Zauberberg'. *Zeitschrift für ärztliche Fortbildung* 62 (1965): 82–9.

Virchow, Christian. 'Geschichten um den "Zauberberg" '. *Deutsches Ärzteblatt* 64.5 (1967): 263–5.

1970s

Schretzenmayr, Albert. 'Der Zauberberg in Farbe. Einführung zum 1. Sommerkongreß in Davos vom 20. Juli bis zum 8. August 1970'. *Deutsches Ärzteblatt* 67.13 (1970): 1034–42.

Virchow, Christian. 'Wiedersehen mit dem "Zauberberg" '. *Deutsches Ärzteblatt* 67.1 (1970): 61–5.

Saueressig, Heinz. 'Literatur und Medizin. Zu Thomas Manns Roman "Der Zauberberg" '. *Deutsche Medizinische Wochenschrift* 99.36 (1974): 1780–6.

1980s

Justin, Renate G. 'Medicine as Business and Patient Welfare: Thomas Mann Dissects the Conflict of Interest'. *Literature and Medicine* 7 (1988): 138–47.

1990–2000

Virchow. *Medizinhistorisches um den 'Zauberberg'. 'Das gläserne Angebinde' und ein pneumologisches Nachspiel.* Augsburger Universitätsreden. vol. 26. Augsburg: Universität Augsburg, 1995.

——'Thomas Mann und "the most elegant operation" '. *Vom 'Zauberberg' zum 'Doktor Faustus'. Die Davoser Literaturtage 1998.* ed. Thomas Sprecher. vol. 23. Thomas-Mann-Studien. Frankfurt am Main: Klostermann, 2000. 47–62.

Carter, Richard. 'The Mask of Thomas Mann (1875–1955): Medical Insights and Last Illness'. *Annals of Thoracic Surgery* 65 (1998): 578–85.

Naef, Andreas P. 'William E. Adams: Thomas Mann and the Magic Mountain'. *The Annals of Thoracic Surgery* 65.1 (1998): 285–7.

Dekkers, Wim, and Peter van Domburg. 'The Role of Doctor and Patient in the Construction of the Pseudo-Epileptic Attack Disorder'. *Medicine, Health Care & Philosophy* 3.1 (2000): 10.

Gesler, Wil. 'Hans Castorp's Journey-to-Knowledge of Disease and Health in Thomas Mann's *The Magic Mountain*'. *Health & Place* 6 (2000): 125–34.

Notes

1. Thomas Mann, 'Vom Geist der Medizin', *Deutsche Medizinische Wochenschrift* 51.29 (1925): 1205–6, 1205. Unless stated otherwise, all translations are mine, and the original is given in parentheses or in the footnotes. Quotations from Mann's letters are cited with date and correspondent in brackets.

2. Letter of 5 July 1919 to the neurologist Gustav Blume.
3. See the chronological overview in Appendix A.
4. Sander L. Gilman, *Disease and Representation: Images of Illness from Madness to Aids* (Ithaca: Cornell University Press, 1988) 7.
5. Renate G. Justin, 'Medicine as Business and Patient Welfare: Thomas Mann Dissects the Conflict of Interest', *Literature and Medicine* 7 (1988): 138–47; Wim Dekkers and Peter van Domburg, 'The Role of Doctor and Patient in the Construction of the Pseudo-Epileptic Attack Disorder', *Medicine, Health Care & Philosophy* 3.1 (2000): 10.
6. Wil Gesler 'Hans Castorp's Journey-to-Knowledge of Disease and Health in Thomas Mann's *The Magic Mountain*', *Health & Place* 6 (2000): 125–34, 132.
7. Howard Brody, *Stories of Sickness* (New Haven: Yale University Press, 1987) 5.
8. Peter Conrad, 'Medicalizations', *Science* 258 (1992): 334–5, 335.
9. 'Alle Ärzte und ehemaligen Patienter, die von dem Unternehmen hören, lechzen nach der Satire'.
10. 'In der gesamten schöngeistigen Weltliteratur dürfte kein Analogon dazu zu finden sein, daß ein zweibändiger Roman sich mit einer Überfülle von Fachausdrücken zum großen Teil nur mit der Schilderung einer bestimmten Krankheit und deren Verlaufsformen beschäftigt. Und zwar geschieht das in einer so auffallenden und einseitigen Weise, daß in Anbetracht des überaus großen Leserkreises wie des hohen künstlerischen Rufes des Verfassers auch von ärztlicher Seite zu seinem Werk Stellung genommen werden muß' (Alexander Prüssian, 'Der Zauberberg', *Münchner Medizinische Wochenschrift* [1925]: 696–97, 696).
11. Hermann Schelenz, 'Thomas Mann: "Der Zauberberg" vom Standpunkt des Tuberkulosearztes aus gesehen', *Deutsche Medizinische Wochenschrift* 51 (1925): 831–2, 832.
12. G. Zickgraf, 'Noch eine ärztliche Kritik über den Zauberberg', *Zentralblatt für innere Medizin* 46 (1925): 869–76, 869.
13. Erwin Loewy-Hattendorf, 'Ärztliche Probleme in der modernen Dichtkunst', *Zeitschrift für ärztliche Fortbildung* 22.19 (1925): 603–6, 603.
14. Felix Klemperer, 'Ärztlicher Kommentar zu Thomas Manns "Zauberberg". Ein Beitrag Zur Psychologie der Lungentuberkulose', *Die Therapie der Gegenwart* (1925): 601–6, 602.
15. Prüssian, 'Der Zauberberg', 696.
16. '... und zwar sehe ich den Schaden darin, daß das nichtärztliche Lesepublikum sich aus diesem Roman ein ganz falsches Bild über Heilstätten und das Innenleben in diesen Heilstätten machen wird. Wir haben nichts über den Heilstättenbetrieb zu verheimlichen, und trotzdem werden wir es nie für wünschenswert halten, daß urteilslose Laien Kritik an uns und unsern Kranken üben werden' (Schelenz 1925, 832).
17. Dehoff, 'Der Zauberberg (Kritisches Referat)', *Die Tuberkulose* 4 (1925): 42–5, 45.
18. Charles E. Rosenberg, 'Framing Disease: Illness, Society, and History', in Charles E. Rosenberg and Janet Lynne Golden (eds), *Framing Disease: Studies in Cultural History* (New Brunswick, NJ: Rutgers University Press, 1992) xiii–xxvi, xvi.
19. Ibid., xxi.

20. Injection of air, or a more slowly absorbed gas such as nitrogen, into a pleural space to collapse the lung.
21. Alexander Prüssian, 'Ärztliche Reiseeindrücke aus Arosa und Davos', *Münchner Medizinische Wochenschrift* (1920): 939ff.
22. Dehoff, 'Der Zauberberg', 44.
23. '... sein Dienst ist Lebensdienst, sein Wille Gesundheit, sein Ziel die Zukunft. Damit ist es ärztlich' (Mann, 'Von Geist der Medizin', 1205).
24. 'Daß es uns Ärzten Nutzen bringt, liegt auf der Hand. Vielfache Anregungen gehen von ihm aus ...' (Klemperer, 'Ärztlicher Kommentar zu Thomas Manns "Zauberberg" ', 605).
25. 'Kritik darf meines Erachtens jeder üben, und wenn sie in dieser feinen Weise geübt wird, dann sollte man sich vielmehr besinnen, ob die Ursachen der Kritik nicht vorhanden und abzustellen sind' (Zickgraf, 'Noch eine ärztliche Kritik über der Zauberberg', 875).
26. '... einen sehr ernsten Appell an das Gewissen der Ärzte, ihre Kranken vor dem psychisch schädigenden Einfluß dieses Milieus zu bewahren' (Margarete Levy, 'Bemerkungen zum "Zauberberg" von Thomas Mann', *Deutsche Medizinische Wochenschrift* 51 [1925]: 1166).
27. 'Statt mit dem Eindruck der einheitlichen Persönlichkeit einen Rückhalt zu gewähren, vermehrt des Hofrats geistvoller Cynismus die sittliche Verwirrung und seinem Scharfblick entgeht vollkommen der geistige Ruin seiner Schutzbefohlenen, ja sogar das widerwärtige Treiben seines Assistenzarztes, der die scheinbare Schärfung der Sinne für die letzten Dinge ausnutzt, die Kranken über spiritistische Wirrnis in erotische Erörterungen und bedenklichste psychoanalytische Experimente hineinzuziehen; auch das ein Beispiel des psychischen Abgleitens solcher Kranken' (Hellmuth Ulrici, 'Thomas Manns "Zauberberg" ', *Klinische Wochenschrift* 4.32 [1925]: 1575).
28. 'Die medizinische Literatur über den Zusammenhang von Psyche und Lungentuberkulose ist bisher nur sehr spärlich, während Laien schon seit langer Zeit dieses Problem mit größtem Interesse verfolgt haben ... Hier sollte die Arbeit der Ärzte, eine vernünftige Psychotherapie, neben und mit der eigentlichen medizinischen Therapie einsetzen. Dazu fordert der Roman von Thomas Mann geradezu heraus, und deshalb sollten die Ärzte ihn nicht als einen gegen sich gerichteten Angriff betrachten, sondern als Mahnung zur Erkenntnis und Einsicht' (Levy, 'Bemerkungen zum "Zauberberg" von Thomas Mann', 1166).
29. Rosenberg, 'Framing Disease', xxii.
30. 'Den mächtigen Einfluß körperlichen Leidens auf die seelische Entwicklung und die korrumpierende Wirkung vergeblichen Ringens gegen haltloses Versinken und gegen den Verlust der Persönlichkeitswerte zu zeigen, bedarf der Dichter der gesellschaftlichen Zustände [...]' (Ulrici, 'Thomas Manns "Zauberberg" ', 1575).
31. 'Die Tuberkulosekrankheit und ihre Anstaltsbehandlung ist eine Gefahr für die Psyche des Kranken, führt zu einer seelischen Verwirrung und Entgleisung, in welcher der Gesundheitswille verloren geht und das "junge Volk verlumpt" ' (Klemperer, 'Ärztlicher Kommentar zu Thomas Manns "Zauberberg" ', 603).

32. Otto Amrein, *Die Tuberkulose in ihrer Wirkung auf Psyche und Charakter* (Basel: Schwabe, 1919). I am indebted to the library of the *Ärztlicher Verein* in Hamburg (*Ärztekammer Hamburg*) for making a copy of Amrein's treatise available to me.

33. Ibid., 6.

34. '... so muß auch nicht vergessen werden (Toxinwirkung hin oder her), daß die Psyche der Patienten auch durch eine falsche *Auffassung und Einstellung* des Leidens [*sic*] mitbeeinflußt werden kann' (Ibid., 10).

35. Klemperer, 'Ärztlicher Kommentar zu Thomas Manns "Zauberberg" ', 603.

36. 'Die glänzendste Bestätigung und Rechtfertigung des Psychologen Thomas Mann schließlich finde ich in einem Buche von Prof. Erich Stern (Gießen) über die "Psyche des Lungenkranken", das vor kurzem erst erschienen ist – Monate nach Manns "Zauberberg"; ob und wieweit es von diesem beeinflußt ist, weiß ich nicht. In seinen Kapiteln "Die Psychologie des chronisch Lungenkranken" und "Der Einfluß des Sanatoriumslebens auf den Kranken" geht Stern vollkommen mit Thomas Mann parallel, kommt zu den gleichen Schlüssen und Erkenntnissen wie dieser' (Klemperer, 'Ärztlicher Kommentar zu Thomas Manns "Zauberberg" ', 604).

37. Erich Stern, *Die Psyche des Lungenkranken: Der Einfluß der Lungentuberkulose und des Sanatoriumslebens auf die Seele des Kranken* (Halle: Marhold, 1925).

38. 'Daß wir den Kranken behandeln sollen und nicht die Krankheit ...' (Klemperer 1925, 605).

39. Arthur Kleinman, *The Illness Narratives: Suffering, Healing and the Human Condition* (New York: Basic Books, 1988).

40. 'Es ist nicht die rein physische Lungentuberkulose; es ist jene seelische Komponente, die [sich], vielleicht mit jeder tuberkulösen Disposition oder Primärinfektion verbunden, durch die Sanatoriumsatmosphäre zu üppiger Fülle entfaltet und nun ihrerseits zu einem leisen, aber unermüdlichen psychophysischen Antriebsmotor des körperlichen Krankbleibens, des Kränkerwerdens, zu einer immer unübersteiglicheren Barrikade vor der Genesung wird. Die systematische Lähmung des anti-tuberkulösen Gesundungswillens durch das Kurmilieu; die systematische Züchtung der tuberkulösen Krankheitsindolenz durch das Kurmilieu: das ist die Zauberberg-Krankheit' (Willy Hellpach, 'Die "Zauberberg"-Krankheit', *Die Medizinische Welt* 1.38 [1927]: 1425–9, 1427).

41. '...den Befallenen in dieser Umwelt und damit in seiner Krankheit festzuhalten' (Hellpach, 'Die "Zauberberg"-Krankheit', 1427).

42. '... der Kranke darf dem Arzt nie zum bloß wissenschaftlichen Fall werden, der Kranke soll vom Arzt geheilt werden, mit oder ohne Wissenschaft, mit viel oder mit wenig Wissenschaft' (Willy Hellpach, 'Die Heilkraft des Geistes', *Schweizerische Medizinische Wochenschrift* 60.25 [1930]: 573–9, 577).

43. '... der Genesende muß vom Arzt loskommen ... sich den Menschen und Dingen der gesunden Lebenssphäre zukehren' (ibid., 575).

44. Klabund, *Die Krankheit: Eine Erzählung* (Berlin: E. Reiss, 1917).

45. Randall McGowen, 'Identifying Themes in the Social History of Medicine', *The Journal of Modern History* 63.1 (1991): 81–90, 84.

46. Thomas Mann, 'Zur Begrüßung Gerhart Hauptmanns in München [1926]', *Gesammelte Werke*, vol. X (Frankfurt am Main: Fischer, 1990) 215–20, 217.

47. Fromm, 'Symphonia Pathologica. Zum 80 Geburtstag von Thomas Mann, dem Nosographen unserer Epoche, am 6. Juni 1955', *Pharmazeutische Zeitung* 100 (1955): 597–9.

48. R. Stein, 'Vom Geist der Medizin – und vom Geist der Literatur. Vier Jahrzehnte Zauberberg', *Zeitschrift für ärztliche Fortbildung* 62 (1965): 82–9.

49. Heinz Saueressig, 'Literatur und Medizin. Zu Thomas Manns Roman "Der Zauberberg" ', *Deutsche Medizinische Wochenschrift* 99.36 (1974): 1780–6.

50. '. . . ist schließlich ein Krankheitsgeschehen, das sich besonders eignet, den Menschen und die Gesellschaft in ihrer Beziehung zur Krankheit zu charakterisieren' (ibid., 1780).

51. '. . . die Symptomatologie und Psychologie der Zauberbergkrankheit, die uns Ärzte heute mehr denn je interessiert' (Albert Schretzenmayr, 'Der Zauberberg in Farbe. Einführung zum 1. Sommerkongreß in Davos vom 20. Juli bis zum 8. August 1970', *Deutsches Ärzteblatt* 67.13 [1970]: 1034–42, 1035).

52. Schretzenmayr literally writes that, with regard to social welfare, social policy and psychology, the novel is 'highly topical and explosive material in the battle between the advocates of state welfare and the champions of the greatest possible freedom for doctor and patient' ('ein hochaktueller sozialpolitischer, sozialmedizinischer und psychologischer Zündstoff im Kampf zwischen den Befürwortern einer Staatsmedizin und den Verfechtern einer möglichst weit gehenden Freiheit von Arzt und Patient', 1036).

53. 'Thomas Mann hat recht! Ärzte und Sozialpolitiker sollten den Roman zum zweitenmal lesen, gerade heute – am Vorabend vor den entscheidenden Reformen der sozialen Krankenversicherung! Die Lektüre könnten den Reformern die Augen öffnen: Förderung der Selbstverantwortung des Gesunden und des Kranken für seine Gesundheit und seine Gesundung ist das Antibiotikum gegen die moderne Kontamination mit der Zauberberg-Krankheit' (Schretzenmayr, 'Der Zauberberg in Farbe', 1036).

54. Richard Carter, 'The Mask of Thomas Mann (1875–1955): Medical Insights and Last Illness', *Annals of Thoracic Surgery* 65 (1998): 578–85.

55. Ibid., 578.

56. The full post-mortem report is printed with annotations in Thomas Sprecher and Ernst O. Wiethoff, 'Thomas Manns letzte Krankheit', *Thomas Mann Jahrbuch* 10 (1997): 249–76. Among other details it reveals that – unlike generations of literary scholars – the presiding anatomist Professor Hedinger did not dissect Mann's brain. For another celebration of Mann's last medical rites cf. Hans Helmut Jansen, 'Letzte Krankheit und Tod von Thomas Mann (1875–1955)', *Hessisches Arzteblatt* II (2002): 651–4.

57. Carter, 'The Mask of Thomas Mann', 583f.

58. Ibid., 583.

59. Gerd Bucerius's words about the revealing insights offered by Mann's diaries.

60. One of the first to write knowledgeably about Mann's diseases was the Davos pneumologist Christian Virchow ('Geschichten um den "Zauberberg" ', *Deutsches Ärzteblatt* 64.5 (1967): 263–5; *Medizinhistorisches um den*

'Zauberberg'. 'Das gläserne Angebinde' und ein pneumologisches Nachspiel. Augsburger Universitätsreden, vol. 26, Augsburg: Universität Augsburg, 1995; 'Thomas Mann und "the Most Elegant Operation" ', *Vom 'Zauberberg' zum 'Doktor Faustus'. Die Davoser Literaturtage 1998*, ed. Thomas Sprecher, vol. 23, Thomas-Mann-Studien (Frankfurt am Main: Klostermann, 2000) 47–62; 'Wiedersehen mit dem "Zauberberg" ', *Deutsches Ärzteblatt* 67.1 (1970): 61–5). Writing about the operation for lung carcinoma that Mann underwent in 1946 in Chicago, Andreas Naef puts Mann the patient in illustrious company by stating that the lobectomy performed on him by Professor William E. Adams deserves to be added, along with Nelson's leg amputation, the empyema drainage on King George V and others, to the list of 'historically famous operations' ('William E. Adams, 'Thomas Mann and the Magic Mountain', *The Annals of Thoracic Surgery* 65.1 (1998): 285–87, 285).

Part II
Framing and Imagining Madness

7
A Little Bit Mad/Almost Mad/Not Quite Mad? Eccentricity and the Framing of Mental Illness in Nineteenth-Century French Culture

Miranda Gill

In 1894 Paul Moreau, the alienist and son of the considerably more famous alienist Jacques-Joseph Moreau de Tours, published a short work entitled *Les Excentriques*.[1] Plagiarizing substantially from existing medical literature, in particular his father's analysis of eccentricity from 1859,[2] the work narrates episodes of incomprehensible yet generally harmless behaviour, such as eccentric journeys, marriages, duels, and testaments. One doctor commented that it looked like little more than selected highlights from the daily newspapers,[3] and indeed Moreau blames the press for feeding an 'epidemic' of eccentricity by implicitly encouraging readers to emulate the bizarre actions they read about in the *fait divers* (22–4). His conclusion, however, suddenly strikes an alarming note. Whilst in times of political stability such episodes are of little social import, during periods of unrest 'the peaceful eccentrics we have just seen will be unleashed and transformed into wild animals, thirsty only for blood and for massacre' (117). Drawing implicitly upon the language of hypnotism, Moreau argues that eccentrics' weak and suggestible personalities make them highly vulnerable to political demagoguery. Alexandre Cullerre's *Les Frontières de la folie*, a popularizing work of psychiatry written three years previously, also treats eccentricity at length.[4] This time, however, his own readership is portrayed as vulnerable to the seductions of the press. Feverishly overheated, they dispute the latest psychiatric diagnoses and resultant commentaries by legislators, journalists, playwrights, and novelists, changing their views with nervous inconsistency (5–6). His text claims to provide this public with 'the notions they lack in order to form their own opinions', replacing such volatility with stable and rational understanding (8). Yet both Moreau's and Cullerre's texts seem fundamentally duplicitous. In pandering to the voyeuristic public interest in problematic cases of madness, they simultaneously disseminate pathogenic narrative material and claim to act as pedagogic palliatives to its consequences.

Such covert fascination characterizes the trajectory of eccentricity in French culture, from its pre-history in eighteenth-century French and English discourses of psychological oddity[5] to this fashionable presence on the *fin-de-siècle* psychiatric scene. In contrast with well-known categories of borderline insanity such as monomania and hysteria, eccentricity has received almost no attention in historical accounts of French psychiatry. Arguably, however, the category merits the title 'the elusive insanity' as much as monomania,[6] for it constantly calls into question the very boundary between health and illness. Eccentricity also provides a paradigmatic case study of nineteenth-century attempts to negotiate the boundaries between norm and anomaly, concepts which play a central role in the medical disciplines of teratology and physiological pathology as well as psychopathology. During the course of the nineteenth century, Canguilhem and Foucault have both argued, the medical profession replaced the structuring division of health and disease with that of normal and pathological, and in turn attempted to define the second pair through quantitative measurements, supposedly objective and value-free. Normality was framed in terms of a statistical biological norm; conversely, departure from this norm through excess or deficit was labelled morbid and pathological. Since the normal nonetheless assumed a qualitative and normative character, the opposition readily mapped on to a realm of purely social norms, creating metaphorical connections with other forms of deviance.[7] This chapter proposes to trace the shifting relationship between eccentricity and mental pathology in the nineteenth-century French cultural imagination. The first section analyses literary and journalistic discourses of eccentricity between 1830 and 1850, which create the cultural and linguistic context for subsequent psychiatric intervention. The second section addresses the psychiatric functions of the medicalization of eccentricity, as well as some key metaphors and narrative structures by which it is framed.

Epidemics of peculiarity

The terms *excentricité* and *excentrique* became current in France in the 1830s, some thirty years after the English equivalents they directly translate.[8] The attempt to find stable definitions, however, is intrinsically problematic. Eccentricity may be defined by means of near-synonyms from an inter-referring semantic network, including *originality, oddity, peculiarity, singularity*, the *bizarre* and the *extravagant*. Dictionary definitions and usage consistently point to an element of hermeneutic frustration: eccentrics are 'strange' and 'bizarre'; in their 'singularity', they fall outside the codes that regulate the interpretation of behaviour. Eccentricity may also be defined in purely abstract and relative terms. Its literal meaning denoting deviation from a centre, eccentricity becomes, in the nineteenth century, a spatial metaphor for behaviour that diverges from a given norm, implying rupture with the conventions underpinning the logic of representation and binding social life as a whole.[9] The concept is therefore particularly fluid, since norms, like the perception of deviance, vary considerably according to context.

As part of ongoing efforts to raise the prestige of the psychiatric profession, Philippe Pinel and his disciple J.-E.-D. Esquirol both sought to purify the language of mental medicine. Specialized and scientific terms, it was thought, should be substituted for terms that had accumulated unpredictable associations through centuries of popular and erudite usage: *folie*, for instance, was to be replaced by *aliénation*, and *mélancolie* by *lypémanie*.[10] Although the term *excentricité* had only two decades to accumulate such a pre-medical linguistic history,[11] its role in literary and journalistic discourses made it far from neutral by the time it came to have wide psychiatric currency. These associations, far from hindering its adoption in medical discourse, contributed to its success as an all-purpose marker of psychological and social deviance.

From the 1830s onwards there were several historical moments when eccentricity was particularly in vogue.[12] This immediately gives rise to mimetic paradox. How can a person defined as individual, original and singular simultaneously be a copy, part of a general trend or even epidemic?[13] A second temporal paradox arises from the first: the normalization of the anti-norm represented by the eccentric suggests the concept of permanent revolution. Rather than the turbulent revolutionary politics of France, though, it was the ideology of English liberalism which first appeared to be the natural context for eccentricity. From the early nineteenth century onwards, English cultural fashions such as Byronism and dandyism had disseminated the values of individualism to a wide audience. Eccentricity, initially associated with both movements, migrated to France shortly after they did. In *Les Excentriques*, Paul Moreau distinguishes between genuine, 'morbid' eccentricity, which he holds to be timeless and universal, and 'imitative' eccentricity, arguing that the latter is responsible for the contemporary epidemic of eccentricity he believes arose in 1889 (26).[14] Whilst his distinction and chronology are evidently mistaken, his perception of the role of imitation in the propagation of eccentricity is not.

In an 1834 article which combines the genres of essay, fantasy, and travel writing, the French journalist and critic Philarète Chasles describes eccentricity as an instance of the 'inviolable power of the *individual self*, the cult of this *self*' in English culture.[15] The article places its French readership in a strangely marginal position, portraying the francophobic opinions of an imaginary English eccentric named Wordem. A collector and self-styled historiographer of eccentricity, Wordem entertains the narrator with his substantial library of 'heteroclite' English eccentrics and their exploits. Repeatedly expressing anxiety that English eccentricity will be lost through contact with the Continent, and the flattening effect of civilization, he contrasts it with French conformism: 'for you, *originality* is a synonym of madness; for us, it is a compliment and an honour' (506). Wordem's conception of eccentricity is disingenuous: he admits that the English eccentric may be influenced by journalism's dissemination of eccentric acts and characters (530). Moreover, in spite of his denial that eccentricity is related to insanity, he employs terms like 'semi-dementia' and 'nuances of madness' which gesture beyond the binary opposition between madness and sanity, and invents a taxonomy of eccentricity which anticipates later psychiatric classifications, as well as suggesting the concept's semantic elasticity:

    I.   Religious eccentrics
    II.   Adventurer eccentrics
   III.   Erudite eccentrics
   IV.   Original women
    V.   The bizarreness of poets
   VI.   The originality of painters
 VII.   Bourgeois originalities
VIII.   Famous eccentrics
  IX.   The biographies of English eccentrics, etc. (510–11)

Eccentricity, the departure from the norm, is portrayed as both normal and, paradoxically, normative in England, a nation of eccentrics in which the right to psychological difference appears as natural as the right to property or religious non-conformism. The alienist John Conolly, writing shortly before Chasles, discusses the condition under the significant heading 'Inequalities, weaknesses, and peculiarities of the human understanding, which do not amount to insanity'.[16] He cautions attempts to police the boundary between the madman and the eccentric: it is 'repugnant to every idea of that rational freedom which all ought to enjoy, that a man should not do as he chooses with his time, or his property, so long as he does not inflict direct injury on others' (139). The view that eccentricity is incompatible with French culture is still voiced in France twenty years later, whilst in Britain, the ideology of liberalism remains associated with the praise of eccentricity, notably in the writings of John Stuart Mill.

The eccentric as monomaniac and bohemian

Even during this early stage in the evolution of eccentricity in France, however, there are signs of naturalization and integration with pre-existent psychological categories. In *Le Dessin de Piranèse*, an essay from 1833, Charles Nodier attaches quite different connotations to the term.[17] Two anecdotes illustrate 'the imagination that has attained the highest possible degree of eccentricity' (159). A wealthy Italian bachelor, after having the interior of his castle decorated in imitation of a fantastically labyrinthine drawing by Piranesi, retires to the dungeon where he slowly and deliberately starves himself to death; a brilliant but reclusive young man, who withdraws to live amongst his mechanical contraptions, kills himself during an experiment. The latter was culled from the *Anecdotes de médecine*, portrayed as a substantial archive of such stories collected by *médecins philosophes*. Nodier carefully nuances their view that insanity is the sole explanation, relating eccentricity to the higher cultural purposes of martyrdom and asceticism:

> The explanation I seek is that of this strange type of madness which, leaving intact all the other faculties of a great mind, has no other purpose than to inflict horrendous tortures upon the material clothing of the soul. [. . .] This mystery is great and sublime, for it encompasses the whole secret of man's destination. (161)

As this suggests, Nodier uses the term 'eccentricity' to denote a masochistic variant of monomania. During the 1830s, this concept was the locus of the most advanced and intense debate in French *médecine mentale*, forming the first major attempt to popularize the view that insanity need not be complete, nor affect all mental faculties simultaneously.[18] Dissatisfied with contemporary medical definitions, however, Nodier proposes his own in an essay entitled *De la Monomanie réflective* ('On Reflexive Monomania').[19] He differentiates between 'explicit monomania', a medical issue; 'militant monomania', a legal issue; and 'reflexive monomania', the more complex form which afflicts the eccentric characters of his anecdotes as well as many other gifted and highly cultivated individuals (48–9). The duality of the condition is repeatedly highlighted: if channelled properly, it may result in heroic achievement, but if the subject is meditative and isolated from society, it will lead to the introverted insanity of the *fou intime* or 'private mad-man' (54). Hence, given the contemporary social context, the condition usually ends in suicide. The reflexive monomaniac, whose symptoms closely resemble those of melancholia, is described in terms of the Janus' head: 'a coin, struck in one sole motion of the coining press, showing on one side the immortal figure of the great man, and on the reverse the infirm head of a maniac' (53). Eccentricity is a malady of excessive individualism; but the tragic element of social and psycholog-ical difference does not – just as for the German Romantic movement which deeply influenced Nodier – detract from its valorization.

Himself a keen collector of rare books, Nodier was fascinated by the psychological dynamics of bibliomania, a specific subcategory of mono-mania. His text *Bibliographie des fous: de quelques livres excentriques* ('A Bibliography of Madmen: On Some Eccentric Books') provides a guide to some of the strangest literary productions of past ages, initiating a lengthy literary tradition.[20] The title gestures towards a significant rela-tionship between madness and eccentricity, yet fails to define its nature, partially displacing the enigma of eccentric minds on to their literary productions. The appeal of eccentric texts derives precisely from such incomprehensible qualities: like their authors, they amaze and con-found those who attempt to read them. The association of eccentricity during this period with monomania – generally understood in terms of the *idée fixe* and obsessional pursuits, including collecting – remains strong. Balzac, for instance, uses the terms 'eccentric', 'monomaniac', and 'original' almost interchangeably in the following passage from *Cousin Pons*, his tragic novel of an obsessive collector:

> Of all the cities in the world, Paris is the one which harbours the greatest numbers of such strange figures [*originaux*], so devoted to their particular religion. The eccentrics in London always grow tired of their enthusiasms in the end, just as they grow tired of life itself, whereas your Parisian monomaniac goes on living with his fantasy in blissful spiritual concubinage.[21]

The concept of the collection functions on several levels, reflexive as well as literal. Eccentrics may collect obsessively; their own literary products may be collected in libraries of eccentric works; and they themselves may constitute psychological specimens. The collection is an organizing principle that attempts to create order and generality amidst a proliferation of singularities.[22] Its literary form, the library, has naturally elicited interest in critics inclined towards poststructuralism,[23] whilst its visual corollary, the 'gallery' of eccentrics, evokes the fairground freak show and its assorted monstrosities, staged for the voyeuristic appraisal of an ambivalent audience.

One such gallery is that provided by the writer and critic Champfleury's text *Les Excentriques* (1852).[24] Eccentricity is viewed above all as metropolitan spectacle for the *flâneur*, a 'free performance lasting the whole day long' (4). Drawing on the visual metaphors of the realism movement, the text aims to sketch its singular subjects. Champfleury also intermittently invokes medical rhetoric, calling for instance for the expansion of popularizing psychiatric narratives (102–3), and deploying metaphors of dissection (9). Yet he avoids sustained classification or analysis of the relationship between madness and eccentricity, despite the fact that many of his subjects have either been incarcerated or display symptoms of contemporary psychiatric conditions (hallucinations, delusions of persecution, disruptive outbursts). Only his terminological qualifications foreshadow future medical interest in gradations of insanity: his subjects are 'a little bit mad', 'almost mad', 'not mad [. . .] but scarcely any better', and, occasionally, go 'beyond the limits of eccentricity'.[25]

Champfleury's subsequent preface attempts to counter criticism of the first edition, aimed at 'the strangeness of the characters, their lowly situation, and above all the unhealthy side of their minds' (1). Socioeconomic marginality and mental deviance, both occasioning bourgeois distaste, are difficult to separate. Like dandyism, another English import, eccentricity loses some of its associations with the aristocracy when naturalized into French culture.[26] This descent in social hierarchy becomes particularly acute in the aftermath of the failed 1848 revolution. Hence Balzac can suggest in 1837 that it is necessary to be rich to be an eccentric, and in 1846 that eccentricity is a malady which only afflicts great households, on both occasions associating eccentricity with the English aristocracy;[27] yet in 1856 Champfleury terms his subjects 'true bohemians' (8), situating them within the disreputable geographical and imaginary space of Parisian Bohemia. Visionaries and utopians, preoccupied by extraordinary schemes to improve society, his eccentrics signal an important feature of the French political scene during the 1840s: the potential link between radicalism and a variety of mystical sects, including freemasonry, Swedenborgianism, Martinism, and Mesmerism.[28] The religious eccentric is often implicated in highly temporal debates. The conjunction also occurs in Nerval's collection of biographical narratives published in final form in 1852 as *Les Illuminés, ou les précurseurs du socialisme* ('The Illuminate, or the Precursors of Socialism'). 'I wanted to paint certain philosophical *eccentrics'*, he announces in the preface.[29] In spite of an acute difference in tone and intention, Champfleury and Nerval's 'galleries' both emphasize the link between eccentricity, idiosyncratic mysticism, and social reform, situating their subjects on the very margins of society.

In summary, the concept of eccentricity evolves significantly during the period 1830–50. Initially associated with English culture, it is rapidly integrated with pre-existent French discourses of psychological and social difference, and also comes to have quite distinct associations of its own. Whilst many commentators focused on male eccentricity, the term 'eccentric' was also applied to disparate categories of deviant women, including bluestockings, wealthy courtesans, spinsters, socialists, and bored aristocrats. Eccentric women engendered particularly ambivalent emotional responses, for they were invariably positioned in relation to male fantasies and anxieties about the enigmatic nature of 'la femme'. Contemporaneous literary depictions of eccentricity, together with the strongly related concepts of singularity and originality, are also highly varied: they include, for instance, Stendhal's unconventional and 'incomprehensible' female characters Mathilde de La Mole and Lamiel, the exhibitionist romantics and dandies of Gautier's short stories, Balzac's mystics and monomaniacs, particularly in the *Études philosophiques*, and Nerval's adventurers. Popular fiction and the *roman-feuilleton*, such as Ponson du Terrail's *Rocambole* and Alexandre Dumas' *Le Comte de Monte-Cristo*, also exploited the enigmatic qualities of eccentricity for dramatic effect. A high degree of porosity is evident between fictional and essayistic texts, the latter often using novelistic methods to capture their readers' attention. The terms 'eccentricity' and 'eccentric' evidently remain in circulation in literary and journalistic discourses after the 1850s, but from this time onwards, the attempt to capture eccentricity moves from general discourses of social and psychological observation into the hands of the professionals.

'An equivocal, fluid, uncertain quality': the psychiatric net tightens

This increasing interest in eccentricity occurs during a crucial juncture in the evolution of the psychiatric profession, for which three related reasons may be suggested. First, the dominant paradigm of Pinel and Esquirol, which tended to view madness from a moral and social perspective, was increasingly challenged from the 1850s by the paradigm initiated primarily by B.-A. Morel. Frequently described as organicist and biological, and ascribing madness to hereditary pathologies of the nervous system, this new framework made the concept of degeneration the hermeneutic master key to a whole network of pathologies; furthermore, it repudiated Pinel's 'moral treatment', since insanity was held to result from incurable physiological defects.[30] The differences between the two paradigms should not be overstated: a distinct physiological focus is present in discussions of monomania prior to 1850, whilst a strong moral and spiritual awareness underlies B.-A. Morel's theories of decline. A change of conceptual focus nonetheless forms part of the self-description of many psychiatrists during the latter part of the century. Second, the 1850s witnessed an expansionist movement in French psychiatry. Having gained professional confidence through attaining a near-monopoly in the treatment and analysis of full madness, or psychosis, psychiatrists turned their attention to mastering various types of 'partial' or 'incomplete' madness, following upon the earlier incursions of monomania into this realm. The physiologist Claude Bernard provided theoretical justification for such expansion. Situating the pathological on a continuum with the normal, his theories undermine the idea that a binary opposition separates disease from health, madness from sanity.[31] Finally, the degeneration model encouraged the blurring of distinctions between mental, physiological, moral, and social deviance. The normal–pathological opposition itself is 'conceptually isomorphic with so many other binary terms that regulate the perception of social life: moral–immoral, criminal–honest, sane–insane, violent-passive'.[32] To this must be added the opposition between French classical and Romantic aesthetics, since the classical values of harmony, proportion, and moderation are central to Claude Bernard's framing of normality in terms of equilibrium, whilst Romanticism, like the pathological (and eccentricity) is associated with heterogeneity, rupture, and intensity.

In this context, eccentricity, a central example of such a problematic liminal state, was a natural candidate for psychiatric attention. Though never so prevalent in psychiatric discourse as hysteria and related nervous conditions, eccentricity fulfilled some of the same conceptual functions. A peculiarly elastic term, it may be used in a very wide sense to encompass borderline insanity as such, even the entire realm of neurotic disorders including hysteria;[33] but it is often employed in a more restricted sense, denoting various non-psychotic conditions. Conceptual vagueness arises from constant terminological slippage, and distinctions between *an* eccentric, the concept of eccentricity, eccentricities, and eccentric behaviour are blurred. Many subcategories of the insane may commit eccentric acts: 'an imbecile may simultaneously be an eccentric', and is probably other things as well, Cullerre complains (51). Indeed in both popular and psychiatric discourse the personal noun 'eccentric' is often used interchangeably with others such as the mono-maniac, the original, the *illuminé*, the degenerate, the *déséquilibré*, and the *détraqué*. The process of renaming serves to side-step actual analysis, creating an alarming degree of category flux. Linguistic proliferation and the creativity of popular language undermine attempts to achieve scientific neutrality, creating networks of subliminal associations.

Eccentricity must be recognized and named on the basis of potentially minute disturbances of mental and physiological norms. Claude Bernard's theories again influence psychiatric discourse: his model of equilibrium, often taken as the first modern elaboration of homeostasis, stages the body in constant efforts to maintain its 'milieu interne' or internal environment, composed of a number of physiological norms. Bernard famously argues that 'equilibrium results from a continuous and *delicate* compensation, established as by the most *sensitive* of balances' [my italics].[34] Discerning such subtle variations in the sphere of psychiatry results in increasing use of Bernard's metaphors of delicacy, together with a heightening of the rhetoric of interpretative skill which, it has been argued, characterized the profession from the outset.[35] Deviation from the norm may occur in any semiotic system: ways of feeling, willing, imagining, and judging, for example, or modes of dress, walking, speaking, and writing.[36] The psychiatrist thus styles himself as sensitive interpreter of signs that are 'delicate to grasp hold of and trace out'.[37] Tantalizingly 'equivocal, fluid, and uncertain', however, eccentricity flees and slips away at any attempt to classify and circumscribe it.[38] Implicitly drawing upon the opposition between artist and scientist, then, psychiatrists repeatedly evoke the intuitive finesse of the former, contrasting it with the outmoded belief in binary oppositions and the simplistic pursuit of 'mathematical delimitations' and 'fixed and precise boundaries'.[39]

Nineteenth-century French psychiatry nonetheless spent much energy constructing, and revising, its taxonomic systems, and these provide the main context for the analysis of eccentricity. As the century drew to a close, Cullerre looked back upon a series of terminological variations upon Pinel's theme of *folie raisonnante*, all attempting to define incomplete madness (25–7). A proponent of the organicist model, Cullerre reads the tradition in terms of a narrative of incipient chaos, in which categories proliferate: *(mono)manie raisonnante, folie des actes, folie lucide*, moral insanity, *folie avec conscience*. The endless play of naming and renaming borderline madness, his chronology implies, served as a substitute for real analysis, the perpetual refinement of terminology only making matters less certain. 'No-one was satisfied with the ideas and classifications of his predecessors', he writes; 'far from advancing towards a scientific solution, one felt that the problem was worsening, becoming more muddled and entangled' (27). Only the success of the biological model of J.-J. Moreau de Tours and B.-A. Morel, he holds, finally created conceptual unity.

More taxonomic effort was put into distinguishing the wider category into which eccentricity fitted than subdividing the category of eccentricity itself. Cullerre proposes a basic distinction between 'eccentric ideas' and 'eccentric acts' (121), which in many ways rephrases Trélat's influential division between 'madness of speech' and 'madness of acts' in *La Folie lucide* (1861).[40] One important diagnostic consequence, under either distinction, is the positing of a dialectic between explicit morbidity, which is easily 'readable' from the trail of astonishment and scandal it leaves in its wake, and concealed morbidity. It might seem likely that non-experts would be as capable of recognizing eccentricity as the doctor, given their intuitive grasp of the social norms from which eccentrics deviate. And indeed psychiatrists frequently appeal to readers to have recourse to their own personal experience, the use of generic 'one' and 'we' marking out a realm of assumed self-evidence. 'Everyone can make, in relation to the circle of facts he has himself observed, the individual applications these last reflections suggest', writes Morel in a typical comment (543n1); 'ECCENTRICITY. – This mental disposition is assuredly too well known not to have been noticed throughout history, by whatever name it was called at the time', declares Paul Moreau, unwittingly imitating the structure of an entry from Gustave Flaubert's posthumously published *Dictionnaire des idées reçues*.[41]

Overwhelmingly obvious, eccentricity would appear to present no diagnostic difficulties. Yet eccentrics endowed with intellectual and rhetorical brilliance are also represented as adept at concealing their condition, frustrating the interpretation of family, friends, and colleagues. Whilst skilled at creating an impression of normality, they are nonetheless liable to violent outbursts in which the underlying pathology emerges, in scenes of cathartic unveiling reminiscent of the popular melodrama.[42] As a sense of all-pervasive social menace intensifies towards the end of the century, borderline insanity is framed as a condition that frequently escapes detection. Eccentrics are 'a hundred times worse than veritable madmen',[43] since their morbidity may propagate unobserved, and they leave their families with no legal redress. Legal medicine repeatedly discusses the difficulties posed when the seemingly sane use rational means to justify 'eccentricities' like unsuitable marriages and capricious testaments.[44] The eccentric is therefore placed in a contradictory position, held to be both familiar and recognizable, and exotically, even duplicitously, alien. The psychiatrist, in turn, increasingly promotes a hermeneutics of suspicion verging on paranoia.

The evolution of eccentricity may also be charted through its close relationship with monomania. In *La Psychologie morbide* (1859), J.-J. Moreau de Tours formulates the concept of the *état mixte* or 'mixed state' (205–6), exemplified by the eccentric. He sharply distinguishes the mixed state from monomania: the latter entails the mere 'juxtaposition' of healthy ideas with a single complex of obsessive and diseased ideas, without total interpenetration; the mixed state, in contrast, is evoked through a range of suggestive imagery of inextricable fusion. Melting and the formation of metallic alloys represent the inseparable nature of health and disease (213–18), whilst the resultant composite entity is described in terms of Horace's monster (217). Like the physiological anomaly, the eccentric is formed of seemingly irreconcilable elements and provokes uneasily hybrid responses. The intensely emotive concept of moral monstrosity, associated with the deviant behaviour of eccentrics, is later transposed into physiological terms with the advent of teratological theories of insanity. These attribute psychological instability to physiological defects or 'monstrosities' of the nervous system.[45]

Morel is well known for his devastating criticisms of the monomania doctrine during 1853–54. He nonetheless, perhaps surprisingly, advocates retaining the term to describe eccentrics: 'it is these men I would like above all to see qualified as *monomaniacs*'.[46] The term is redeployed in the service of his own system, but rather than implying that eccentricity, like monomania, can be localized and thus potentially contained, his writings suggest that it functions as an index of further perturbations of the nervous system, the smoke which indicates future conflagration. Indeed Morel subscribes to J.-J. Moreau de Tours' view that '*madness* and *eccentricity* are two *pathological* states with a common origin' (188), namely heredity. Morel narrates the case history of a banker who, since childhood, has suffered from periodic outbursts of eccentric behaviour: 'the diverse anomalies of mind and sentiments revealed in the acts of these eccentric men', he concludes, 'are in fact intimately linked to the hereditary neuropathic element' (532). The eccentric forms part of the class of hereditary madmen who have descended only to the first level of *dégénérescence*. The terms 'eccentric' and 'eccentricity', however, are used so widely in Morel's medical writings that they may appear inter-changeable with insanity as such, his personal usage tending to stress the propensity to violent and extravagant behaviour.[47]

The distance travelled since the widespread equation of the eccentric with the monomaniac and victim of the *idée fixe* during the 1830s is notable. Whilst both are forms of 'incomplete' madness, the idea of a single locus of mania, without any relationship to other faculties, was progressively abandoned in organicist psychiatry. The eccentric there-fore comes to stand as emblem of both the invisible circulation of noxious 'germs' in the human nervous system, and the subterranean circulation of deviance in the modern metropolis. The conceptual vagueness promoted by the degeneration system, however, has signifi-cant drawbacks. Disease may be multitudinous, 'an infinite network of diseases and disorders, and the patterns of return and transformation between them'.[48] Yet its aetiology remains monolithic: degeneration and heredity. The overwhelming nosological coherence of the degener-ation paradigm eventually undermines its interpretative power, for it is unable to grasp particularity and specificity. Precisely the same may be said of eccentricity. Its polymorphous properties, and its ability to evoke multiple forms of deviance, are a distinct advantage in an era of per-ceived national vulnerability, leading directly to 'whole underworlds of political and social anxiety'.[49] But this very elasticity means that it is in danger of coming to signify nothing in particular. The demise of both the psychiatric use of the term and the degeneration paradigm shortly after the turn of the century are, significantly, contemporaneous.

On the brink: the narrative dynamics of eccentricity

Claude Bernard's model of homeostasis implies a narrative of constant, subtle adjustments, as well as sudden ruptures in which the environ-ment suddenly changes, followed by a new process of adjustment. The degeneration paradigm is based upon a central and obsessive narrative trajectory of decline. Taken together, these two models, in which decline is framed in terms of progressive loss of equilibrium, have important consequences for eccentricity. Decline involves temporality, and therefore narrative patterning. In narratives of degeneration, eccen-tricity is the sinister harbinger of full disintegration, the eccentric a 'superior degenerate' occupying only the first rung on the ladder of decline.[50] But if eccentricity is 'madness in an embryonic state',[51] at what precise moment is full madness born? At what point is psychological equilibrium thought to shift, however subtly, into definitive disequilibrium? Several narrative alternatives exist.

The fall may be abrupt. Describing the fate of 'degenerate eccentrics', Tardieu writes:

> Thus they hasten to enter into a process of degradation: since they find neither in their conscience nor in their judgement any brake which could restrain them, since they are quickly repulsed from the society of honest and sensible people, they fall from level to level right down to the lowest level of abjection. (153)

This description of decline exemplifies the concept's metaphorical fluidity. Heavily over-determined, the 'fall' is charged with connotations at once moral, religious, biological, social, and economic. Those in the eccentric's social circle are, here, credited with intuitive discernment of the pathological.

Yet there is also a model of slow and insidious decline. Its time-span may be that of an individual lifetime: B.-A. Morel argues that many eccentrics finish their existences in suicide, the progressive weakening of their faculties, imbecility and dementia, or full madness (532). It may take even longer; elsewhere, he represents it occurring over four generations, of which the second represents a disposition to eccentricity.[52] Signs may thus be read in one member of a family, and conclusions drawn about the likely fate of another. Imperceptible decline is conducive to anxieties about the invisible spread of social decay, and eccentrics are represented insidiously gnawing at the heart of society.

Third, the fall may be perpetually warded off. J.-J. Moreau de Tours views the decline in panoramic, transgenerational terms:

> Just as a state of real madness may only be reproduced through heredity in the form of eccentricity, and may only be transmitted from forebears to descendants with a diluted complexion, if I may speak in this way, its colour more or less softened, it is also the case that a state of simple eccentricity in the parents, a state which does not go beyond a certain strangeness of character and singularity of mind, may become, in the children, the origin of true delirium. (187)

Narrative uncertainty remains: madness may unpredictably recede from one generation to the next, trapping the family in a perpetual dialectic of contamination and dilution. Moreau de Tours multiplies such racial metaphors: eccentrics are 'the cross-breeding of the races transported into the moral order', and 'true intellectual half-castes' (211). Social and colonial anxieties are occasioned by the threat of impurity, the disruption of clear category-divisions by an indeterminacy at once visual, conceptual, and temporal. This type of perpetual balancing may also operate on the level of the individual. Cullerre describes a state of instability and nervous disequilibrium which is 'not yet illness' but 'no longer health' (21). His comments posit a type of indeterminate narrative limbo in which the eccentric is poised. A range of suggestive metaphors evokes the eccentric's efforts to avoid the narrative closure of full insanity: on the brink of collapse, the mind still struggles to preserve its equilibrium. Legrand du Saulle, for instance, describes the borderline psychiatric case in terms of architectural structure: 'in many cases, if the *self* has swayed, it has not yet fallen to the point at which it is no longer anything but a ruin' (53). Paul Moreau takes this homeostatic terminology to a theatrical extreme. 'The eccentric is a perpetual candidate for madness, but he does not fall into it; he stops on the brink of the abyss' (6), he writes. Or, elsewhere, eccentrics 'hold themselves in equilibrium on the tightrope between madness and reason, leaning to the right, leaning to the left, but not falling' (20). The mind's ability to ward off external and internal threats creates agonising narrative suspense.

Finally, there is an unexpectedly optimistic narrative structure. In the 1830s, Nodier had argued that eccentricity, given the right social circumstances, may result in glorious achievement. Subsequent psychiatric discourse repeatedly reasserts a potential link with creativity, albeit ambivalently, since although the genius is frequently eccentric, not every eccentric is a genius (the physiological 'monster' is, after all, supremely original). Retrospective psychiatric histories attempt to reinterpret the psychological 'evidence' provided by the repositories of history, biography, and literature, in the light of contemporary scientific theories of the mind.[53] J.-J. Moreau de Tours, for instance, discerns eccentricity in numerous artists, religious visionaries, and thinkers, and suggests that childhood eccentricities may be a characteristic of those later to become great men.[54] The tradition culminates in euphoric passages verging on the genre of the praise of folly. The psychiatrist Benjamin Ball asserts that those afflicted by borderline madness are often more intelligent than others; relentlessly energetic, 'their brains swarm with absolutely novel ideas'; civilization itself depends on them in order to move forward (95).[55] Cullerre likewise claims that, were it not for the 'grain of madness' they provide, the civilized world would perish from an excess of mediocrity (9–10). Although there is some dissent – Morel, in particular, is characteristically pessimistic as to the ability of the 'partial genius' to escape his or her underlying morbidity (259) – psychiatry theoretically carves out a small space in which divergence from the norm is viewed as permissible, even beneficial to society as a whole.

The merits of (dis)order

This brief overview of the historical trajectory of the concept of eccentricity in the nineteenth century suggests three main conclusions. First, eccentricity is one example of a number of psychiatric categories reframed with imagery drawn from Claude Bernard's models of equilibrium and gradation. The condition necessitates skilful interpretation and threatens to remain, in the final instance, undecidable. This potential diagnostic indeterminacy is closely related to the affective ambivalence that the eccentric elicits, recalling Nodier's image of the Janus' head. When perceived as expressing a normal degree of individual difference, eccentrics may elicit considerable admiration, appearing enviably free to enact the secret wishes of their more constrained bourgeois observer. When perceived as pathologically defective, they may arouse the defence mechanisms of the same observers, creating responses of anxiety, disgust, or horror, all of which may be displaced through ridicule. The simultaneous presence of positive and negative responses creates considerable emotional tension in many nineteenth-century observers.

Second, the eccentric is a hermeneutic puzzle, a symbol of the enduringly enigmatic nature of the mind in an era in which positivism constantly claims to unveil, decipher, and expand the boundaries of rational knowledge. Like Jean Baudrillard's metaphor of the strange attractor, eccentrics remain opaque.[56] They function as partially blank signifiers within the interpretative economy of the period, able to bear a variety of contradictory meanings.

Finally, the vocabulary of homeostasis with which eccentricity is framed still provides a useful metaphorical frame within which to envisage its social and psychological function during this period. In an increasingly regulated society, the individual freedom to differ may be viewed either as dangerously destabilizing or as a necessary 'grain' of chaos, preventing civilization from stagnating. This ambivalence translates directly into political terminology, representing the clash between liberalism and the politics of self-defence driving French nationalism, the latter particularly acute after defeat in the Franco-Prussian War. The eccentric thus mediates dialectically between two extremes – oppressive over-regimentation and anarchic chaos – which exist on a number of different symbolic levels.

Several methodological consequences follow. Historical analysis need not exclude synchronic analysis. The subsequent metamorphoses of eccentricity in the twentieth century may result in the equally vague and contestable categories of contemporary psychiatry, a discipline that often prefers to ignore the genealogy of its concepts. The nineteenth-century pre-histories of 'borderline personality disorder' and 'psycho-pathic personality', for instance, are constituted by many of the taxonomic categories used during this period to frame eccentricity.[57] The clinical psychologist David Weeks demonstrates an equal lack of disciplinary reflexivity when attempting a 'scientific investigation' of eccentricity, taken to signify creative and healthy non-conformism.[58] His enterprise, which relies upon subjects identifying themselves as eccentric, is evidently contentious: the label 'eccentric' has functioned as a subtle form of social control during much of its history, and been applied to subjects quite unwilling to acquiesce in the process. Suffering and the stigma of social exclusion have played a central role in the term's evolution, and persistent semantic association cannot simply be ignored. Furthermore, defining eccentricity in atemporal and essential-ist terms (albeit by reversing the values with which it was previously associated in psychiatric discourse) necessarily fails to account for its linguistic functions and its role as social construction. Formalist literary criticism also risks anachronism. Daniel Sangsue's study of nineteenth-century eccentric *narratives* avoids dealing with the psychological aspects of eccentricity, instead focusing on a number of French experi-mental narratives from the first part of the nineteenth century that use devices such as parody and narrative reflexivity to break with the con-ventions of fictional realism. His work nonetheless reinstates mental processes at the level of the text itself (narratives are shown, for instance, defying received opinion, and drawing attention to their own singularity), but the values he discerns are unmistakably those favoured by poststructuralist literary critics rather than by nineteenth-century writers.[59] Like Weeks, Sangsue persistently attempts to write the nega-tive axis of eccentricity out of the term's history. Eccentricity has under-standable attractions for the many strands of postmodernist thought that valorize difference, alterity, and singularity.[60] But the retrospective 'discovery' of such concepts at work in literary history fails to respect the genuine alterity of nineteenth-century writers, and is unable to account for the complexity and ambivalence of their contemporaries' response. Finally, the study of a diverse range of sources, including journalistic, theoretical, legal, and medical texts, is required in order to grasp the term's intriguingly polysemic properties.

Notes

Unless otherwise indicated, all translations from the French are my own.

1. Paul Moreau, *Les Excentriques: étude psychologique et anecdotique* (Paris, 1894).
2. Jacques-Joseph Moreau de Tours, *La Psychologie morbide: dans ses rapports avec la philosophie de l'histoire* (Paris, 1859).
3. Jules Dallemagne, *Dégénérés et déséquilibrés* (Paris, 1895) 593.
4. Alexandre Cullerre, *Les Frontières de la folie* (Paris, 1888).
5. On the eighteenth-century history, see Michèle Plaisant (ed.), *L'Excentricité en Grande-Bretagne au 18e siècle* (Lille: U Lille III, 1976) and Roland Mortier, *L'Originalité: une nouvelle catégorie esthétique au siècle des Lumières* (Geneva: Droz, 1982).
6. See Jan Goldstein, *Console and Classify: the French Psychiatric Profession in the Nineteenth Century* (Cambridge: Cambridge University Press, 1987) 169–78.
7. Georges Canguilhem, *The Normal and the Pathological*, trans. Carolyn R. Fawcett and Robert S. Cohen (New York: Zone, 1989) 39–46, and Michel Foucault, *The Birth of the Clinic: an Archaeology of Medical Perception*, trans. A. M. Sheridan Smith (London: Tavistock, 1976) 34–6. See also Robert A. Nye, *Crime, Madness and Politics in Modern France: the Medical Concept of National Decline* (Princeton: Princeton University Press, 1984) 46–8.
8. Jean-Pierre Leduc-Adine, 'A Propos de Courbet, un champ sémantique: l'excentrique', in R. Mathé (ed.), *Actualité de l'histoire de la langue française, méthodes et documents*, (Limoges: UER, 1984) 149–54.
9. Joseph Margolis, 'Reinterpreting Interpretation', *The Journal of Aesthetics and Art Criticism* 47 (1989): 245.
10. See Goldstein, *Console and Classify*, 99 and 156–7.
11. The term was used intermittently in psychiatry from the 1830s: see, for example, François Leuret, *Fragmens psychologiques sur la folie* (Paris, 1834).
12. Daniel Sangsue plausibly posits two post-revolutionary vogues following 1830 and 1848: *Le Récit excentrique: Gautier – de Maistre – Nerval – Nodier* (Paris: José Corti, 1987) 33. Leduc-Adine suggests the period 1840–1870: 'A Propos de Courbet, un champ sémantique', 152.
13. See Sangsue, 'Vous avez dit excentrique?', *Romantisme* 59 (1988): 41–57 (53–5).
14. Paul Moreau also holds, however, that the imitative eccentric's impressionability derives from hereditary, hence morbid, weakness of personality.
15. Philarète Chasles, 'Les Excentriques', *Revue des deux mondes*, 1 September 1834: 509.
16. John Conolly, *An Inquiry Concerning the Indications of Insanity* (London, 1830).

17. In Charles Nodier, *De Quelques phénomènes du sommeil* (Paris: Castor astral, 1996).
18. See Goldstein, *Console and Classify*, 152–96.
19. In Charles Nodier, *L'Amateur de livres* (Paris: Castor astral, 1993).
20. On the subsequent tradition, see André Blavier, *Les Fous littéraires* (Paris: Cendres, 2001).
21. Honoré de Balzac, *Cousin Pons*, trans. Herbert J. Hunt (Harmondsworth: Penguin, 1968) 146.
22. See Juan Rigoli, *Lire le délire: aliénisme, rhétorique et littérature en France au XIXe siècle* (Paris: Fayard, 2001) 192–205.
23. See Meryl Tyers, *Critical Fictions: Nerval's* Les Illuminés (Oxford: Legenda, 1998), 69–82.
24. Champfleury [Jules Husson-Fleury], *Les Excentriques* (1852; Paris, 1877).
25. Ibid., 107, 157, 239, 208.
26. Emilien Carassus, *Le Mythe du dandy* (Paris: Colin, 1971) 33, 82.
27. Balzac, *La Comédie humaine*, 7 vols (Paris: Seuil, 1966), VI, 424, and V, 20.
28. See Lynn Wilkinson, *The Dream of an Absolute Language: Emanuel Swedenborg and French Literary Culture* (Albany, NY: State University of New York, 1996) 8, 113–15.
29. Gérard de Nerval, *Oeuvres complètes*, 3 vols (Paris: Gallimard, 1984–93) 2: 885.
30. See Castel, 149–56.
31. See Goldstein, *Console and Classify*, 332–3. Influences on this aspect of Bernard's thought include Broussais and Comte: see Canguilhem, *The Normal and the Pathological*, 47–64.
32. Nye, *Crime, Madness and Politics in Modern France*, 48.
33. Cullerre, *Les Frontières de la folie*, 226.
34. Quoted in Joseph Schiller, *Claude Bernard et les problèmes scientifiques de son temps* (Paris: Cèdre, 1967) 173; on equilibrium, see 172–200.
35. See Rigoli, *Lire le délire*, 19–33.
36. J.-J. Moreau, *La Psychologie morbide*, 211; Dallemagne *Dégénérés et déséquilibrés* 592.
37. Ambroise Tardieu, *Étude médico-légale sur la folie* (1872; Paris, 1880) 152.
38. Cullerre, *Les Frontières de la folie*, 25.
39. Henri Legrand du Saulle, *La Folie devant les tribunaux* (Paris, 1864) 54.
40. Ulysse Trélat, *La Folie lucide étudiée et considérée au point de vue de la famille et de la société* (Paris, 1861) xii–xiii.
41. Paul Moreau, *La Folie chez les enfants* (Paris, 1888), 207.
42. See Trélat, *La Folie lucide*, 6–15.
43. Tardieu, *Étude Médico-légale sur la folie*, 152.
44. See Legrand du Saulle, *La Folie devant les tribunaux*, 48–62, and *Étude médico-légale sur l'interdiction des aliénés et sur le conseil judiciaire* (Paris, 1881) 406–13.
45. See Charles Féré, *La Famille névropathique: théorie tératologique de l'hérédité et de la prédisposition morbides et de la dégénérescence* (Paris, 1889) 19–21.
46. Bénédict-Auguste Morel, *Traité des maladies mentales* (Paris, 1860) 531n1, quoting from his own *Études cliniques* (Paris, 1852–53).
47. Rigoli, *Lire le délire*, 199.
48. Daniel Pick, *Faces of Degeneration: a European Disorder, c.1848–c.1918* (Cambridge: Cambridge University Press, 1989) 50.
49. Ibid., 10; see also Nye 132–70.
50. Dallemagne, *Dégénérés et déséquilibrés*, 592.

51. P. Moreau, *La Folie chez les enfants*, 207.
52. Quoted in Cullerre, *Les Frontières de la folie*, 31.
53. See Michael Finn's essay in this volume.
54. J.-J. Moreau, *La Psychologie morbide*, 218–27 and 542–4.
55. Benjamin Ball, *La Morphinomanie; Les frontières de la folie; Le dualisme cérébral; Les rêves prolongés* (Paris, 1885) 95.
56. Jean Baudrillard, *The Transparency of Evil: Essays on Extreme Phenomena*, trans. James Benedict (London: Verso, 1993).
57. See G. E. Berrios, 'European Views on Personality Disorders: a Conceptual History', *Comprehensive Psychiatry* 34 (1993): 14–30.
58. David Joseph Weeks with Kate Ward, *Eccentrics: the Scientific Investigation* (London: Stirling University Press, 1988).
59. Sangsue, *Récit.*
60. See, for example, Thomas Adam Pepper, *Singularities: Extremes of Theory in the Twentieth Century* (Cambridge: Cambridge University Press, 1997).

8
Retrospective Medicine, Hypnosis, Hysteria and French Literature, 1875–1895

Michael R. Finn

The demise of hysteria as a reputable medical diagnosis in the 1880s and 1890s and its eventual 'dismemberment' by doctors such as Joseph Babinski[1] are generally attributed, in the first instance, to the success of the Nancy medical school in advancing its theses regarding suggestion. Suggestion, argued Dr Hippolyte Bernheim and his colleagues, played an important role in preparing Jean-Martin Charcot's Salpêtrière hysterics for public exhibition of their symptoms. If hysteria's behaviours had been 'cultivated' by the staff of La Salpêtrière, then the ailment, in its four-stage, Charcot-dictated form, did not exist. But success in the 'quarrel' of hysteria, as it has been called,[2] depended also on the ability of La Salpêtrière to maintain not just medical but public credibility vis-à-vis its positions. Two Charcot-led initiatives, little studied up until now in this particular context, clearly produced a contrary effect in the reading public's mind and contributed, in some measure at least, to the waning of La Salpêtrière's authority.

In the mid-1870s, doctors associated with Charcot began a campaign to integrate demonic possession and hypnosis into the diagnostics of hysteria. They were convinced that the possessed of history – ecstatics, mystics, demonics – were simply the hysterics of 1880. And, secondly, some of them became convinced that hypnotism (or 'magnetism' in the more usual pre-1880 terminology of the time) was not simply a technique for producing an altered mindstate, but a neurosis equivalent to hysteria. Needless to say, these attempts at a medical reformulation of historically charged concepts such as possession and magnetism met with some resistance. This essay will attempt to explore that resistance and the evolution of certain aspects of the popular understanding of hysteria in France in the period 1875–95 by comparing the content and framing of a set of medical narratives with literary and journalistic narratives that also address possession and hypnosis.

Our discussion will centre around three main areas of negotiation. First, we will examine the treatment of the sexual and the erotic in medical and fictional narratives. In spite of, or perhaps because of, the abundant erotic content of stories of demonic possession, doctors exercised careful self-censorship in discussing them, often interpreting sexual references as evidence of repressed desire. For their part, novelists construed references to erotic relationships in real terms and their narratives brought into focus not only the relationships of priests and nuns, but also those of doctors and their female patients. Second, we will assess some of the various modes – explanatory and supportive, sarcastic and debunking – in which works of popular fiction represented hypnosis and hysteria during the Salpêtrière's heyday. Perhaps surprisingly, even those works that propose to celebrate the scientific advances in the understanding of nervous ailments also read as attacks on aspects of Charcot's theories. And in evaluating the impact of these fictional portraits, we will briefly investigate a third question. Certain doctors – in their scientific writings, but also in their fiction – depicted hypnosis not as a circumscribed, medical phenomenon, but rather as a gateway to the investigation of the paranormal. The scientific urge to investigate – plus a powerful dose of personal creativity – thus combined to challenge La Salpêtrière's science from within.

Beginning in 1874 (although there were some earlier studies which we will mention in due course), a group of French medical men began to resuscitate, re-tell and re-frame a set of historical texts that recounted the demonic possessions and religious ecstasies of the sixteenth, seventeenth and early eighteenth centuries. The medical and scientific purpose of their work was clear: to identify, root out and explain, from among the many superstitious and supernatural elements in these stories, the concrete indications of disease. In a way, of course, the doctors were simply extending into the past the practice of the case history, presenting in clear, editorialized form, for the benefit of the modern reader, accounts of the emotional and psychic upheavals in the lives of nuns and priests.

These exercises in the historical reconfiguration of disease became popular in parallel with the campaign to convert mesmerism and magnetism into a medical phenomenon – hypnotism. Viewed from today's perspective, we might consider that hypnotism and demonic attacks had something in common: the notion of domination and control. The mystical/demonic possession of the nun usually had some relationship to her priest and confessor, and the 'possession' of the hypnotized subject or hypnotized hysteric (usually female) depended in some way on her doctor or magnetizer.

Although the idea of retrospective medicine is associated with the Charcot school, it owes its existence more to earlier nineteenth-century doctors and their preoccupation with defining abnormal mental states. In attempting to distinguish between genius and madness, many found it convenient and persuasive to extend the diagnostic frame backwards and examine what seemed to be well-documented cases of genius accompanied by neuroses. Louis-Francisque Lélut is a case in point. In his study of Socrates (1836), subtitled 'application de la science psychologique à l'histoire', he wrote famously that because of their hallucinations both Socrates and Pascal were incontrovertibly mad.[3] But it was in particular Dr Louis Calmeil's two-volume study *De la folie considérée sous le point de vue pathologique, philosophique, historique et juduciaire* (1845) that set the stage for 'retrospective medicine' as such, for he examined many of the demonic possessions that would preoccupy later doctors and identified them, in anticipation of Charcot and Paul Richer, as variants of hysteria, instances of 'hystéro-démonopathie'.[4] Dr Gabriel Légué continued on this path, focusing on one instance of mass possession in his medical thesis, *Documents pour servir à l'histoire médicale des possédées de Loudun* (1874). He then produced a follow-up volume that enjoyed great success among readers who sympathized with its priest-protagonist, condemned to the stake by possessed nuns, *Urbain Grandier et les possédées de Loudun* (1880). This study drew an even wider readership when re-edited in 1884 by the naturalist publisher Charpentier.

In 1880, using information he had gleaned as an intern at La Salpêtrière, Dr Charles Richet published a set of three important articles in the *Revue des Deux Mondes*, the first titled enticingly 'The Demonics of Today'.[5] These essays preview much of the retrospective material in Dr Paul Richer's extremely influential *Études cliniques sur la grande hystérie ou hystéro-épilepsie* (*Clinical Studies on Hysteria Major or Hystero-Epilepsy*, 1881; second, expanded edition, 1885).[6] It was Richer's tome and the co-authored Charcot–Richer volume *Les démoniaques dans l'art* (*Demonics in Art*, 1887) that brought the expression 'médecine rétrospective' into currency. These volumes take their cue from an 1869 article by Émile Littré, by training a doctor, as well as the originator of a dictionary, 'Un fragment de médecine rétrospective' ('A Fragment of Retrospective Medicine'),[7] that attempts to demystify and understand as a normal physical phenomenon a thirteenth-century miracle from the Miracles of Saint-Louis.

In *Console and Classify*, Jan Goldstein explains the retroactive extension of hysteria's diagnostic frame in two ways: the Salpêtrière doctors were closely allied with a Republican government intent on removing Roman Catholic influence from hospitals and medicine, and from education in general.[8] More importantly, the four stages of Charcot's 'grande hystérie' had now been promulgated as the universal form of the ailment, 'common to hospital and private practice, valid for all countries and all races'.[9] It was thus a law that could be applied retroactively, and the possessed French nuns of Loudun and Louviers were natural targets for annexation. But these doctors were well-educated men, most with considerable training in languages, literature, philosophy and history. As they combed historical sources on demonology and possession looking for hysteria's symptoms, they unearthed the passionate stories of humans struggling with the forces of good and evil, accounts they found of great human interest, if we are to judge by the extended quotations they provide. One consequence is obvious: the imposition of a single, prescriptive frame on the rich and dramatic narratives of the trials of witches, the dialogues of demons with their exorcists, and the exchanges of possessed nuns with their judges, was bound to shake free narrative elements that would not fit comfortably into a retrospective discourse about hysteria.

The substantial chapter that Dr Paul Richer devotes to hysteria in history in his Charcot-sanctioned *Études cliniques* is formatted in such a way that a reader's attention can never wander too far from the medical objective at hand. The main sections are devoted to the seventeenth-century demonic possession of the daughters of Saint-Ursule in Aix-en-Provence, of the Ursuline nuns in Loudun, and of nuns at the Saint-Louis monastery in Louviers. There is a chapter on the eighteenth-century convulsionaries of Saint-Médard, and on certain instances of religious ecstasies, with special reference to the Belgian stigmatic of the late 1860s, Louise Lateau. The recategorization of all these supernatural events as hysterical attacks means, in Richer's text, that almost every historical citation must itself be framed by cautionary remarks: 'In the following passages', he will typically say, 'it is easy to identify the symptoms of the second period of a major hysterical attack' (811). When a young woman faints, it must be because an examiner has touched 'a hysterogenic point' (841). Much is made of the demonics' body convulsions, frequently qualified as Salpêtrian 'arcs de cercle'. And Richer's text makes widespread use of reader-directing italics to identify the brief sections in long quotations that support his argument.

In this tunnel-vision approach to disease, the psychological and moral content of the nuns' visions are given short shrift. The autobiography of Sister Jeanne des Anges (mother superior of the Ursulines in Loudun), annotated by Drs Légué and Gilles de la Tourette and prefaced by Charcot, is a case in point. Jeanne believes she has been impregnated by the devil and wishes to kill herself, but a powerful force suddenly knocks her to the ground, reminds her of her sin and insists that she rededicate herself fully to God. The doctors' comment on all this is that suicidal tendencies are fairly frequent in hysterics and that Jeanne's acute attack was followed by 'aural and visual hallucinations'.[10]

There is one subject about which Richet and Richer remain totally orthodox, and that is the ability of female hysterics to fabricate sexual innuendo. The two propose that the sexual repression of the nunnery must be the source of claims by religious women that they have been physically possessed by demons or demonically impregnated. Richet looks at accusations against the secular priest Gaufridi from Aix, father Urbain Grandier of Loudun, father Boulé of Louviers, and the Jesuit priest Girard also of Aix but who was put on trial later, in 1730. In every case, without exception, the female accuser is judged to be delirious: 'A nun, hysterical and mad, accuses her confessor, father Girard, a Jesuit, of having cast a spell over her and seduced her' (859). In each instance the bare statement of these 'facts' shows the ridiculousness of the woman's claim.

Yet what confounds the reader is the doctors' admission that in a number of these cases, the nun may indeed have been seduced by her priest. Gaufridi, says Richet, possibly did sleep with his accuser Madeleine de la Palud. Yes, Father Gérard probably did seduce and impregnate Catherine Cadière: 'Gérard was capable of libertinage, of "spiritual incest" toward his penitent, as they used to say in those days. So be it! But frankly, do we have the right to burn someone at the stake for such an offence?' (860). At the trial of the handsome, magnetic Grandier, evidence was given – some of it no doubt prejudiced or self-interested – that he had frequently had intercourse inside his church with women of the town. He had definitely enjoyed an affair with a girl in her late teens who afterwards entered the Loudun convent.[11] It is clear that the man was more of a voluptuary than a sorcerer, and yet even given the abundant evidence about his reputation, no credence is given by Richer or Richet to his accusers' claims of abuse.

In spite of the clear anti-clerical bias of these retrospective medical texts, the doctors always seem to take the side of the priests against the women. Should one be burned at the stake for having seduced one's spiritual charge? No doubt the punishment exceeds the crime. But these medical psychologists see no relationship between the feeling of moral degradation that a spiritually centred woman felt at losing her virginity to her spiritual advisor, and female accusations that the priests were fallen angels, evil incarnate, demons in fact. The physical contorsions and convulsions that may have been the somatization of the woman's attempts to rid herself of her 'demons' were the only factor that caught the attention of these visually attuned men. And the very use, by a nun, of terms such as 'bewitched' or 'possessed' – terms entirely authentic and appropriate within the culture of the time – was sufficient to relegate her claim to the realm of the hallucinatory.

Readers and writers of the 1880s had their own acquired narrative frames, and one of the most firmly established was the tale of the imagined sexual exploits of cloistered nuns and priests supposedly committed to chastity. Both Richer and Richet are, of course, aware of their readers' potential attraction to the salacious, and it is no doubt, in part, a certain medical 'correctness' that has them downplay the sexuality of the historical texts. But medical sensitivity on this point had another source. As one reader has put it, the authors of retrospective medical studies perceived 'a continuity in their patients'[12] between the sixteenth and nineteenth centuries, but – sympathetic with the position of accused clergy because it might resonate with their own – appeared to deny a similar continuity between the role of the historical cleric and the modern-day doctor. An 'incomplete analogy' was created, and a number of journalists and novelists began to rework the themes of these retrospective studies with results sometimes unforeseen by the doctors.

L'hystérique (1885), by the Belgian novelist Camille Lemonnier, is a relentlessly unforgiving portrait of a stigmatic, the Beguine convent in which she resides, and a duplicitous, ferociously sensual priest whose heredity includes priests and torturers who were members of the Inquisition. One commentator suggests that the model for Lemonnier's priest/nun duo, the abbé Orléa and sister Humilité, is Michelet's *La sorcière* (*The Witch*) and his story of Father Girard and La Cadière there,[13] but Lemonnier was also familiar with the central sexual protagonist of retrospective medicine, Urbain Grandier, and father Orléa is in his mould:

> Then [Orléa] tasted the dark joy of sensing [Sister Humilité] lose herself in the monstrous madness of his unquenchable male desire [. . .], of reinflicting on her the effects of the famous possessions in which Grandier and others had excelled. She was his animal, his prey, the

machine-like being that he pestered in the nerves, in the soul, hurling her down or lifting her up at his pleasure. (189)

The depiction of Orléa's magnetic, almost occult power over the nun and his determination to extract every possible pleasure, including sadomasochistic sex, from her, challenges the retrospective medical readings of Grandier's lust as innocuous. In fact, the ambivalence of the medical perspective on sexuality is personified in the inept physician Basquin. He appears to believe that Sister Humilité's affliction is genitally based, suggesting that marriage would cure her, but is too reticent to broach the question of sexuality openly with those around her. A letter which the novelist Joris-Karl Huysmans wrote to Lemonnier after reading *L'hystérique* points up another confusion in the public mind: is Sister Humilité truly a hysteric simply because she has religious visions, and is the title *L'hystérique* really appropriate? Huysmans' view is that authentic stigmatics, 'lunatics of Christ',[14] exist.

As much as Charcot and his colleagues wanted to purge hysteria of its traditional sexual connotations, sexual issues were always associated with La Salpêtrière and their prevalence contributed to an undermining of the credibility of the 'grande hystérie' syndrome as put forward by Charcot.

Magnetism and hypnotism

In these same late 1870s and early 1880s, psychologists and doctors began to reassess the history and reconfigure the meaning of another type of 'possession', that of the magnetized or hypnotized subject. Richer's *Études cliniques* state Charcot's case: 'hysteria and hypnotism are close relatives' (505). What is the connection? The muscular contractions, paralyses and anaesthesias of hypnotized and hysterical subjects are similar; one can pierce the arm of each with a pin and cause no pain. And many hysterics appear to be, while awake, in exactly the same state of somnambulism that the hypnotized display. Hypnotism is thus the artificially triggered version of spontaneous hysteria; they represent the twin halves of the same 'névrose'.

Charcot was now provided with an intellectually satisfying equation: 'grande hystérie' with its four fixed stages on the one hand, 'grand hypnotisme' with its three (catalepsy, lethargy, somnambulism) on the other. But in this transfer from the paranormal to the medical, a number of grey areas remained. What was the public to make of the mind-reading and mental telepathy that seemed to be part of traditional magnetism?

Magnetism was, of course, alive and well as Charcot's conversion attempts began. There had been scores of periodicals devoted to the subject since the time of Mesmer's French student, the marquis de Puységur, a number of them founded in the 1840s. There was another flurry in the 1860s[15] and again, during this period from 1875 to 1885, in which religion and spiritualism were preoccupying the reading public, a wave of interest in hypnotism swept over France. Hector Durville became editor of a new *Revue Magnétique*, founded in 1878, and in 1879 the Société magnétique de France established its *Journal du Magnétisme*, naming as its supporters 'a society of magnetizers and doctors'. In 1877 Edmond de Goncourt inserted a 'hystérique magnétique' named Alexandrine Phénomène into his novel *La fille Élisa*. From 1880 onwards, almost every issue of the prestigious *Revue Philosophique* carried an article on hypnotism, and in 1882, the Belgian magnetizer Donato took Paris by storm. In 1884, the major magnetizers in vogue, in addition to Donato, were listed as the Italian Alberti, the Dane Hansen, and the Hungarian Welles.[16] And in 1885, Dr Georges Gilles de la Tourette conducted a poll on magnetism in Paris and found that there were about 40,000 practising subjects, some 500 hypnotists' offices, and 20 journals specialized in the field.[17] What may perhaps have created the ultimate confusion among observers was the involvement of doctors in public hypnotism demonstrations. *Le Voltaire* of 22 April 1887 reports one such event during which Dr Lucien Moutin conducted hypnotic experiments before a huge crowd that would have made even Donato proud.

Even well-disposed doctors contributed to a blurring of the understanding of hypnotism/hysteria. Charles Richet first became an important player in the medical debate upon the publication of an article entitled 'Du somnambulisme provoqué'[18] ('On Induced Somnambulism'). His essay proposed that a medical person such as himself could in fact 'magnetize' patients and instruct them to act in various unorthodox ways. He was especially interested in the way his patients seemed to develop a second personality when hypnotized. A key and seemingly unremarkable aspect of his hypnotic practice was that most of his subjects were perfectly healthy individuals. When, in 1877–78, Charcot and his team themselves began employing hypnosis to experiment with their patients at La Salpêtrière, they would rapidly make the claim that only the most serious hysterics were hypnotizable. Richet thus found himself on the wrong side of a debate with the most powerful motor of the medical establishment at this time.

In 1884, at a crucial moment in the hysteria debate, Richet again undermined the Salpêtrière position and gave comfort to its enemies by republishing a set of essays in which he had argued that normal individuals could be hypnotized.[19] Early in the year, Dr Hippolyte Bernheim and the Nancy lawyer Jules Liégeois had struck a double blow against Charcotian hysteria by calling attention to the role of suggestion in hypnosis and possibly in hysterical states themselves. The former published *De la suggestion dans l'état hypnotique et dans l'état de veille* (*On Suggestion in the Hypnotic and in the Waking State*), a set of case studies examining (mostly) non-nervous individuals who had been hypnotized and instructed successfully to commit various dubious acts or 'experimental crimes'. Liégeois looked at many of the same cases from a legal viewpoint,[20] opening up a major debate on the legal responsibility of subjects told to commit crimes post-hypnotically. The theme became an immediate favourite of pulp novelists and added a note of unwanted spice to La Salpêtrière's outwardly rational conflation of hysteria and hypnosis.

Paul Ginisty, the literary critic for *Gil Blas*, co-authored a novel entitled *L'Idée fixe* (1885), in which a young man gradually implants the idea of imminent death in a friend's mind so that he can possess the fellow's wife. The friend does in fact die, but the wife subsequently has the criminal prosecuted for the murder. In Hector Malot's *Conscience* (1888), a doctor, anxious after killing a usurer, hypnotizes his own wife to find out if she knows he is the guilty party. It was, however, Jules Claretie's *Jean Mornas* (1885) that became the classic novel of post-hypnotic suggestion. Mornas, a graduate of medical studies and La Salpêtrière, is unable to develop a practice in Paris and lives an embittered existence, forced to survive on minor research and writing projects for others. He develops a friendship with Lucille (the Christian name of the magnetizer Donato's most famous subject), a woman of weakened nervous disposition whom emotion can sometimes reduce to a somnambulistic state. Mornas realizes that he can hypnotize her and use suggestion to have her commit a robbery that will make him rich. But he is eventually found out by two enterprising doctors who re-hypnotize Lucille and wring the truth from her.

In spite of Claretie's close personal connections with La Salpêtrière – he had in fact participated in Dr Gilles de la Tourette's experiments with hypnotized patients and had been the voluntary victim of a suggested 'crime' – and in spite of an impressive apparatus of references to real medical research on hypnotism and hysteria, his novel could only be read as an assault on La Salpêtrière. The inordinate emphasis the story places on the central idea of the Nancy school, suggestion, comes at a time when the connection between suggestion and hysteria had become a minefield, and the sensationalist focus on the criminal potential of mind control, the latter connected in the public mind to telepathy and the old idea of a magnetic fluid, reasserted the paranormal and non-medical face of magnetism.

The fictional representation of hypnotism could thus lead in a number of directions, most of them inimical to La Salpêtrière's positions. And here again, we encounter the intriguing figure of Dr Charles Richet who, under the pseudonym of Charles Epheyre, published two novels that reinvest possession and medical hypnotism with a paranormal aura. His novel *Possession* (1887) recounts a rivalry between two Russian women, Marie-Anne and her cousin Sacha, for the love of the officer Stéphane. Marie-Anne asks Sacha to tell Stéphane that, whatever happens, she will one day be his. The text then reminds the reader of the meaning of the title: 'An incarnation, or a possession, happens when a dead person returns for a few days or hours to inhabit the body of a living person!' (97).

Stéphane gradually falls in love with the charming Sacha, they marry and leave for an Italian honeymoon. In Venice, Sacha is suddenly possessed by the spirit of Marie-Anne, who has died in the interim. She explains to Stéphane: 'I won't harm you, my dear friend. Sacha's soul has become numb . . . and it is I, I, your beloved Marie-Anne who has plunged her into a deep sleep to take advantage of her body and her voice. I wanted to tell you of her treachery' (243). Stéphane, now unhinged, shoots the spirit-woman, whereupon the spell vanishes. Finding himself alone, he commits suicide.

Soeur Marthe (1890) is the drama of a young doctor-magnetizer who is caught up not with the positivistic aspects of science but with the mysteries of the human psyche, rather like Richet himself. While visiting a childhood friend at the latter's estate in Plancheville, Laurent is introduced to sister Marthe, a novice nun suffering from tuberculosis but also described as 'une névrosée' ('a neurotic', 27). As he begins to play Gounod's *Ave Maria* for her, Marthe falls into a hypnotic trance, speaking in a wholly different voice, and reveals that she is Angèle de Mérande, a headstrong, passionate version of Marthe with the same family name.

Laurent is troubled by Angèle's psychic powers: she can in fact read his mind and gives several proofs of it. He would like to run off with her but is wary: 'There was a lot of talk, at the time, in newspapers and in the courts, of seduction under hypnotism' (87). Post-hypnotic suggestion is again involved: the magnetizer instructs Angèle that her Marthe-side will be cured and will live. She then falls into a semiconscious lethargy from which he cannot rouse her, and from that moment on, whatever his hypnotist's tricks (barking loudly at Marthe that she become Angèle), only Marthe remains. The passionate woman he knew is lost, and yet if Marthe is to live, her spirit-sister Angèle must logically disappear.

The argument could certainly be made that Richet was one of the leaders of a kind of 'fifth column' within the medical community, confirming through his fiction the popular notion that magnetism/hypnotism and parapsychological phenomena such as mind-reading, mental telepathy and even spirit life were part of a continuum. And the adepts of the magnetizing movement in France were certainly pleased to note the attendance at their public rallies of a man who was director of the *Revue Scientifique*.[21] Medical biographies note that Richet won the Nobel Prize for Physiology in 1913 for his discovery of anaphylaxis, but more rarely do they report that he was the inventor of the term 'métapsychique', one of the fathers of the parapsychology movement in France, president of the anglophone Society for Psychical Research in 1905, and co-founder, along with the spiritualist and astronomer Camille Flammarion, of the Institut Métapsychique International, of which he was president from 1930 until his death in 1935.

Erotic overtones are carefully downplayed in Richet's fiction, as they were in his medical texts, but, as we saw in Camille Lemonnier's *L'hystérique*, most fiction that chose to represent hysteria and possession reinstated the sexual component which medical narratives would embed in a different manner. Hypnotism in particular, with its aura of the magnetic, is a figure of male domination and control which almost by definition eroticizes fictional narrative and thus serves to dislodge the medical perspective.

'Magnétisme', a Maupassant short story published in 1882, is an example of this tendency. In it, Charcot is presented as a dreamer whose explanations of inexplicable nervous states resemble religious pronouncements rather than scientific judgements. The story itself is the tale of lust shared telepathically in which the narrator succeeds in sleeping with a woman he barely knows because she appears to have had exactly the same obsessive dream about him that he has had about her.

An earlier bestseller by the prolific Jules Claretie can only be read as a challenge to La Salpêtrière's medical and moral authority because of the way it eroticizes the medical gaze. *Les amours d'un interne* (*The Loves of an Intern*, 1881) takes the reader inside La Salpêtrière into the service of a fictional Dr Fargeas, co-director, along with Charcot, of the hospital's nervous diseases section. The love affairs portrayed – and there are many – involve mostly the interns and the female staff plus a group of ancillary characters working at the hospital – artists, sculptors and photographers. Mathilde Mignon, a beautiful model who has been seduced and abandoned, has a hysterical attack and is hospitalized in the nervous diseases section. Her convulsed form is described hungrily: 'the body of the poor child [was] twisted in an arc, and this frail body, with its charming grace, this young body with its pure forms, rose in a curve so that, beneath her shift, one saw the outline of her round breasts, erect, her stomach which seemed swollen, and her finely shaped legs, white as marble' (239). She is later seen naked, thighs spread (248).

One of the interns, Pedro, is in hot pursuit of an androgynous visiting Russian beauty, that is until she defiantly bares her chest and reveals that, as a member of the self-mutilating Skoptzy sect, she has cut off her breasts (312). Another intern, Finet, is the most accomplished hypnotist among his fellows, showing off by magnetizing one of the hospital workers, the towering Lolo, at the drop of a hat. One evening as he is attending the opera, he suddenly remembers that he has left her mesmerized with her hands stretched out over her head for more than five hours. Finet's interest is not only playful. When he hypnotizes Lolo during parties at his apartment, his thoughts are all about control. Not only can he touch her without her knowledge, but he may also direct her thoughts to his advantage: 'When she was in a cataleptic state, he would suggest to her whatever ideas he wanted' (145). Finet's weakness for mind control in particular makes a reader think of claims that certain Salpêtrière doctors who were also accomplished hypnotists, such as Puyfontaine and Albert Ruault, 'spent too much time with their patients'.[22]

The theme of sexual abuse of a female subject under hypnosis was to become more firmly rooted in the public mind as the decade progressed. In *Le Temps* of 30 March 1887, Hugues Le Roux recounts a rape outside the hospital. The attack was committed by a student doctor working on a nervous diseases ward on a patient whom he had magnetized. Doctors[23] and the lawyer Jules Liégeois[24] discussed similar cases. Even the medical men of fiction, as we have seen in Richet's novella *Soeur Marthe*, are wary of the relationship with their hypnotized patients because of court cases where hypnotizers have been charged.

Even more apparent than the sexual undercurrents in *Les amours d'un interne* is the author's scientific ambition, the desire to provide a comprehensive account of La Salpêtrière's activities in the field of retrospective medicine and hypnotism. The interns discuss Mesmer, magnetism and medical hypnotism; hysterical figures in Italian art; father Urbain Grandier, the possessed nuns of Loudun and the convulsionaries of Saint-Médard; modern-day stigmatics like Louise Lateau and the question of religious ecstasies. That Claretie is already familiar with the material in Richer's *Études cliniques* is evident, but the scepticism voiced by sympathetic characters – the photographer and plasterer/moulder Mongobert, the spiritualist/sculptor Platoff – introduces a discourse that runs counter to the medical narrative. Even if possessed or ecstatic nuns can be termed hysterics, one of the Catholic interns still believes in the supernatural nature of certain possessions. Mongobert is bored by the so-called 'discovery' that Renaissance painters were painting hysterical fits rather than moments of demonic possession. And he is openly dubious about the connection between hysteria and hypnotism. Perhaps most damning is the fact that the interns, even in group session, are unable to define the hysteria they are treating (103). Thus, in spite of its apparent good intentions, the novel problematizes many of the medical findings it discusses.

It is in the life and writings of a female novelist, the decadent Rachilde (1860–1953), that the counterpoint of medical theory about and popular understanding of these subjects is played out in its rawest form. Marguerite Eymery acquired her pseudonym Rachilde during a family ouija-board session, where she *pretended* (it is she who says she pretended, the family was not so sure) to adopt the spirit voice of a long-dead Swedish nobleman and recount his life. Always conscious of this aura of possible 'possession', and intensely aware of her problematic heredity (her mother would be interned in a psychiatric hospital for a time), Marguerite labels herself a nervous hysteric and describes in an autobiographical text suicide attempts and two important hysterical attacks, the second taking place when she was about 22 years old and attempting to ward off the advances of an older writer to whom she was attracted.[25] She was attended at this point by one of the best-known hysteria specialists in Paris, Dr Charles Lasègue.[26] We know little about their actual meeting and exchange, but Rachilde reports that her attack was followed by a two-month paralysis of the legs. In a sense, she now became, through her body, a medium for the canonic medical discourse of the time, exhibiting one of hysteria's most representative symptoms, anaesthesia of a body part. But a few years later, two of her novels reflect both a loss of confidence in the Salpêtrian version of hysteria and a female reaction against the scientific pretensions of medical hypnotism and hysteria research in general.

In Rachilde's *A mort* (*To the Death*, 1886), the destiny of the heroine Berthe Soirès, manipulated by the off-again, on-again affections of two men, is mirrored in the two sessions of salon magnetism that serve as bookends to the narrative. For the benefit of a cross-section of attending bourgeois, a doctor puts a 16-year-old girl into a trance and has her hang from the ceiling, suspending herself from a cord she holds in her teeth. The medical community thus seems to prefer to view women as circus performers whom they coach. And the text proposes that men are wedded to theories of magnetism 'out of sadism, sadism in a latent state that makes them want to rape sleeping girls without, however, allowing them to succeed' (230). Hypnotism is but another figure of male control, and the deep-running argument of the novel is that so-called respectable medicine and charlatanesque science converge in this one important aspect, the masculine desire for domination.

Written just a few months later, *La marquise de Sade* reverses the terms of *A mort*: the female is no longer the victim. She has now learned how to use scientific and medical knowledge (in addition to sex) in order to damage or eliminate men. Mary Barbe executes a sexually abusive doctor-uncle by allowing him to inhale chemical fumes while unconscious. She exhausts and murders her brute of a husband over a period of time by administering doses of poison mixed with a powerful aphrodisiac. A number of medical men and scientists appear as hapless characters in the text, especially a nerve doctor named Marscot, the name sounding suspiciously like Charcot:

> Marscot described his miraculous procedure of beating a drum which later, if he was allowed to experiment, would enable him to hypnotize dozens of nervous young girls (whom he would, by the way, never attempt to cure), knocking them off their feet like decks of cards. He was content to observe the curious manifestations of catalepsy without a thought for anything further. Girls and dogs existed to serve as common objects of suffering (200).

And towards the end of the novel, Mary becomes an almost male doctor-figure in the experimental, Salpêtrière mode. She treats an emotionally delicate young medical student who is prone to nosebleeds like a patient, informing him of a few facts about anatomy and then, as though he were the hysteric, continually sticking him with pins to test his resistance to pain and check for anaesthetized zones.

Let us summarize. Certainly, the active role played by some doctors in exploring the extra-medical aspects of hypnosis undermined La Salpêtrière's position concerning the link between hypnotism and hysteria. Sitting on the boards of magnetism journals, attending or leading public demonstrations of hypnotism, stubbornly exploring the possible paranormal associations of hypnotism, all these caught the attention of the public and authorized non-scientific interpretations of hysteria itself. But it was the very claim that hypnosis was a subset of hysteria which was the real disaster for Charcot. Traditionally, this disaster has been seen, in medical terms, as the victory of one school over another. It was the persuasive argument of Dr Hippolyte Bernheim and his colleagues from Nancy, that hysteria was a condition artificially cultivated through suggestion, which led to its eventual defeat as a medical diagnosis.

But the fiction we have examined shows the extent of another credibility gap – a gap in the cultural understanding of hysteria in the 1880s caused by a confusion over competing narratives of sexuality. The reading public was clearly aware that medical texts had broached the sexual face of hysteria, and Charcot's statement that 'it is always the genital thing . . . always . . . always!' was well known. Those who followed hysteria research were thus frustrated at the medical profession's reluctance to acknowledge the full story. Rachilde's female gaze on this point does not differ substantially from that of Jules Claretie. Each interprets medical hypnotism and research on female hysterics as suspect: they serve either as covers for symbolic rape or as devices for experimentation as opposed to therapy. And indeed, it was a desire to round out a *theory* of disease that helped launch the medical investigation of religious ecstasies and magnetism in the first place. The attempt to impose a medical frame on demonic possession and magnetism contained, therefore, the seeds of its own defeat. The public imagination saw in the resulting narratives not tales of scientific progress but a thematics of eroticism drawn from the eternal human drama of sexual attraction, domination and submission.

Notes

Unless otherwise indicated, all translations from the French are my own.

1. Joseph Babinski, *Démembrement de l'hystérie traditionnelle: pithiatisme* (Paris: Imprimerie de la Semaine Médicale, 1909).
2. Pierre-Henri Castel, *La querelle de l'hystérie* (Paris: Presses Universitaires de France, 1998).

3. See Juan Rigoli's discussion of this point in his *Lire le délire* (Paris: Fayard, 2001) 328 n12.
4. Charcot's conflation of hysteria and mystical possession was also anticipated by about 40 years in the medical thesis of Alexis Favrot, *De la catalepsie, de l'extase et de l'hystérie* (Paris, 1844). See Mary Donaldson-Evans, *Medical Examinations* (Lincoln, NE: University of Nebraska Press, 2000) 42.
5. The articles are 'Les démoniaques d'aujourd'hui', *Revue des Deux Mondes (RDM)*, 15 January 1880: 340–72, 'Les démoniaques d'autrefois. I. Les sorcières et les possédées', *RDM*, 1 February 1880: 552–83, and 'Les démoniaques d'autrefois. II. Les procès de sorcières et les épidémies démoniaques', *RDM*, 15 February 1880: 828–63.
6. My references will be to the second edition (Paris, 1885).
7. *Philosophie positive* 5 (1869): 103–20.
8. Jan Goldstein, *Console and Classify: the French Psychiatric Profession in the Nineteenth Century* (Cambridge: Cambridge University Press, 1987).
9. Charcot's introduction to Richer, *Études cliniques*, p. viii.
10. I have borrowed this example from Jean Céard's article 'Démonologie et démonopathies au temps de Charcot', *Histoire des Sciences Médicales* 28, 4 (1994): 339.
11. See Roland Villeneuve, *La mystérieuse affaire Grandier: Le diable à Loudun* (Payot, 1980) 19, and Michel Carmona, *Les diables de Loudun. Sorcellerie et politique sous Richelieu* (Paris: Fayard, 1988) 74.
12. Sarah Ferber, 'Charcot's Demons: Retrospective Medicine and Historical Diagnosis in the Writings of the Salpêtrière School', in M. Gijswijt-Hofstra et al. (eds), *Illness and Healing Alternatives in Western Europe* (London: Routledge, 1997) 129.
13. See Eléonore Roy-Reverzy's introduction to the *L'hystérique* (Paris: Nouvelles Éditions Séguier, 1996) 9, and Michelet, *La sorcière* (Paris: Didier, 1956) II, chapters X–XII.
14. Huysmans, *Lettres inédites à Camille Lemonnier* (Paris: Droz/Minard, 1957), quoted in *L'hystérique*, 226.
15. *La Revue magnétique* was established in 1844 and *Le magnétiseur spiritualiste* in 1849. Joseph Gérard, not always an accurate observer, also mentions *Philanthropico-magnétique* (1840), *Mesmérisme* (1844) and *Jury-magnétique* (1847) in his *Le magnétisme appliqué à la médecine* (Paris, 1864) 25–6. In the 1860s *Le magnétisme*, later *Revue des sciences magnétique, hypnotique et occultes*, appeared in 1862 and *La revue magnétique, journal des malades* in 1869.
16. Dr Fernand Bottey, *Le 'magnétisme animal'. Étude critique* (Paris, 1884) 259.
17. On his website (http://pierrehenri.castel.free.fr), Pierre-Henri Castel provides an update of the 'Chronology and Historical Bibliography' of hysteria published in his study *La querelle de l'hystérie* (Paris: Presses Universitaires de France, 1998). The entry regarding Gilles de la Tourette's investigation is listed in the update for the year 1885.
18. *Journal d'anatomie et de physiologie normale et pathologique* 11 (1875).
19. *L'homme et l'intelligence: fragments de physiologie et de psychologie* (Paris, 1884).
20. In his memoir presented to the Académie des Sciences morales et politiques, *De la suggestion hypnotique dans ses rapports avec le droit civil et le droit criminel* (Paris, 1884).

21. As does Édouard Cavailhon, a promoter of magnetism and derider of Charcot, in *La fascination magnétique* (Paris, 1882) 31–2.
22. Castel, *La querelle de l'hystérie*, 55 n1.
23. For example, Dr Ladame, 'L'hypnotisme et la médecine légale', *Archives de l'anthropologie criminelle et des sciences pénales* 10 (1887): 293–335, 520–59.
24. See chapter 14, 'Crimes commis contre les somnambules', of his extremely informative *De la suggestion et du somnambulisme dans leurs rapports avec la jurisprudence et la médecine légale* (Paris, 1889).
25. See the preface to her novel *A mort* (Paris, 1886).
26. Lasègue had written a ground-breaking article on anorexia and was interested in the simulative and theatrical aspects of hysteria. He had also authored a paper on the dual personality of hysterics. See the collection *Écrits psychiatriques*, ed. J. Corraze (Toulouse: Privat, 1971).

9
From Private Asylum to University Clinic: Hungarian Psychiatry, 1850–1908[1]

Emese Lafferton

> Previously, there was no science of psychopathology [in Hungary] ... [whereas] in the Western countries of Europe, mental pathology – in spite of the fact that for a long time it had been a step-child of medicine – had grown into a fully-developed, large, ramifying tree by the middle of this century, which, with its dense foliage, kept the mental patients who were enjoying rest under its shade free from the attacks and sufferings that prejudice, superstition, ignorance and malevolence had directed against them in the past centuries.[2]

The development of Hungarian psychiatry in the nineteenth century was belated compared with Western Europe. For political and economic reasons, modernization started relatively late in the country, before a period of remarkably energetic progress in the second half of the nineteenth century. This essay focuses on this period and has two main aims. Firstly I give a necessarily brief account of the birth and early development of Hungarian psychiatry, a topic hitherto unexplored by historians. At the centre of this study are two types of institutions which characterized the period: the asylum and the university clinic. Secondly, I reconstruct distinctive models of the psychiatrist, the mental patient, and the doctor–patient relationship framed within these institutional settings. Using a case of hysteria and hypnosis from the 1880s, I shall demonstrate the mutual relationship between medicine and social and cultural thinking, and the extent to which the medical framing and imagining of these phenomena was informed by prevalent social values while psychiatry's normative function in the medicalization of deviant behaviour simultaneously reinforced socially sanctioned boundaries distinguishing normal from abnormal, acceptable from deviant, and healthy from pathological.

The first madhouse and a comprehensive theory of mental illness

From the second half of the eighteenth century onwards, the most significant problem facing the treatment of the mentally ill in Hungary was the narrowly focused one of establishing a national asylum. Endeavours emerged from different quarters: the Austrian imperial court, high-ranking church authorities, aristocratic circles, and medical professionals. Partly because of clashing interests and, more significantly, lack of money, the establishment of a national public institution was not realized for another century. Thus, around 1800, at a time when the 'trade in lunacy' was flourishing in England, and when reforms of the custodial asylum opened a new, hopeful era of therapeutic asylums in England and France,[3] Hungary lacked any such mental institutions. Sources reveal that some hospitals, especially those run by Catholic healing orders, took care of the mad, but since no specialized institution existed, most of the insane roamed freely, and were cared for at home, locked up in prisons, or kept on hospital wards without adequate medical attendance. When the first criticisms of the therapeutic asylum were made in the West in the 1850s,[4] Hungarian doctors were still lobbying for a national asylum. Great hopes were invested in it, and even at the end of the nineteenth century psychiatrists retrospectively regarded the opening in 1868 of the Lipótmező national asylum as a sign of the country's arrival in the ranks of civilized and cultured nations.

In psychiatrists' accounts from around 1900 it is a general topos that the 'father' of Hungarian psychiatry was Ferencz Schwartzer (1818–89), owner and director of the first 'modern' private madhouse, 'the cradle of mental-pathological studies in Hungary'.[5] Schwartzer's students – the doctors who gained their first experience at his private asylum – later became holders of key posts within Hungarian medical and psychiatric circles (including the first medical staff at subsequent state lunatic asylums, the first lecturers in psychiatry at the Medical Faculty, and directors of psychiatric hospital wards).

The Catholic Schwartzer family was of German origin, and could boast of eminent descendants in the sciences and among tradesmen: they were master coopers and wine merchants, and two sons excelled in philanthropy and became influential educators of defective children at the Vác institute for the deaf and dumb.[6] Clearly, entrepreneurial spirit and an interest in mental deficiency ran deep in the family. Ferencz Schwartzer studied at the Vienna medical faculty and, for a while, worked there at the mental ward of the Allgemeines Krankenhaus. He then travelled widely in Europe funded by the Hungarian state, visiting lunatic asylums in the hope of using his experience to establish a national public state asylum in Buda, for which he enthusiastically lobbied. His efforts proved unsuccessful, so in 1850 Schwartzer founded his own private madhouse. This was moved to Buda two years later, where it functioned as the family's private enterprise till 1910. Originally designed for 60, the asylum was gradually enlarged and, by 1863, could house 120 patients.

In 1858, after eight years of experience with mental patients at his own institution, Schwartzer published *General Pathology and Treatment of Psychic Disorders, with Forensic Psychology*. The book was immediately hailed as 'a new testament on the heavenly altar of our national language, . . . a generous guide in an untrodden oasis, . . . a fresh spring in a bleak desert'.[7] The work has since been widely celebrated as the first comprehensive book on mental pathology written by a Hungarian in the mother tongue. In the title, Schwartzer introduced the term 'psychic disorders' (or 'disorders of the soul'), and used it as synonymous with mental pathology throughout the book. He defined mental pathology as the 'long and feverless process of the pathological confusion of psychic powers, which robs man of his capability to think and act freely concerning his own well-being, care and responsibility'.[8]

Schwartzer's book is a remarkably late example of an age-old comprehensive medical theory. His unfolding conception of mental illness reveals a holistic view of the patient recognizing an inseparable unity of mind and body, and an understanding of mental illnesses in their complexities. Although not explicitly spelt out by the author, the cohesive force behind his view of mental disorders is the explanatory potential of humoural pathology, the powerful theory that had characterized medical thinking from ancient times till the late-eighteenth century (and even later), with its complex view of the human being integrated into the universe. Schwartzer describes the internal world of the individual as an elaborate economy of all the bodily processes, powers, fluids, heat, upon which the external world exerts its influence. Illness visits the human body when the internal economy is disturbed, the balance is overthrown, or when external forces strengthen certain pathological processes within the body. Physical therapy conforms to this understanding, and it is the reconstruction of the balance of internal powers and fluids that brings about healing.

Elaborating on the aetiology of mental disorders over the course of a hundred pages, Schwartzer identifies physical and psychic predisposing and precipitating factors, and offers a wide range of physical and psychic treatments. The elimination of possible organic causes, blood-letting, a variety of cold and warm baths, purges, refreshing drinks, sedative substances, and the manipulation of the body with hunger, thirst and pain constitute the physical treatments he proposes to restore health. Psychic healing – or, as he explicitly calls it after Pinel and Esquirol, moral treatment – is more complex, and centres around the idea of the asylum. In the theory of moral treatment as well as in ideas of the therapeutic asylum contemporary to Schwartzer, the asylum itself is turned into a therapeutic tool, or, in Roy Porter's words, a 'therapeutic engine' – a machine to restore the insane to health.[9]

The notion of the asylum as a therapeutic tool, together with the moral (psychic) and physical treatment, was intended to achieve the 'complete systematic re-education of the individual',[10] leading patients back to their families and to society at large. The doctor was 'striving to give them back to the circle[s] that nature assigned for them, but from which upbringing, fate, their own leanings or aversions removed'.[11] Within the asylum, 'the first step is to accustom them to order, and not to allow the neglect of duties, otherwise many would die of hunger and filth. Therefore we have to encourage the patient to wash himself every day, dress up properly, get up and go to bed in time, and urge him to do physical exercise.'[12]

The gendered occupational and social activities offered at Schwartzer's private institution, with its emphasis on industriousness, work, and the strict daily routine, suggest that life within the walls reflected every-day social life and dictated social norms prevailing in the outside bour-geois world. Work and amusements were central preoccupations that constituted part of the treatment. Because of the patients' higher social status,[13] it is unsurprising that so much emphasis was laid on exercising the intellectual faculties (including the study of history, the natural sci-ences, geography, and the solving riddles), as well as amusements (such as chess, cards, dominoes, music, travel, and theatre). Women listened to music, played instruments and chess. Their work included rending, plucking, needlework, reeling, knitting, and the cleaning of furniture, rooms and clothes. While Schwartzer allowed patients to choose their own occupations, he placed a great stress on the importance of on industriousness, and made sure that patients of all social status took part in the cultivation of gardens. In his view, it was tantamount to 'strengthen domestic virtues and increase . . . contentment within the more genteel'.[14]

Moral treatment did not consist of 'master strokes'; rather, it was based on a 'rational order' which pertained to everyone, and aimed at the pacification of the spirits, which had a great effect on the clarity of cognition. The patients placed 'under serious discipline, were compelled to follow an ordered life and diet, which obliged them to consider their situation'. This was supposed to bring them back to reason, and the conditions to kindle their longing for their previous life: Schwartzer believed that 'From deprivation arises his desire for freedom and the wish to see his relatives'. Thus, psychic treatment built on the constant 'serious and loving' reminder of the patient of his own rationality to increase 'real moral freedom and self-restraint'.[15]

The case of Katalin N., the 40-year-old wife of an artisan, published by Schwartzer's assistant doctor, Károly Bolyó, demonstrates the duality of physical and psychic treatment. After Katalin N. murdered her five-month-old child, she was diagnosed mad, and said to be suffering from religious melancholy with hallucinations. Bolyó stated that her treatment was both 'medical and psychic', the first including the increase of metabolism and the function of the bowels with medication, and fighting insomnia with opium, which also affected her moods positively. The opium was given in 'cure cycles', a few days' increasing, then decreasing doses, followed by a few days' interval, over and over for six weeks. She was assigned plenty of walking in the garden, and a cold 'rain' shower every three days. The psychic treatment consisted of introducing order and cleanliness into her life, and diverting her attention away from her crime. Her needs for 'noble entertainment' such as music and chess were satisfied. Bolyó emphasized that 'the doctor's authority had to be bolstered', while the patient was kept under 'constant surveillance'. The woman was eventually claimed to have been completely cured of her disease.[16]

Crucial to the idea of the therapeutic asylum professed by Schwartzer was the specific view of mental illness and the doctor–patient relationship that had prevailed in the theory of moral therapy since about 1800. According to this, the insane were seen as children: mental illness was 'a condition that resembles childhood, the early exaggerated conditions of childhood'. At the centre of the family formed by these disturbed children of nature stood the doctor, 'who . . . is the spirit of the institution'. Like the paterfamilias, he ruled over the household, and emerges from Schwartzer's description as an authoritarian, charismatic figure with a huge influence on and control over his patients. 'The doctor has to impose punishments, but also has to give rewards.' He has to be the patients' 'benevolent protector', his speech to them had to be 'consoling, ... friendly, but serious', flowing from 'a good heart'.[17] Isolation in the asylum greatly exposed the patient to the doctor, who thus elicited greater obedience.[18]

The doctor's art consisted of a mastery of control over the patient's psyche and a manipulation of fear without resorting to physical coercion. 'The attention of raging mad people cannot be fixed, in order to make them hear and follow reasonable propositions. The essence of psychic healing is to get the mastery over [the patients'] attention, govern their rationality, and gain their trust.' Fear 'makes them willing to listen and follow the given advice'. In a doctor–patient relationship 'the fearless and courageous' patients had to be 'tamed, and our vigilance can practice ... such a power over them, that they become intimidated and tremble, and yield to those, who are skilful enough to demonstrate power before them'.[19] The doctor's charisma was thus supposed to replace physical coercion; or rather, physical coercion was substituted by a form of psychic coercion.

Schwartzer was praised for introducing a 'no restraint' policy in his asylum, an ideal professed by many of his assistant doctors who subsequently became the directors and head doctors at large public asylums.[20] Schwartzer stated that the institution refrained from anything that would increase pain or fear even in the most restless patients, and he permitted the use of the straightjacket only in the most extreme cases.[21] In an 1858 article published in the *Orvosi Hetilap* ('Medical Weekly'), Schwartzer's assistant doctor, János Lyachovics, described the case of S.E., a 19-year-old Jewish shop assistant who suffered from mania, and who was screaming night and day for ten days 'during which he was of course kept in a straightjacket, tied to the bed'. Lyachovics mused disbelievingly over how the English could apply the 'no restraint' system with their raging and destructive patients.[22] Bolyó reported the case of a female patient who was calm during her admission and first observation. However, after the doctor left she developed a raging madness and attacked a nurse, tearing off the nurse's cloths and beating her up, until the nurses were able to put a straightjacket on her. Diagnosed as suffering from mania, the patient was subsequently tied to her bed, isolated and forcefully fed with special tools – 'the most difficult and unpleasant, but necessary procedure', Bolyó conceded.[23] Resort to some form of physical coercion was thus occasionally seen as necessary.

In the subsequent decades several public asylums were opened, often headed by doctors who had gained their first experience under Schwartzer. But just as in western countries, within one or two decades of their establishment large state asylums had revealed the inadequacies of the therapeutic asylum.[24] They were overcrowded with numerous hopeless cases, the death-rates were high, and there was little time available for individual patients. Although Schwartzer emphasized individual treatment, expressing great concern for the 'patient's entire mental personality', subsequent asylums could not cope with the flow of paralytic and alcoholic patients, and the large numbers made personal therapy impossible. While lobbying for further asylums continued well beyond the turn of the century in Hungary, increasing disappointment encouraged psychiatrists to look for alternatives outside the large asylum, in other types of institutions and psychiatric practices.

New hopes were invested in the university clinic and academic research.[25] By this time, anatomical and histological research had come to the fore throughout Europe. The expansion of research schools, teaching hospitals, and the increasing availability of scientific equipment made clinical and laboratory experiments possible and desirable. Germany was leading the way in what Shorter called 'the first biological psychiatry'[26] with its numerous research institutes, which – from the 1870s onwards – also had a strong influence on Hungarian psychiatry.

From this period, Hungarian psychiatry became especially open to and receptive of foreign ideas. Translations ensured that influential western theories were available, and numerous articles published in the medical weeklies show that foreign ideas and developments were discussed by Hungarian psychiatrists who read widely in foreign languages. Furthermore, after acquiring their diploma at the Budapest or Viennese medical faculties, many young Hungarian doctors who became prominent psychiatrists visited renowned western centres of research. Top of the list were Meynert's institute in Vienna and Westphal's centre in Berlin, which excelled in brain and histological research, and Charcot's ward at the Salpêtrière, whose physiological, neural, and hypnosis research attracted doctors from all over the world.

Thus, Schwartzer's outdated comprehensive theory was soon replaced by more contemporary ones, although elements of his ideas and therapeutic solutions survived for decades. However, in no subsequent general textbooks published in Hungary in the second half of the nineteenth century do we find such a complex view of mental illness and related physical and psychic treatments as in Schwartzer's work. What followed was fragmentation: breaking insanity down into well-outlined, distinct disease forms and searching for the remedies specific to each. While the model of the charismatic, patriarchal figure of the alienist was transported to the public asylums (for instance, by Gyula

Niedermann, formerly Schwartzer's assistant doctor, and director of Lipótmező state asylum between 1884 and 1899), over the following decades it went through transformations and resulted in a more balanced relationship between doctor and patient based on their mutual co-operation in new forms of psychiatric practices (for instance, hypnosis research and experimental psychological research) conducted in new types of institutions, such as the clinic, or the observation ward.

University teaching and academic research: the department and the clinic

The issue of university teaching in psychiatry had been discussed by doctors from the middle of the nineteenth century and gained further significance following the rise of new institutions. In order to secure the recruitment of new generations of psychiatrists, to set alternative career patterns, and to strengthen the sense of belonging to the same trade, members of the new profession had to gain legitimacy within the Medical Faculty, and had to work out a curriculum to define the expert field of psychiatry. As early as the 1850s Schwartzer had realized the importance of psychiatric knowledge and practice for general practitioners since, as he argued, they were supposed to at least recognize the earliest signs of mental disease and were in the position of sending these patients to hospital. General knowledge in the field was also important since, in the process of declaring someone mentally deranged in court, the state required expert opinion by two general doctors with medical diplomas. Thus Schwartzer's 1858 textbook, as well as general works in forensic medicine, all argued for the practical education of doctors in mental pathology.

While repeating these concerns from the beginning of the 1870s, the eminent psychiatrist Károly Laufenauer (1848–1901) stressed another, purely scientific claim as well: psychiatry as an exact science was lagging behind because it was not included in university teaching, and there were no possibilities for academic research.[27] Psychiatry's relationship with medicine had been fraught with problems from the beginning and this presented obstacles in establishing it as a separate medical science. These problems centred around questions of objectivity and scientific method. While mental pathology was often dismissed as subjective and lacking hard scientific foundations,[28] Laufenauer believed that, by connecting mental pathology to academic research in neuro-pathology and brain anatomy, this scientific status could be established. In his reflections on this period of the history of psychiatry in Hungary, Erno

Moravcsik (1858–1924), the best clinician of the period and author of many textbooks in mental pathology and forensic psychiatry, acknowledged the role that earlier asylums had played in the history of the discipline. He nevertheless stated that in this period, 'the scientific foundation and further development of psychiatry were connected to the establishment of university clinics', whose furnishing, equipment, and larger doctoral staff finally made academic research possible.[29]

It was Laufenauer who established histological and neurological research in Hungary and succeeded in introducing the systematic study of mental pathology in the medical curriculum.[30] Laufenauer studied medicine at the Medical Faculty in Budapest. From 1873, he worked for three years at the Schwartzer asylum, and he then spent a year studying with the great figures of the German-language schools of neurophysiology: Meynert in Vienna and Westphal in Berlin. He worked for three years at the Lipótmező mental asylum, and from 1881 continued to practise at Saint Roch Hospital. After tireless lobbying from the 1870s, the Department of Mental Health and Pathology was finally established in 1882 at the Medical Faculty, with Laufenauer as head.

The original model was Griesinger's ideal of a medium-sized clinic connected to the department in the vicinity of other medical clinics, collecting mostly acute cases for patient presentation and undertaking academic research. This model was introduced at many German universities from the mid-1860s. Since Griesinger's model of a separate clinic was not realizable for financial reasons until 1908, the psychiatric observation ward at Saint Roch Hospital was attached to the department.[31] Subsequently the Viennese neuropathologist Meynert's influence was the most considerable in starting neuropathological research.[32] In 1884, Laufenauer's mental observation ward was expanded with the opening of a small nerve-clinic which consisted of a room with 12 beds for nervous patients and a small laboratory for conducting neurological research.

The ward had a variety of functions. There was a constant flow of patients, and, unlike asylums, the ward also treated outpatients, most of them presenting with nervous problems. Ward statistics from the year 1885 show that 327 of the 813 patients treated throughout the year (that is, around 40 per cent) were referred to other institutions, which demonstrates that the clinic served as a centre for the redistribution of patients.[33] Considering the large annual number of patients and the small number of beds, we can conclude that the average time patients spent on the ward was considerably shorter than the time spent in asylums. While all chronic cases were quickly moved on through transfer, it was mostly the acute psychiatric cases (including forensic cases) who were retained and used for experimentation and as teaching cases at the ward.

The main role of the university clinic, however, lay in the fact that it allowed for the development of academic research in the anatomy, chemistry, and physiology of the brain and the nervous system, and thus was instrumental in the appropriation of the neurological sciences by psychiatry. In Hungary, brain and neural research were rooted in two distinct areas. These were first conducted within the field of internal medicine, and even by the turn of the twentieth century, some of the eminent neurologists who also performed psychiatric clinical practice identified themselves primarily as internists; the best-known of these was Ernő Jendrássik. The other area was psychiatry.[34] As Moravcsik reminisced: due to this new interest in neural research from the 1870s, mental pathology clinics transformed into laboratories of the healthy and pathological anatomy and histology of the central nervous system. The influence of Meynert, Westphal, Wernicke, Ebbinghaus and other excellent representatives of the anatomical and experimental psychophysiological investigation became influential in Hungary and gave rise to its own areas of research.[35]

Laufenauer and his assistant, Károly Schaffer, are seen as the fathers of modern neurology in Hungary, combining clinical practice in nervous disorders with patho-anatomical studies at the university clinic. While Laufenauer, with his experience of asylums, was from an older generation of neurologically-orientated psychiatrists, Schaffer embodied the new type of researcher with his primary preoccupation in focused study: he conducted brain-histological research at the clinic, and prepared fine excisions which he tirelessly studied under the microscope. Schaffer's absorption in his brain sections and histological research illustrate the decline of interest studying the 'whole' patient. In a sense, these new kinds of studies reduced the patient to the brain, the nerves, and the nervous system.

Neuro-physiological interest also led doctors to conduct research in areas such as hypnotism, where they were often preoccupied with physiological experiments rather than therapy. From the middle of the 1880s, the two most prominent psychiatrists in pioneering hysteria and hypnosis research were Laufenauer and Jendrássik. Laufenauer's treatment of the hysterical patient Ilma, and Jendrássik's hypnotic experiments with her, reveal how their work framed hysteria and the hypnotized hysterical patient, and give insights into the nature of such research and the doctor–patient relationship.[36] Accounts of hypnosis and hysteria give rise to a peculiar and strong image of the patient and demonstrate the gendering of the conceptual frame of medical discourse, as will be discussed in the next section.

Framing the disease hysteria

Ilma was treated by Laufenauer in 1885 and Jendrássik in 1887, and became the star hysterical patient in Budapest medical circles at a time of rapidly growing European interest in hypnosis research. In the mid-1880s, Laufenauer published several articles on hysteria, and Jendrássik experimented with hypnosis with Ilma for nine months, publishing his findings in several papers (his great interest in hypnosis stemming from his visit to Charcot's ward at the Salpêtrière in 1885). After living in a convent for 16 years, Ilma had escaped and established an independent life for herself. She dressed in men's clothes, forged documents to seek jobs, became a petty thief and a swindler, and showed an open attraction for girls. In 1885 Laufenauer observed Ilma and gave his expert opinion on her mental state: concluding that she was suffering from hysteria, he exempted her from legal responsibility. Ilma's case contained many examples of female social deviance, and was the most elaborated, lengthy first case of hysteria that Laufenauer published in the medical weeklies. Thus it offers a compelling example of how hysteria could be framed by the medical community.

In the nineteenth century, the medical concept of hysteria and its social meanings were intricately intertwined. The medical/psychiatric conception of hysteria was informed by commonsense views on woman's nature, the female body and deviant social behaviour. Contemporary textbooks on mental illness made much of the enormous influence of female biology on the integrity of mind and the morality of women. At the same time, social behaviour (especially socially deviant forms of behaviour) constituted a central aspect of the medical description of hysteria. Thus, Ilma's cross-dressing and alleged lesbianism become inseparable from her disease. Laufenauer's description of Ilma's conditions and course of disease combines the usual somatic and neurological symptoms of hysteria (which included frequent acute seizures, convulsive fits, headaches, faints, twitching, tonic and 'clonic' convulsions, reflex and sensory problems) with constant references to her deviant social behaviour.[37]

The psychiatric description portrays Ilma as a restless, sleepless, deceitful liar, a lesbian constantly thinking of how to trespass into forbidden territories, rather than a helpless patient in need of treatment.

Laufenauer constructs the image of the nervous and uncontrollable woman. His medical thinking and descriptions are saturated with social meanings, and register social anxieties surrounding cross-dressing and female homosexuality. In his concluding psychiatric opinion, Laufenauer highlights the causative relation between hysteria and deviancy: 'her common sense and consciousness are enlightened not by judgement and reason, but by the animal instinct leading towards a perverse way of living and a perverse sexual instinct'.[38]

Ilma's factual life becomes the psychiatric 'novel' of medicalized deviance. In the convention of the nineteenth-century novel, female cross-dressing was the symbol of individuality, of female aspirations and rebellion. It stood for the power to transcend the constraints imposed on women in society. In Ilma's life, it was the male garment that made her 'invisible' as a woman. Establishing her independent life also required money and fake documents. Stealing and forgery are thus the necessary crimes accompanying Ilma's cross-dressing. The choice of a deviant lifestyle enabled her to invade parts of the public sphere closed to decent and respectable women and proved to be an effective means of establishing economic and personal independence. It is this power of Ilma, this socially deviant behaviour, that is being medicalized: the psychiatrist uses the socio-medical argumentation not simply to exempt her morally and legally, but to find her problematic from the medical/psychiatric point of view. Psychiatry here takes on the normative function and via the medicalisation of deviant behaviour reinforces the boundaries distinguishing normal from abnormal, acceptable from deviant, and healthy from pathological.

The dissected, headless frog, or the hypnotized body

In Jendrássik's descriptions of the hypnotic experiments with Ilma, the body of the hypnotized hysteric appears as *deceived and deceptive* at the same time.[39] On the one hand, the senses entirely mislead and betray the hypnotized person to experience phenomena which do not really exist. When suggested to experience anaesthesia, Ilma does not feel the piercing pain of a needle thrust into her arm to the bone. When told to be deaf to the horrible noise of the drum, she does not hear it, when told to be blind, she sees nothing but darkness around. On the other hand, Ilma *appears* to feel the heat that no one else can feel, she *seems* to see unwritten letters, hear the silent sounds. With this betrayal of the senses, the body of the patient loses its ability for defence, for self-preservation, and finally may even become self-destructive. When told not to breathe, 'for a long time her chest and abdominal wall remained motionless, her face turned pale, and her body started to shiver, when finally there was some *inspiratio*'.[40] When told to vomit, the hypnotized body cannot stop emptying the contents of the stomach. And when, during cruel and outrageous experiments, the woman's skin was touched with an ordinary object which was suggested to be a heated piece of metal, the body produced serious burns that caused considerable pain and took more than three weeks to heal.

The body of the hypnotized patient is shown to lack 'normal' contact with the world around it: with the senses disturbed, an 'objective' perception of the world through the body becomes impossible. The most frequent phenomenon among hysterics and hypnotized women was the *hyperexcitabilité neuro-musculaire* – that is, an increased reflex sensibility combined with frequent involuntary muscular contractions to stimulus. While the senses break down and are no longer able to mediate between the self and the outer world, the body cannot help overreacting to stimuli in an involuntary and uncontrollable way.

Jendrássik, an adherent representative of organic psychiatry, sought to find the key to the hypnotic state in the structure of the brain. In his thinking, the hypnotic state is characterized by the functional incapability of the brain to judge, compare and associate – the active and productive mental capabilities traditionally regarded as male that are missing in the hypnotized person. While hysteria had been traditionally seen as the intensification of the female nature, the same is true of the hypnotized patient, who becomes an uncontrollable body with deceptive senses, lacking any power of the mind. The presumed unity of the mind, soul and body in the healthy and normal person is exchanged here for a breach between them. Although Jendrássik criticized Hyppolyte Bernheim for comparing a hypnotized person in the lethargic phase to a headless, dissected frog, with the connotations of his theory of the hypnotic state, Jendrássik in fact reproduced this parallel.

The 'construction' of the hypnotized person in the experimental setting, regardless of their actual gender, appears to be a creature endowed with capabilities commonly regarded as female – while at the same time lacking male/human characteristics. This experimental result is then turned into psychiatric knowledge by the case being included in medical weeklies and the theoretical findings built into general textbooks. Jendrássik – consciously or unconsciously – translated social values and beliefs into the language of science in order to explain a complex phenomenon, while at the same time successfully strengthening these notions and values. Laufenauer and Jendrássik's examples thus reveal that medical theory construction and the framing of disease is greatly informed by social values and demonstrates the mutual dependence between medical and general social discourses.

Such an image of the patient as arises from Jendrássik's account could not be further distanced from the image to be found in Schwartzer's theory or in subsequent works by alienists. There, the holistic view of the individual patient, the scrupulous study of their bodily and psychic phenomena was meant to be instrumental in healing. Here, the fragmentation of the person and the body of the patient was to reveal new information on the bodily processes and function of the brain and the nervous system. In these later cases, the psychiatrist still poses as the powerful figure, which suggests an uneven power relationship between doctor and patient: his unappeasable curiosity and enchantment with the experiments push him to unacceptable lengths, producing much pain to the patient. However, as I have discussed elsewhere,[41] the doctor–patient relationship in an experimental setting is, in fact, much more complex. The patient could retain certain power, partly because of the doctor's vested interest in the success of the experiments and his fears of the patient's dissimulation. As the most important contributor to the success of the experiments, the patient's attitude and willingness to partake in the experiments was very important. Furthermore, patients could creatively use the knowledge gained in the psychiatric setting for their own benefit, and they often followed clear strategies. In Ilma's case, convicted as a petty criminal, her choices were either to go to prison or to let the doctor exploit her high suggestibility and contribute to the hypnotic experiments – the joint project of doctor and patient.

Great hopes in vain?

By the 1890s there was widespread disillusionment with regard to the usefulness of neural research from a practical psychiatric point of view. While most mental pathology textbooks from the 1880s included the discussion of neurological findings related to certain disease forms, in his book published in 1890, Salgó justified his almost complete neglect of neurological and histological explications with the verdict that 'all the great hopes that a decade earlier still surrounded pathological and anatomical studies were in vain'. He believed that 'the anatomical basis of mental illnesses is still an undiscovered area, and it is still the question of the future if it will ever be mapped.'[42] He admitted that anatomical research had produced some knowledge about the functions of the central nervous system, but this still added little to the development of mental pathology, and brought doctors no closer to therapy.[43] Salgó spoke up for alienists, who found it crucial to shift the attention to the brain and nerves back to the living patient and the manifestations of his illness.

A debate between Salgó and Laufenauer at the 1900 National Congress of Psychiatrists highlights the rivalry between the asylum and the university clinic. In discussing what kind of psychiatric knowledge and experience students should acquire during their university studies, the asylum doctor Salgó spoke for alienists. He claimed that exclusive medical practice at the university clinic was insufficient for students since the long-term observation of patients was impossible: most patients were retained there only for a short time, very rarely for the entire period of their mental illness. This, in addition to the administrative and forensic aspects of the psychiatrist's work, he asserted, could only be studied in depth at the asylum.[44] Laufenauer rejected this idea, downplaying the necessity of student medical practice at asylums. He realized that the failures witnessed during the last years of the nineteenth century had shattered both the traditional asylum and the histological research centres. Neither the treatment in overcrowded asylums, nor the narrow attention on neural research which, for a while, vindicated exclusive scientific status for itself at the expense of clinical investigation, had brought much success in the treatment of patients.[45] In Laufenauer's mind, the solution was the integration of different psychiatric approaches. Thus, he emphasized the combined teaching of mental and nervous disorders at the clinic, 'since the two disciplines are inseparable', believing that a doctor without a sound basis in nervous disorders and neurology could in no way grasp mental illnesses.[46]

Laufenauer played a more important role in this phase of the history of Hungarian psychiatry than any other of his colleagues. His extensive knowledge and varied experience in different types of institutions made him open to new approaches. Shortly before his death he supported Pál Ranschburg, one of the first Hungarian representatives of experimental psychology, in setting up a Wundtian laboratory at the university clinic.[47] Finally, Laufenauer's endeavour to achieve the integration of clinical research and neurology was realized in 1908, seven years after his death, with the establishment of the large, separate, modern University Clinic of Mental- and Neuro-pathology in Balassa Street, Budapest, close to the other university clinics. The new clinic was considerably larger than the previous one (160 beds instead of 40), which made the long-term observation and treatment of both mental and nervous patients possible. Furthermore, it was equipped with modern laboratories where Schaffer could continue his research and establish his neurological school.

The head of this new clinic was Laufenauer's former student and colleague Ernő Moravcsik. He was Kraepelin's most prominent Hungarian follower, and the clinical trend he represented 'rehabilitated' the patient by embracing a more holistic view. He reformed patient observation and produced lengthy case studies, with the description of the patient's condition at the time of admission ranging from between 10 and 30 pages, and the report on the course of disease often exceeding 60 pages and including the detailed account of matters such as dreams, doctor–patient dialogues, and association-experiments with reaction times.[48] At the clinic, Moravcsik used methods of experimental psychology, and he supported the first representatives of psychoanalysis at a time when other psychiatric circles despised the new movement. The new university clinic thus served integrative functions in a period of fragmenting psychiatric practice, and at least temporarily put an end to the rivalry between the traditional asylum and the former university clinic.

From private asylum to university clinic

Hungarian psychiatry went through a period of remarkable development during the second part of the nineteenth century. After the appearance of the first small private asylum in 1850 and Schwartzer's antiquated views as presented in his 1858 book (the first 'modern' Hungarian work on mental pathology), and in the flourishing times after the political compromise with Austria in 1867, state psychiatric institutions and hospital observation wards mushroomed. The gradually emerging psychiatric profession proved open to new influences, which was seen as fundamental in developing a Hungarian psychiatry, which in turn was understood as a symbol of Hungary taking its rightful position among civilized nations.

By the 1880s Hungarian Psychiatrists were quick to adopt the latest German, French, British and Swiss ideas and theories. Biographies of eminent Hungarian doctors show that increasing numbers of them visited outstanding centres of research throughout Europe, and cultivated good personal and professional relationships with foreign psychiatrists. In the second part of the nineteenth century, Hungarian psychiatric history shows broadly similar trends to those that could be observed in the

West (although further detailed study is necessary to show its idiosyncratic features). The failure of the therapeutic asylum and the strong
influence of German organic psychiatry gave rise to the university clinic
and neuro-pathological research from the 1870s, marking a decline in
personal therapy and a loss of interest in the concept of the living
patient that had been the focus of asylum psychiatry. From the 1890s,
disillusionment over the practical application of neurological sciences
for therapeutic purposes sharpened the rivalry between the asylum and
the small university clinic. By this time, the former represented over-
crowdedness and the desperate use of sedatives, while the latter was criticized for an inadequate approach to mental patients, and neither could
show much therapeutic success. The new, large university clinic opened
in 1908 fulfilled an integrative function by supporting diverse organic
and psychological approaches, and succeeded in nurturing clinical psychiatry represented by Kraepelin in Germany.

The various institutional settings, from which I have singled out the
asylum and the university clinic, together with their distinct practices
and views of the psychiatrist's role, helped to frame different models of
the doctor, the patient and their relationship. In the early private mental asylum where moral therapy was professed in the 1850s and 1860s,
the asylum community was framed as a family which mirrored the
familial hierarchy cherished in society. The doctor was posing as a patriarchal figure while the patient was seen as a child into whose life the
doctor (re)introduced order and discipline. Mental illness was understood as a childlike state, and treatment consisted of a mastery of control over the deluded childish psyche and a manipulation of fear. The
doctor–patient relationship was thus characterized by very uneven
power-relations.

The fragmentation in institutions and views on mental illness, as well
as the new emphasis put on alternative functions of the profession (like
academic research), brought about a multiplication of the frames within
which new models of the doctor and the patient emerged by the end of
the nineteenth century. From these, I have given examples for the new
type of researcher conducting histological and anatomical studies, and
the hypnotist interested in physiological experiments. The first, with
his preoccupied focus on brain sections and histological research,
reduced the patient to the brain, the nerves and the nervous system,
with little sign of interest in the living patient, or the holistic view professed by asylum doctors. The second example showed a different sort
of fragmentation of the patient's person and body. The kind of physiological experiments with hypnosis described above demonstrate the

primacy of experimentation over treatment where the unity of the mind, soul and body of the person was sacrificed. While these experiments still show the enhanced power of the doctor over the patient, doctors in such experimental settings were more exposed to the patients, since success greatly depended on the latter's contribution.

With its manifold social functions and increasing 'presence' in society, it is not surprising to find that, by the end of the nineteenth century psychiatry gained cultural monopoly over a number of issues related to the hygiene of everyday life as well as a 'healthy' society. Mental illness penetrated everyday life not only by becoming a reality for a growing number of patients and their relatives in the emergent institutions. The fact that the mental illnesses of eminent politicians, poets, painters, and doctors were widely discussed in the mass media (the best early example is the madness of the eminent aristocrat politician, Count István Széchenyi, from the middle of the century) and that there was a growing popular scientific literature on the topic, all led to psychiatric thinking becoming pervasive in the wider public imagination by 1900. However, probably even more influential was the literary production of the era which provided numerous descriptions and stories related to madness. Partly due to urbanization, the strengthening of the bourgeois middle classes, and the impact of the French novel, there was an increasing preoccupation with insanity in Hungarian literature from the mid-nineteenth century onwards.

Influenced by Eugène Sue's *Les Mystères de Paris* (1842), two popular novelists of the period produced novels under similar titles. Lajos Kuthy's (1813–64) short stories and novel *Hazai rejtelmek* ('Hungarian Mysteries', 1846–7) as well as Ignác Nagy's (1810–54) *Magyar titkok* ('Hungarian Secrets', 1844–5) portray the growing urban life of Pest with all the crimes of the underworld, miseries of the poor and scandals of the bourgeoisie and the wealthy.[49] Madness and secrets are the indispensable keys to these works. Mór Jókai (1825–1904), the greatest, most popular and prolific Hungarian novelist of the period, produced numerous novels which included stories about madness. As early as his first novel *Hétköznapok* ('Everydays', 1846), he wrote of a young heroine abducted by a man and forced to live with him, who later goes mad after childbirth. In his novels from the late 1860s we find more and more characters with deep inner conflicts, split mentality and double lives that echo contemporary psychiatric literature on nervousness and insanity. Madness is constructed as a form of social critique in several works: in his late novel *Öreg ember, nem vén ember* ('It's Not Age That Counts', 1900) the engineer hero's career and life is destroyed by business machinations and ends in madness, while in *Enyim, tied, övé* ('Mine, Yours, His', 1875) Áldorfai is first enriched by investing in railway shares, then becomes obsessed with money and is ruined. The heroes of both novels end up in lunatic asylums.[50]

Many poems and ballads by the celebrated poet János Arany (1817–82) also take up the topic of madness, whilst another highly popular and productive novelist, Kálmán Mikszáth, regarded *Beszterce ostroma* ('The Siege of Beszterce', 1894) as his favourite novel. In this the eccentric hero closes off his lands from the modern world of the late nineteenth century and lives in the illusion of being the last lord, waging war with the help of his peasants, his obsession growing into a mania. The short stories and novels by Gyula Krúdy (1878–1933) and Géza Csáth (1887–1919) likewise illustrate the turn-of-the-century mentality of psychiatry, with the latter author also being a psychiatrist practising psychoanalysis.

Hungarian literature of the period thus elaborated on the topic of madness and was reflexive of psychiatry. Many writings register fears surrounding the legitimate functioning of asylums and air the suspicion that families could use it as a place to dump their unwanted relatives. Other writings, however, served the critical function of putting a mirror to society by casting light on social conditions and changes that were perceived as dangerous to the individual. In some of these, the asylum is shown as the only 'normal' retreat, the only source of peace in a mad society. In a manner similar to the increasing popular psychiatric writings of the late nineteenth century, novels also castigate 'civilizational forces' and blame the spread of nervous disorders on overexertion for the sake of social advancement, on speedy industrialization, on the demands of business and the financial system, and on pauperism. Just as in contemporary asylums and at observation wards, nervous and insane heroes are recruited from all strata of society. We can read about simple peasant girls or urban maids gone mad after being seduced and then cast off by their landlords, and about swindlers and petty thieves (like Ilma) caught up in different psychiatric institutions, but also about distinguished male members of the urban elite who become slowly deranged by their debaucherous lifestyles (and who in fact populated asylums as patients suffering from paralysis progressiva). Asylum statistics and psychiatric textbooks thus form only one type of documentation concerning nineteenth-century treatment and understanding of insanity, while other forms of cultural production reveal the complex world of psychiatry and madness deeply embedded in a modernizing society.

Notes

1. I am grateful to George Rousseau, John Forrester, Natsu Hattori and the editors for their encouragement and comments on this essay. I wish to thank the librarians of the Semmelweis Library for the History of Medicine, Budapest, for their kind help in my research.
2. László Epstein, 'Magyarország elmebetegügye' ['Mental Health Care in Hungary'], *Gyógyászat* ['Medicine'] 38 (1897): 582.
3. For general histories of madness and psychiatry, see Roy Porter, *Madness: a Brief History* (Oxford: Oxford University Press, 2002) and Edward Shorter, *A History of Psychiatry: From the Era of the Asylum to the Age of Prozac* (New York and Toronto: John Wiley and Sons, Inc, 1997).
4. Porter, *Madness*, 120.
5. See Epstein, 'Magyaroszág elmebetegügye', 582, and Kálmán Pándy, *Gondoskodás az elmebetegekről más államokban és nálunk* ['The Care of Mental Patients Abroad and at Home'] (Gyula: Corvina, 1905) 383–4, and Ernő Moravcsik, 'A psychiatria fejlődése hazánkban az utolsó 50 év alatt' ['The Development of Psychiatry in Our Country During the Last 50 Years'], *Orvosi Hetilap* ['Medical Weekly'] 1 (1906): 38–42. In fact, the very first private asylum was opened by Jenő Pólya in 1840, but it only treated a few patients and was closed within a year.
6. On the Schwartzer dynasty, see the booklet Nándor Horánszky, *A Schwartzer-család a magyar tudományos életben: Bibliográfia* ['The Schwartzer Family in Hungarian Scientific Life: Bibliography'] (Budapest: Plantin Kiadó, 2000).
7. János Lyachovics, 'Könyvismertetés: Schwartzer Ferenc: A lelki betegségek általános kór- és gyógytana' ['Book Review: Ferenc Schwartzer: General Pathology and Treatment of Psychic Disorders'], *Orvosi Hetilap* ['Medical Weekly'] 29 (1858): 460.
8. Ferencz Schwartzer, *A lelki betegségek általános kór- és gyógytana, törvényszéki lélektannal* ['General Pathology and Treatment of Psychic Disorders, with Forensic Psychology'] (Budapest, 1858) 22.
9. Porter, *Madness*, 100.
10. Schwartzer's assistant doctor, János Lyachovics, 'Töredékek a budai magán őrüldéből' ['Fragments from the Buda private madhouse'], *Orvosi Hetilap* ['Medical Weekly'] 12 (1857): 187.
11. Ferencz Schwartzer, *A Budai Magán Elme- és Ideggyógyintézet tudósítója és tizenkét évi működésének eredménye* ['Report on the Buda Private Mental and Nerve Institute and its 12-year Operation'] (Buda, 1864) 9.
12. Lyachovics, 'Töredékek', 187.
13. My calculations based on the first fourteen-year statistics of the asylum show that 57 per cent of patients belonged to 'the more educated class', 37 per cent to the middle class, and only 6 per cent came from the lower classes. See Schwartzer, *A Budai*, 12.
14. Schwartzer, *A Budai*, 9.
15. Schwartzer, *A lelki*, 95, 8.
16. Károly Bolyó, 'Tudósítás Schwartzer tr. budai magán őrüldéjéből' ['Reports from Schwartzer's private madhouse in Buda'], *Gyógyászat* ['Medicine'] 17 (1861): 348–52.
17. Schwartzer, *A lelki*, 122–3.

18. Ibid., 93.
19. Ibid., 122–3.
20. See Pándy, *Gondoskodás az elmebetegekrűl*, 369 and János Fekete, 'Intézetünk megalapítása és müködése 1900–ig' ['The Foundation of Our Institute and Its History until 1900'], *Az Országos Ideg- és Elmegyógyintézet 100 éve* ['Hundred Year Anniversary of the National Institute for Nervous and Mental Diseases'] (Budapest, 1968) 73, 74, 77. In large public asylums, 'no restraint' was recommended by the Interior Ministry only in 1900. See the Ministry of Interior's *Magyarország elmebetegügye az 1900. évben* ['Mental Health Care in Hungary in 1900'] (Budapest, 1901) 11.
21. Schwartzer, *A Budai*, 9.
22. János Lyachovics, 'Töredékek a budai magán őrüldéből' ['Fragments from the Buda private madhouse'], *Orvosi Hetilap* ['Medical Weekly'] 6 (1858): 85–8.
23. Károly Bolyó, 'Tudósítás Schwartzer tr. budai magánőrüldéjéből' ['Reports from Schwartzer's private madhouse in Buda'],' *Gyógyászat* ['Medicine'] 26 (1861): 558–9, 578–9.
24. See Porter, *Madness*, 89–123 and Shorter, *A History of Psychiatry*, 33–69.
25. See Tibor Győri Nádudvari, *Az Orvostudományi Kar története, 1770–1935* ['The History of the Medical Faculty'] (Budapest, 1936) 62–3, 613; Béla Kollarits, István Joó and Géza Bajza (eds), *Magyarország gyógyintézeteinek évkönyve, 1934* ['Yearbook of Hungary's Hospitals'] (Budapest, 1935).
26. Shorter, *A History of Psychiatry*, 69.
27. Károly Laufenauer, 'Néhány szó a hazai elmekórtani oktatás tárgyában' ['A Few Words on Teaching Mental Pathology in Hungary'], *Orvosi Hetilap* ['Medical Weekly'] 45 (1876): 90.
28. See Jakab Salgó, *Az elmekórtan tankönyve* ['Textbook of Mental Pathology'] (Budapest, 1890) 1–2.
29. Moravcsik, 'A psychiatria', 38.
30. For Laufenauer, see the memorial speeches: Ernő Moravcsik, 'Emlékbeszéd Laufenauer Károly felett' ['Remembering Károly Laufenauer'], *Orvosi Hetilap* ['Medical Weekly'] 4 (1906): 82–95; Károly Schaffer, 'Laufenauer Károly jelentősége' ['The Importance of Károly Laufenauer'], *Orvosi Hetilap* ['Medical Weekly'] 9 (1928): 243–7.
31. Laufenauer, 'Néhány szó', 91–2.
32. For German and Austrian university and biological psychiatry, see Shorter, *A History of Psychiatry*, 71–81.
33. *Orvosi Hetilap* ['Medical Weekly'] 5 (1886): 134–5.
34. See Károly Schaffer, 'Az elme- és idegkórtannak egymáshoz való viszonya és fejlődése. A constitutio fogalma [The Relationship of Mental- and Nervous Pathology, and Their Development. The Concept of Constitution],' *Orvosi Hetilap [Medical Weekly]* 7 (1925): 132–7.
35. Moravcsik, 'A psychiatria', 36.
36. For a detailed and lengthy reconstruction of Ilma's case, see Emese Lafferton, 'Hypnosis and Hysteria as Ongoing Processes of Negotiation: Ilma's Case from the Austro-Hungarian Monarchy', *History of Psychiatry* 50 (2002): 177–96; 51 (2002): 305–27.
37. Károly Laufenauer, 'Hystero-epilepsia; lopás és okmányhamisítás [Hystero-Epilepsia; Theft and Forgery],' *Orvosi Hetilap [Medical Weekly]* 31 (1885): 70–1.

38. Laufenauer, 'Hystero-epilepsia', 75.
39. Ernő Jendrássik, 'A suggestióról' ['On Suggestion'], *Orvosi Hetilap* ['Medical Weekly'] 23 (1888): 746–9, 781–5.
40. Ibid., 747.
41. Lafferton, 'Hypnosis and Hysteria', 177–96, 305–27.
42. Jakab Salgó, *Az elmekórtan*, iii–iv.
43. Ibid., 3.
44. Jakab Salgó, 'Az elmegyógyászat oktatásáról' ['On Teaching Mental Pathology'], in László Epstein (ed.), *Első Országos Elmeorvosi Értekezlet Munkálatai* ['First National Congress of Psychiatrists'] (Budapest: Pallas, 1901) 85–8.
45. This criticism can also be found in Moravcsik's account of the history in the period: see Moravcsik, 'A psychiatria', 38–42.
46. See Laufenauer's response to Salgó in Salgó, 'Az elmegyógyászat', 87.
47. Csaba Pléh, *A lélektan története* ['The History of Psychology'] (Budapest: Osiris, 2000) 277.
48. See Ferenc Pisztora, 'A 100 éves budapesti Pszichiátriai Tanszék és Klinika kezdeti időszaka' ['The Early Phase of the Hundred Year Old Budapest Psychiatric Department and Clinic'], *Ideggyógyászati Szemle* ['Neurological Review'] 36 (1983) 206.
49. I am grateful to Anna Fábri for her suggestions.
50. See also his *Akik kétszer halnak meg* ('Those Who Die Twice', 1881).

Part III

The Patient's Narratives and Images

10
Patients and Words: a Lay Medical Culture?

Philip Rieder

The chronology of medical history is generally organized around medical discourses and the evolution of 'scientific' knowledge. The position or role of the patient has long been ignored or, at best, inferred from medical knowledge, past or present. Roy Porter's call, almost twenty years ago, for the development of a history of medicine from the patients' perspective has done little to transform this way of considering the medical world of the patient in history.[1] Events such as the invention of the clinic and the discovery of the world of the infinitely small, structure the way in which medical history and the history of the patient are written. In fact, a now-famous article written well before Porter's call, Nicholas Jewson's 'Disappearance of the Sick-man from Medical Cosmology (1770–1870)',[2] offers a model explaining the evolution of the patient's role through history and contributes to shaping the way patient's history is thought of today. And yet, in the aftermath of Porter's appeal, much was reported and published on individual or family relations to health in the past. Roy and Dorothy Porter have produced a particularly extensive book based on patients' lives, strategies and stories.[3] Through their research and that of many others, some knowledge about the general reality of patients' situations, apprehensions and strategies has now been accummulated.[4] It is no longer possible to claim that, as Roy Porter wrote in his initial article: 'We lack a historical atlas of sickness experience and response'.[5] We now have an atlas albeit, as suggested in Porter's initial proposition, a descriptive one.

   One of the main characteristics of what can be considered as 'patient history' is that the figure studied extends beyond the 'doctor's patient' or the user of medical services. The very title of Porter and Porter's book, *In Sickness and in Health*, signals the scope of the subject.[6] The 'patient' discussed, as it is the case in the following pages, is not only the client of any given healer, but the individual as he or she deals with health-related issues. Plotting a course somewhere between Barbara Duden, in her remarkable investigation into body history, and Françoise Loux and Philippe Richard in their appraisal of traditional proverbs, the approach chosen in this essay is hermeneutic.[7] The aim is to demonstrate the importance of focusing on lay discourse in order to understand lay medical culture and the historical potential of that particular culture in apprehending past medical realities. The material used comes from an important series of sources (mainly diaries and letters) relating to patients in the region around Lake Geneva in the eighteenth century. The patients considered here do not represent all strata of society: they all write, read and are well read. Among those discussed below are two famous natural historians, Charles Bonnet (1720–93) and Horace-Bénédict de Saussure (1740–99), two well-known writers, Jean-Jacques Rousseau (1712–78) and Isabelle de Charrière (1740–1805), and a series of less well-known figures: the village clergyman Théophile Rémy Frêne (1727–1804), a Genevan housewife, Jeanne-Mary Bellamy (1725–85), and a series of patients of the famous Swiss physician Samuel-Auguste Tissot (1728–97).

Existing contributions to 'patient studies' constitute a logical starting point for the purposes of this text. In most cases, the processes of reconstruction, tale-telling and publishing have induced social historians and other commentators to assimilate the disorders of the past into diseases meaningful today. Phrases such as 'we can tentatively identify as'[8] or 'perhaps what we would call'[9] such and such a disease, appear regularly in even the best historical discourse and are deemed necessary in order to render complaints intelligible to contemporary readers. On the other hand, historians regularly refer to present-day medical specialists in order to ascertain what is actually happening in different discourses about the body. Until recently, it was indeed necessary to refer to biomedical knowledge in order to 'understand' past pathological conditions. In 1968, for instance, Marjorie Nicolson and George Rousseau refer to no less than 5 specialists in their study on Alexander Pope and opt for an all-embracing diagnosis: 'kyphoscoliosis'.[10] In so doing, they attribute an important interpretative role to contemporary medical culture both in understanding their texts and Pope. The means that the 'interpreter's' role in transcoding discourses is certainly not neutral.[11] Naming is important to understand the 'real' object discussed, the disease itself, and, as Charles Rosenberg quite rightly asserts, naming is a distinctive feature of our culture.[12] But was it so in the past? This problem may be considered in the same manner as a well-known methodological danger, that of considering all medical practices of the past in the light of present-day knowledge: the confrontation of past acts with present knowledge leads historians to consider the former dangerous or, at the best, useless.[13] In this particular perspective, positive transformations in illness are seen as resulting from what is known as the Placebo effect or, more simply, the natural evolution of the sick person's state.[14]

Labels and patients

In order to reach beyond common knowledge and to achieve a deeper understanding of pathological labels in the past, it is thus necessary to avoid contemporary medical categories. At the same time, and for similar reasons, it can be argued that past scholarly medical knowledge can also bias the interpretation of lay discourse. By purposefully rejecting both contemporary and past medical knowledge as interpretative categories, it should be possible to build an approach closer to the sources themselves, an investigation of the words used by the patients. The exploration conducted in the following pages is far from comprehensive. Its modest aim is to isolate a series of characteristics of lay discourse. The first point that should be made is that in letters, diaries and other texts written by patients, the relationship between illness and the name of any given disease is rarely explicit. In fact, in letters to Tissot, many patients refer to the doctors' names for disease with a certain reserve. In one example, a M. Magelli, established in the town of Fribourg, in a letter addressed to Tissot, discusses the illness of a women aged 50, who had previously 'suffered from a long illness which the physicians call an effusion ('épanchement') of bilious humour'[15] and in another letter to Tissot Marie Agier, living in Geneva, compares her present complaint to a previous 'long disease that Mister Tronchin called an inflammation in the peritoneum'.[16] In other cases, the names given by physicians describe different phases in the sick person's career. 'The gentlemen', comments Elisabeth Develay in a letter concerning her husband's long illness, previously known as a 'slight catarrhal fever', and referring to the doctor's visit, 'named his illness at that time a slight inflammation of the chest, a "peripneumonie" and a discharge of bile'.[17] And these are just two episodes in a long illness, clearly understood as evolving over time, if not as a series of different complaints. Many names describing a sick person's state are assimilated to physicians' jargon, and rarely have the ontological meaning one would expect today. Some lay actors are overtly critical of professional opinions and feel competent to voice their own interpretation. For example, the village minister Théophile-Rémy Frêne plays an important role in his wife's health during their married life (1758–1803). This entails negotiating at different moments with a variety of healers, among whom was the physician Dr Friedrich-Ludwig Watt (1737–after 1803). In an evening in 1800, at the age of 58, Mrs Frêne loses her wits and behaves in an incoherent and alarming way. The next morning, from his country vicarage, Frêne addresses a letter to Watt, established in Bienne, a small town in the neighbourhood. The physician sends a few remedies and promises a visit for the next day. When he finally gets to see Mrs Frêne, she is already on the mend. Watt assures her husband that there is no 'danger' and explains the crisis as resulting from an 'attack of indigestion'. In a very matter-of-fact manner, Frêne adds his own comments concerning the episode in his diary: 'For my part, I think it was a violent attack of the nerves, due to the fact that my wife had been doing too much spinning with her arms in the air', an exercise to which she was not accustomed.[18] Dis-ease is almost systematically given meaning and the latter is regularly found in the patient's past. Patients, or those close to patients, have the best knowledge of these all-important variables. Their interpretation is, as suggest the cases related here, paramount and they do not hesitate to voice their disagreement with physicians' explanations.

It is clear from the evidence given here that it is quite common for lay figures to engage in negotiations with physicians. This attitude comes easily to well-read patients, such as the famous natural historian Horace-Bénédict de Saussure, who was in the habit of writing to well-known practitioners about the health of his close relatives. Among these, his sister, regularly reported to be ill, is sometimes mentioned. As a young spinster, she is involuntarily involved in a literary scandal: in January 1773, the periodical *Correspondance littéraire*, written by Grimm, associates her presence at Ferney with a bout of strangury suffered by Voltaire.[19] The disapproval of the young lady's conduct expressed by Geneva's society and the illness of Miss de Saussure in the following year are clearly related by her family and friends. As winter dawns a year after the event, her brother, clearly worried, mentions her case in a letter to the famous physician and physiologist Albrecht von Haller (1708–77). One of the main problems is a sore ('dartre') – a family complaint from which Saussure himself also suffered. His sister's sore was called by 'M. Tronchin an erysipelatous sore'.[20] But, adds Saussure, 'it is not a dry sore as it flows and sometimes abundantly'. Tronchin is no longer in Geneva and is quite obviously not considered competent in this case. Saussure continues his description: 'At the same time, the blood goes ('se porte') to the head and the upper part of her Body so that her feet are cold and she has a lot of trouble warming them up.' The humours accumulated in the head cause 'severe head aches and a lot of sadness'.[21]

Lay interpretations

Saussure's appreciation of his sister's condition illustrates two important characteristics of lay perceptions of illness. The first appears clearly in the last element of his description. Saussure asserts that the humours accumulated in the head lead to sadness, a symptom of her complaint. It is apparent that, to Saussure, the boundary between the body and the mind are quite clearly porous. In fact, it is worth questioning the validity of the separation between what appear today as two distinct entities. Many patients list among their symptoms terms such as 'agitation', 'prostration' ('accablement'), 'anxiety' ('inquiétude') and 'anguish' ('angoisse'). Agitation and anxiety are very common symptoms, often listed among others:[22] 'Our little Amélie', begins the countess Golowkin in a letter to Tissot, 'has a sore throat, trouble to swallow, a heavy tongue, no sleep, a lot of anxiety and red mouth, tongue and gum.'[23] Such states can be symptoms, or indicators of a future illness: Jeanne-Marie Bellamy Prevost, a contemporary of Saussure, is worried, agitated (often in her sleep) during the year of her diary. She is then 47 years of age and very anxious about the development of her health: agitation and anxiety are among the signs she is attentive to as she awaits a 'Big Illness'.[24] These characteristics are listed next to and carry clearly the same level of meaning as other symptoms. In her case, anxiety and agitation can be read as symptoms and the results of her general situation: the more she worries about her health, the more she is frightened of the effects of her worrying on her health.

Other common appreciations of health hazards, such as the danger of emotions for health or the fact that overheating ('échauffement') can be induced either through bodily or intellectual exertion with the same pathological effects,[25] indicate that health is not just a question concerning the body, or at least not the body as we know it today. This difference can be illustrated through a wide range of lay and medical texts, but the perspective chosen here suggests another means of presenting the distinction: a simple semantic comparison. Today, the body, as defined in a common French dictionary, can be translated as the 'Material part of an animated being' ('Partie matérielle des êtres animés'), thus clearly referring to the physical body. In the fourth edition of the famous *Dictionnaire de l'Académie* (1762), the term means literally 'extensive ('étendu') and impenetrable substance' ('substance étendue et impénétrable').[26] In both eighteenth century dictionaries and discourse, the word body signifies literally the totality of any given man or women, and not just the physical part: it is the self as one is inside, beyond the limit of the skin.[27] Karl Figlio sums up the situation by describing the living body in the eighteenth century as an 'inseparable extension of the self'.[28]

The second feature suggested by the already-mentioned excerpt from Saussure's letter is the internal movement of illness: his sister's humours migrate to her head. The result is clearly opposed to the perception of a coherent or stable illness as we would understand disease today. Internal movement is often reported and generally related to humoural movements, in his case explicitly named, but elsewhere discernible through a series of allusions (verbs and nouns) relating to movement.[29] A flux or related illness (rheum, rheumatism, . . .) are relatively sophisticated expressions of internal humoural displacements. Some are 'felt' or simply related by the patients themselves. During the winter of 1772–73, Mrs Bellamy Prevost is often unwell. In April, she suffers a cold ('rhume'), at first described as 'without cough'. She makes efforts to ignore it.[30] On the second of May, she comments:

> The weather is confused ('s'embrouille'), as is my health, I was not as well as usual last night, I have a pain in the left arm, which becomes acute as soon as I move. I had a lot of trouble getting dressed this morning. Above all, I still suffer from hoarseness, all of this annoys and saddens me, I am afraid of disabilities, I can feel a catarrhal humour rolling here and there.[31]

The correlation between the pain in the arm and the movement of the catarrhal humour is not explicit, but becomes very probable when compared to transformations read or felt by other patients in their own bodies. Some humoural movements go on for years. A young girl was aged six when the first symptoms of a sickness appeared, a simple scab ('gale'). The author of a letter addressed to Tissot more than a decade later summarizes the evolution of her situation:

> Ill advised counsellors suggested mercury frictions on her body. The treatment put a stop to the eruption, but as there was a danger that the humour's course having been interrupted, it may then affect the mass of the blood, and as she complained of severe itching all over her body, warm baths were given to her. These reinstated the

eruption, which became then so strong and so long (it lasted 4 months), that M. Haidelofer, physician at Yverdon, gave her two pills that put an end to the scabies at once. The humours then travelled ('se porter vers'), with violence, to her head, the inside of her nose was particularly affected by spots ('des poutons'). It was decided to bore a hole through her ears and her nose healed. The next year the (same) humour caused another rash of erysipela all over her face. At times it disappeared for one, two or three months

and this situation continued for ten years, until the girl reached her eighteenth year.[32] In many accounts, the movement of humours are clearly isolated. The dis-ease moves, and is often followed by the corresponding displacement of pain.

Patients and words

What then, in lay terms, is diagnosis? Furetière's dictionary suggests that it is either a means to signify a series of symptoms or a method for a physician to recognize the 'nature' of the disease.[33] The first mention of the word in the dictionary of the *Académie française* appears in the third edition (1740), where diagnosis is described as: 'A symptom that indicates the nature of an illness'.[34] Both these definitions are supported by evidence in common lay writing, but the names given by patients suggest a dynamic, fluid or evolutionary perception of dis-ease. The most common words, as it is certainly still the case today, are vague: dis-ease ('mal-aise'), pain and awkwardness ('incommodité') figure among the most used and are not very informative about lay knowledge and interpretations. More interesting are the words used beyond such generalities. For the purpose of this text, only a superficial overview is possible, but even that is sufficient to give a general idea. Among the most common complaints are colds, colics, fevers, inflammations, rheumatisms and dropsys. These terms figure among the terms frequently used and are clearly perceived as passing ills, at least at first. Time is always an important factor in defining what is 'dangerous' – an important concept – and what is not. All these conditions, even a simple cold, carry the potential danger of degenerating into some other, more dangerous illness. By neglecting a cold, for instance, Jean-Jacques Rousseau's condition deteriorates into what he calls a 'flux in the chest' ('fluxion de poitrine'). A clearly 'dangerous' condition.[35] Most of the common complaints listed above are recognized by the patient himself or herself on his or her body, and that with no particular difficulty and very little possible ambiguity: a cold is perceptible thanks to the flux of phlegm, a colic because of its painfulness and the accompanying diarrhoea, a fever is recognized by an initial 'shiver' followed by a quickening pulse, a rheumatism thanks to the accompanying inflammation and a dropsy by the obvious internal accumulation of liquid. Other words describe literally objective realities as they depict visible details: body colour, loss of weight, signs on the skin (erysipela, sores, and so on.).

Patients' discourse can be broken down into numerous other categories of words, some of which are more useful than others in helping us to grasp lay medical concepts. A group, for instance, can be clearly related to internal bodily sensations: the mother (referring to female vapours),[36] nervous affections, biliousness, acrid blood, and so on. The precise meaning of such terms and expressions is difficult to grasp today and the investigation of the situations and sensations concealed behind these words extends beyond the scope of this discussion. The different categories of words listed up to this point are the most apparent, and at the same time the more 'medical' of the words found in the complex narratives of the patients. Other words refer to diseases in a perspective closer to that of today. The names that are more often associated with what can be now understood as clearly identifiable nosological entities are contagious diseases: smallpox, measles and scarlet fever are commonly used, although in many cases the basis of the diagnosis is shaky and regularly proved incorrect. Kitty Fabry, a young Genevese, for instance, catches the measles, although she and her family were convinced that she was immunized thanks to an earlier bout of the disease.[37] A handful of individual diseases are also named. Apoplexy, 'maladie de langueur', gout, asthma and consumption figure among the most commonly used. Each of these terms could potentially be studied individually, and every one of them cover a variety of symptoms and circumstances. But beyond the detailed discussion of each term, their common characteristic is that their usage is not standard. Many patients have only a vague idea of the scholarly definition. The minister Frêne, for instance, observes the multiplication of cases of nervous disorders in the second half of the century, 'also called' he adds in his diary 'the mother or vapours'. The words, clearly distinct in medical texts, are here synonymous.[38] Confusion and imprecision are common in lay texts and are most apparent in the use, as here, of new words. The new vocabulary related to nervous complaints is often used side by side, and with the same logic, as the traditional humoural register: the nerves are fashionable and most certainly liquid.[39] Some patients clearly use the new vocabulary to describe affections that are difficult to describe in other terms.[40] Others are clearly perplexed. Isabelle de Charrière, for instance, although a lot of her time was spent taking care of her health and of those of her friends, and having suffered a lot from her own nerves, remains unsure of their precise meaning. In a letter to a friend about the health of the latter's future husband, she asks: 'Is his regimen not of the sort that could tighten ('tendre') excessively "ce je ne sai quoi" which are called nerves?'[41]

All words used by the laity, no matter how clearly defined, are spun into complex life stories and are most often particularized consequently. Consumption ('phtisie'), for instance, can be associated with the coughing up of blood, and yet many patients do not accept the label so easily.[42] Horace-Bénédict de Saussure's mother, for instance, is ill for long periods of her life and, at different intervals, coughs up blood. Her son is motivated to write to Albrecht von Haller, a physician established in a distant locality, by the danger of his mother being labelled as consumptive – he proceeds to give a detailed explanation of his mother's ills and the medication she had taken over the previous five years, relating a great variety of symptoms (perspiration, spitting, pains, digestion, common bodily evacuations, etc.) – the story is spread over ten pages of the modern edition of their correspondence. The same phenomenon can be observed in other cases.[43] In lay discourse, the emphasis is not on the common aspect of illness, or the similitude between different ills, but rather the particularity of the person and of his or her temperament and constitution.

Singular ills

Considered together, the different groups of words listed so far reveal the complexity of the sickness experience. Interpreting or understanding their usage in different contexts requires detailed investigation: the individual experience, the infinite variations offered by different events conferring meaning, complicate the field. The names given to dis-ease are often integrated into the stories told by patients or their friends and family, stories that often go back a long way and focus on the cause of illness. The importance of the cause is essential for the elaboration of meaning, here cause and diagnosis are often one. The cases of Charles Bonnet and his nephew, Horace-Bénédict de Saussure, as told by the patients themselves illustrate this point in very different ways.[44] Saussure's story is better understood when compared with his mother's complaints mentioned above and also those of his sister. Both of these ladies are valetudinarians most of their lives: they suffer, among other things, from skin rashes and a difficulty to perspire. Horace-Bénédict de Saussure himself suffers from similar complaints.[45] His discretion concerning his own health problems is extreme, to the point that Albrecht von Haller receives an anonymous letter, clearly from Saussure's circle of friends and kin, expressing concern about his reserve on health matters and his habit of self-prescription.[46] There is little to add to Saussure's silence. Such afflictions were poorly regarded in polite society in Geneva[47] and Saussure quite obviously kept his anxiety about his complaints to himself, in his personal notes and short diaries. All considered, Saussure is certainly convinced that he himself was suffering from a hereditary disease which, like his mother before him, he tries to hide as much as possible, possibly in the perspective of his own children's future.

Charles Bonnet's life story is told in his long autobiography, first published in 1948, and can be completed thanks to his voluminous correspondence held today by the Public Library of Geneva. As a child and a young man, his health was good, notwithstanding a slight deafness from which he suffered throughout his life. He discovered natural history as he was preparing to study law and it became his main interest. He made rapid progress and started an important correspondence with one of France's leading natural historians, Antoine Ferchault de Réaumur (1683–1757), and that before even having finished his law studies. Through careful observation, he discovered the mode of reproduction of a variety of aphids. His research lead him to work long hours and within a few years – shortly after his twenty-fourth birthday – his health deteriorated. He lost weight and seemed to be on the verge of a 'maladie de langueur'. The following year, the evolution of his health continued for the worse: 'I could neither read nor write without pain or extreme tiredness.' He notes a 'disturbance' in his eyes without being able to ascertain either the precise location or the cause of the problem. In a series of letters addressed to physicians, he describes the resulting visual deformations, namely filaments that obstruct his vision. Bonnet decides, after having had his eyes examined by opticians and doctors, that his suffering was not due to a cataract.[48] He promptly reduces his usage of the microscope, singled out as the cause of his ills. The relationship between his eye problems and his activities as a natural historian is constantly restated in the following years. In fact, all of his health problems are later reduced to the status of effects of his work and, in contrast to his nephew, he continually repeats this 'fact' all around him: his ills are caused by his activities as a 'homme de lettres'. This can be illustrated in many different contexts, but nowhere better than in his exchange with Jean-Henri-Samuel Formey (1711–97) many years later. The starting point is an injunction by Bonnet to his correspondent to reduce his activities in order to preserve his health, in the course of which he offers his own case as an example of what excessive work can lead to.[49] Formey's answer is surprising. Rather than agreeing with Bonnet, he states that he himself was never better than when working without restraint and he in turn encourages Bonnet to follow his example. Bonnet is shocked and his reaction is illuminating as to the importance of his own interpretation:

A man of letters, who has been writing for more than 26 years on different subjects, most of which are quite abstract, and who can no longer write today without severe stomach troubles which disturb his digestion, which affect his ears and makes him quite deaf, such a man must he continue writing although it is clear that he shall soon be no longer able to produce in this life? Would you prefer to lose a friend before his time or keep him a little longer? Would you take him from a wife, family and friends whom he cherishes and who cherish him in return? And from a homeland to which he is accountable? What I am trying to say is very serious, and if you care for me as I think you do, you will be the first to encourage me to rest . . . I would break the Law of Nature if I did not take the necessary rest. I may rest without shame, I have paid society an honest portion: I gave up the best years of my life.[50]

To sum up, from the patients' perspective, sickness is rarely understood as the effect of a coherent disease – rather, sickness is related to meaning. Meaning is construed by the bodily sensations of the patient, his or her past, and sometimes with the counsel of the practitioner. In a sense, the interpretation of the patient and that of the practitioner need not meet: the practitioner offers counsel, but the understanding is more generally in the patient's hands. This particularity is one of the main reasons why patients are all different – or more precisely singular – in their interactions with ill health. Their singularity can be reduced to the individual apprehension of ill health as it is traditionally related to Galenism – in a sense, already considered, from a learned perspective, a past reality in the eighteenth century.[51] In that light, lay medical culture can be perceived simply as lagging behind the novelties of learned medicine. Yet this proposition can only be maintained if only part of the documentation is considered: the reality of the lay medical world, as suggested in patients' texts, offers a more complex picture. Lay knowledge is not, as one could infer from similarities across time, static.[52] Many accounts show the importance of the circulatory principle of blood in lay interpretations of understanding transformations in health during the eighteenth century and clearly reflect the general adoption of Harvey's principle. At the same time, the vocabulary developed for nervous conditions, used as suggested above, by many patients, conveys what appears to be a new sensitivity and perception of both the self and of health. Furthermore, the interest for anatomy and a 'physiological' understanding of bodily disorders is widespread in the last two-thirds of the century.[53] People such as the country parson Frêne read anatomy books, examine dead bodies and discuss the results of post-mortems with physicians.[54] The history of therapeutics, as yet little explored, may contribute to a better understanding not only of what people used to fight off ill health, but of the evolution of patients' expectations and perceptions of ill health: the patients of the eighteenth century certainly request gentle remedies, coherent with their gentle and sensitive selves.

Beyond a better understanding of the patients' words, what is the incidence of the patient's perspective on social history? The meaning of illness is neither an abstract idea, nor an individual problem. This short investigation of different 'cases' involving patients, practitioners, family and neighbours, makes it clear that these meanings are discussed and negotiated in social contexts. Patients' understanding of complaints or constitutions have important effects on personal decisions and destinies, on social strategies and the social perception of the other. The data exposed in the previous pages suggest that it is possible to reconstruct certain aspects of lay medical cultures and that this knowledge in turn gives way to a new appraisal of the nature of relations with medical practitioners. After all, the practitioner himself or herself is also a 'patient'. Beyond having a 'point of view', and following Colin Jones's stimulating discussion of the necessity to understand the nature and evolution of 'demand' in the medical marketplace, could the patient not be construed as an active social actor?[55]

Notes

1. Roy Porter, 'The Patient's View: Doing Medical History from Below', *Theory and Society* 4 (1985): 175–98.
2. N. D. Jewson, 'The Disappearance of the Sick-man from Medical Cosmology, 1770–1870', *Sociology* 10 (1976): 225–44.

3. Roy Porter and Dorothy Porter, *In Sickness and in Health: the British Experience 1650–1800* (London: Fourth Estate, 1988).

4. For a recent bibliography, see Eberhard Wolff, 'Perspectives on Patients' History: Methodological Considerations on the Example of Recent German-speaking Literature', *Bulletin Canadien d'Histoire de la Médecine* 15 (1998): 207–28; Philip Rieder and Vincent Barras, 'Ecrire sa maladie: les lettres à Tissot', *Tout autour de Tissot*, eds Vincent Barras and Micheline Louis-Courvoisier (Geneva: Bibliothèque d'histoire des sciences, Georg, 2001): 201–22; Raymond A. Anselment, ' "The Wantt of health": an Early Eighteenth-Century Self-Portrait of Sickness', *Literature and Medicine* 15.2 (1996): 225–43.

5. Porter, 'The Patient's View', 181.

6. See also Wolf, 'Perspective on Patients' History', 207–28; Aline Steinbrecher, 'Patientengeschichte. 5. Treffen des Arbeitskreises für Sozialgeschichte der Medizin der Robert Bosch Stiftung in Stuttgart, 9–10 November 1998', *Arbeitsgemeinschaft ausseruniversitärer historischer Forschungseinrichtungen in der Bundesrepublik Deutschland* 77.10.12.1998 (1998): 1–4.

7. Barbara Duden, 'Medicine and the History of the Body', in Jens Hachmunal and Gunnar Stollberg (eds), *The Social Construction of Illness: Illness and Medical Knowledge in Past and Present* (Stuttgart: F. Steiner (Robert Bosch Stiftung, Institut für Geschichte der Medizin), 1992) 39–51; Barbara Duden, *The Woman Beneath the Skin* (Cambridge and London: Harvard University Press, 1991); Françoise Loux, 'Popular Culture and Knowledge of the Body: Infancy and the Medical Anthropologist', in Roy Porter and Andrew Wear (eds), *Problems and Methods in the History of Medicine*, (London and New York: Croom Helm, 1987) 81–97; Francoise Loux and Philippe Richard, *Sagesses du corps. La santé et la Maladie dans les proverbes français* (Paris: G.-P. Maisonneuve et Larose, 1978).

8. Dorothy Porter and Roy Porter, *Patient's Progress* (London and New York: Routledge, 1989) 5.

9. Porter and Porter, *In Sickness and in Health*, 134.

10. Marjorie Nicolson and G. S. Rousseau, *'This Long Disease My Life': Alexander Pope and the Sciences* (Princeton: Princeton University Press, 1968) 7–82.

11. Jean Starobinski, 'La Littérature, le texte et l'interprète', in Jacques Le Groff and Pierre Nora (eds), *Faire de l'histoire nouvelles approches*, t. 2 (Paris: Gallimard, 1974) 176–7 and 180–2

12. Charles E. Rosenberg, 'Introduction', in Charles E. Rosenberg and Janet Golden (eds), *Framing Disease. Studies in Cultural History* (New Brunswick and New Jersey: Rutgers University Press, 1992) xiii.

13. The tension aroused by the incompatibility between past and contemporary nosologies has previously been observed, and yet no satisfactory immediate translation has yet been found. Duden, *The Woman Beneath the Skin*; Jean-Pierre Peter, 'Les mots et les objets de la maladie', *Revue historique* 246 (1971): 13–38; Jean-Pierre Peter, 'Malades et maladies à la fin du XVIIIe siècle', *Annales E. S. C.* (1967): 711–51.

14. For instance, Michael Stolberg, 'La négociation du régime et de la thérapie dans la pratique médicale du XVIIIe siècle', *Les thérapeutiques: savoirs et usages*, ss la direction d'Olivier Faure (Oullins: Fondation Marcel Mérieux, 1999) 364.

15. All translations are my own. Bibliothèque cantonale et universitaire de Lausanne, département des manuscrits (as from now: BCUL) Dorigny, Fonds Tissot, IS 3784/II/144.05.07.24: M. Magelli to S. A. Tissot, Fribourg, 28 May 1793.

16. BCUL Dorigny, Fonds Tissot, IS 3784/II/144.02.06.28: Marie Agier to S. A. Tissot, Geneva, 9 September 1775.

17. BCUL Dorigny, Fonds Tissot, IS 3784/II/146.01.05.03: Elisabeth Antonette Develay (born Gonzabeth) to S. A. Tissot, Geneva, 21 May 1792.

18. Théophile Rémy Frêne, *Journal de ma vie*, eds Carille Gigandet, Pierre-Yves Moeschler and André Bandelier (Porrentruy: Société jurassienne, 1993–1994) 2969–70, February 1800.

19. 'Comme le venin de la calomnie est intarissable, on n'a pas manqué de remarquer que mademoiselle de Sau . . . était revenue à Ferney deux jours avant la strangurie [. . .]; on veut absolument lui attribuer tous les désordres qui arrivent dans l'économie animale dudit seigneur'. Baron de Grimm, *Correspondance littéraire, philosophique et critique adressée à un souverain d'Allemagne, depuis 1770 jusqu'en 1782* (Paris: F. Buisson, 1812) 2: 420.

20. The fourth edition of the *Dictionnaire de l'Académie française* refers to érysipélateux, euse: 'Qui tient de l'érysipèle [tumeur superficielle, inflamma-toire, qui s'étend facilement sur la peau, qui est accompagnée d'une chaleur âcre et brûlante]. *Bouton érysipélateux*'.

21. Horace-Bénédict de Saussure to Albrecht von Haller, Geneva, 11 December 1773, *The Correspondence between Albrecht von Haller and Horace-Bénédict de Saussure*, ed. Otto Sonntag (Bern, Stuttgart and Toronto: Hans Huber Publishers, 1990) 476–7.

22. Agitation, for instance, is regularly listed as a symptom in letters addressed to Tissot. For an example: BCUL Dorigny, Fonds Tissot, IS 3784/II/146.01.03. 18: L. Arthaud to S. A. Tissot, Vevey, 16 January 1768.

23. Countess Golowkin to S. A. Tissot, Monnaz, undated [1766–1767]: M. et Mme William de Sévery, *Le comte et la comtesse Golowkin et le médecin Tissot* (Lausanne, Genève, etc.: Librairie Payot, 1928) 55.

24. *Bellamy*, le 8 mars 1773.

25. Charles Bonnet, for instance, associates the loss of most of his teeth with his excessive application in study, whereas the minister Frêne relates his own teeth problems to excessive work in the fields at harvest time. Charles Bonnet à Albrecht de Haller, Genthod, le 8 mai 1777: *Mémoires autobiographiques de Charles Bonnet de Genève*, ed. Charles SAVIOZ (Paris: Librairie Philosophique J. Vrin, 1948) 84; Frêne, *Journal de ma vie*, 678.

26. *Dictionnaire de l'Académie françoise*, 4th edition (Paris: Bernard Brunet, 1762) and *Le Petit Robert. Dictionnaire alphabétique [et] analogique de la langue française*, eds J. Rey-Debove, H. Cottez and A. Rey (Paris: Société du nouveau Littré, 1975).

27. This definition is close to that of Barbara Duden in her study of the bodies of the women of Eisenach. Duden, *The Woman Beneath the Skin*.

28. Alternatively, the self can be understood as 'extended into a unique and inviolable corporeal volume'. Karl Figlio, 'The Historiography of Scientific Medicine: an Invitation to the Human Sciences', *Comparative Studies in Society and History* 19 (1977): 273 and 285.

29. The importance of internal humoural movement is largely attested. For instance: Duden, *The Woman Beneath the Skin*, Gianna Pomata, *Contracting a Cure: Patients, Healers, and the Law in Early Modern Bologna* (Baltimore and London: Harvard University Press, 1998 (1st edn 1994)); Loux and Richard, *Sagesse du corps*.
30. 'Il faut aller et venir comme si de rien n'étoit, ah vraiment, il y aurait bien à faire si on voulait écouter toute les misères de mon Age, il vaut mieux aller son grand chemin sans faire semblant de les voir.' *Bellamy*, le 30/4/1773.
31. *Bellamy*, 2/5/1773.
32. BCUL Dorigny, IS 378 41/II/144.04.01.01: Anonymous to S. A. Tissot, [Vallorbe], unsigned.
33. 'Terme de Médecine, qui se dit des signes et des symptomes qui donnent l'indication et la connoissance aux Medecins de la nature et des causes des maladies': Antoine Furetière, *Le dictionnaire universel*, 3 vols (Paris: SNL - Le Robert, 1978 (1st edn 1690)).
34. *Dictionnaire de l'Académie Française*, 3rd edn (Paris: Jean-Baptiste Coignard, 1740) 1: 499. As from the 1762 edition, the definition is completed as follows: 'Il se dit des signes & des symptômes qui indiquent la nature et les causes d'une maladie.'
35. Jean-Jacques Rousseau, 'Les Confessions', *Oeuvres Complètes. Les Confessions et autres textes autobiographiques,* ed. Bernard Gagnebin and Marcel Raymond, vol. 1 (Paris: Gallimard, 1959) 293.
36. The same term is used in English: Helen King, *Hippocrates' Woman: Reading the Female Body in Ancient Greece* (London and New York: Routledge, 1998) 34.
37. Albertine de Saussure, 'Journal inédit d'Albertine de Saussure', *Le mois suisse*, 1939–1940, avril 1783.
38. Frêne, *Journal de ma vie*, 772.
39. For instance: BCUL Dorigny, IS 3784/146/34: Anonymous to S. A. Tissot, undated. Tissot also uses nervous terminology in a humoural logic in his book on onanism. Michael Stolberg, 'An Unmanly Vice: Self-Pollution, Anxiety, and the Body in Eighteenth Century', *Social History of Medicine* 13.1 (2000): 4–5.
40. Caroline Sandoz-Rollin fails to understand her own sickness: 'Il n'y a là ni goute ni rhumatisme ni panaris voilà tout ce que j'en sais'. She decides to tell everyone that *'c'est nerveux'*, but adds in a letter to a friend: 'mais je ne sais trop ce que je dis'. Caroline Sandoz-Rollin to Isabelle de Charrière, 12 March [1800], *Isabelle de Charriere. Belle de Zuylen. Correspondance*, ed Jean-Daniel Candaux, C. P. Courteney et al. (Amsterdam and Genève: G. A. Van Oorschot & Slatkine, 1984) 6: 37.
41. Isabelle de Charrière to Caroline Chambrier, [May and October] 1790, ibid., t. 3, 205.
42. The negative appreciation of the term is well known. See, for instance, Susan Sontag, *Illness as Metaphor; and AIDS and its Metaphors* (New York and London: Anchor Books, 1990).
43. In one instance, the symptoms of a teenager, Antoine Louis Lullin, are organized in such a way as to stress elements which are not characteristic of consumption: Philip Rieder, *Vivre et combattre la maladie: représentations et pratiques dans les régions de Genève, Lausanne et Neuchâtel au XVIIIe siècle* (Geneva University: mss dissertation, 2002) 366–73.

44. Other cases lead to similar conclusions: Brigitte Schnegg and Angelica Baum, ' "Cette faiblesse originelle de nos nerfs". Intellektualität und weibliche Konstitution – Julie Bondelis Krankheitsberichte', Helmut Holzhey and Urs Boschung (eds), *Gesundheit und Krankheit im 18. Jahrhunderts*, (Amsterdam: Rodolphi, 1995) 5–17; Sabine Sander, ' "... Gantz toll im Kopf und voller Blähungen ...". Körper, Gesundheit und krankheit in den Tagebüchern Philipp Matthäus Hahns', *Philipp Matthäus Hahn 1739–1790: Aufsatzband* (Stuttgart, 1989) 99–112.

45. Philip Rieder and Vincent Barras, 'Santé et maladie chez Saussure', *H.-B. de Saussure (1740–1799)*, ed. René Sigrist (Geneva: Bibliothèque d'histoire des sciences, Georg, 2001) 501–24.

46. Burgerbibliothek Bern, Correspondance Haller, XVIII 32/66, s.d.

47. Louis Odier (1748–1817), one of Saussure's physicians, is very clear about this point in a text on medical ethics. Musée d'Histoire des Sciences (Genève), Z 92/4: Louis Odier, *Mémoire sur la discrétion médicale* (pour la Société de médecine et de chirurgie), the 2nd of July 1803.

48. Charles Bonnet to Albrecht von Haller, de ma Retraite, the 14th of February 1776, Bonnet 1948, 79.

49. BPU, Ms Bonnet 71: Charles Bonnet to Jean-Henri-Samuel Formey (letter copy), Thônex, the 5th of June 1764.

50. Wellcome Library, London, Charles Bonnet: Charles Bonnet to Jean-Henri-Samuel Formey, Genthod, the 21st of September 1764.

51. See, for instance, Lester S. King, 'The transformation of galenism', in Allen G. Debus (ed.), *Medicine in Seventeenth Century England*, eds Allen G. Debus (London and Berkeley: University of California Press, 1974) 7–31.

52. Compare Mikhail Bakhtin, *Rabelais and His World*, trans. Helene Iswolsky (Cambridge, MA and London: The Massachusetts Institute of Technology, 1968 (1st edn 1965)); Duden, *The Woman Beneath the Skin*; Loux and Richard, *Sagesse du Corps*.

53. See also Colin Jones, 'Montpellier Medical Students and the Medicalisation of 18th-century France', in Roy Porter and Andrew Wear (eds), *Problems and Methods in the History of Medicine* (London and New York: Croom Helm, 1987) 71.

54. A series of private openings suggest that although such events were not systematic, many bodies were opened. Among the few figures presented here, the number of attested post-mortems gives an idea of the phenomenon. The father of the young Lullin, who died after a long pulmonary infection, had the body of his son opened, Charles Bonnet discussed the opening of his mother-in-law's body, Horace-Bénédict de Saussure's body was opened and one of his doctors described the process in a public conference, Jean-Jacques Rousseau's body was also investigated. In his case, as in those of the others listed above, there was no medico-legal basis for the operation. Only the curiosity of those left behind (and in the case of Rousseau, his own request) explain these procedures. Rieder, *Vivre et combattre la maladie*, 718–21.

55. Jones, 'Montpellier Medical Students', 57–80.

11

Framing Samuel Taylor Coleridge's Gut: Genius, Digestion, Hypochondria

George Sebastian Rousseau and David Boyd Haycock

> I am better, than I was. My Spirits are low: and I suffer too often sinkings & misgivings, alienations from the Spirit of Hope, strange withdrawings out of the Life that manifest itself by existence – morbid yearnings condemn'd by me, almost despis'd, and yet perhaps at times almost cherish'd, to concenter my Being into Stoniness, or to be diffused as among the winds, and lose all individual existence. But all this I well know is a symptom of bodily disease, and no part of sentiment or intellect / closely connected with the excessively irritable State of my Stomach and the Viscera, & beyond doubt greatly exasperated by the abruptness & suddenness of my late Transitions from one state to another.
>
> (Samuel Taylor Coleridge, letter to Sir George Beaumont, 1804)[1]

The health – or rather the lack of it – of Samuel Taylor Coleridge (1772–1834) was of considerable and sustained concern to the writer himself and to his family and his friends, and has remained so to his subsequent biographers and critics. Sometimes it has been thought to have been of *too much* interest to him, often curiously so. Earl Leslie Griggs, in the introduction to the first of the invaluable six edited volumes of Coleridge's *Collected Letters*, observed that the correspondence 'may at times contain too much of ill health ... too much of remorse and self-justification'.[2] Indeed, to work through the letters and notebooks is to discover over and over again Coleridge's boundless fascination with his own soul and body, and in particular the focus of his attention on his stomach and bowels. He never overlooked the former but was far more obsessed with the latter. The intestinal tract – stomach, liver, intestines, rectum, the whole of his innards except his penis – proved to be the specific

site of endless curiosity and mystery. Here in the midriff was the key to
his malady, the long disease his life, and its implied antithesis – health –
which he rarely enjoyed. To friends and strangers alike he variously
explained the debilitating disturbances in his body – be it constipation,
flatulence, vomiting, diarrhoea or simply *pain* – according to a long
litany of possible ailments: gout, dysentery, cholera, chronically irritable
bowel or an irritable bladder, influenza, sciatica, rheumatism, cancer,
stone or diabetes. Sometimes he blamed the effects of bad food or bad
weather. But what exactly was it that so endlessly troubled him throughout his life? Was he diseased, or was he pre-eminently hypochondriacal,
as a number of previous critics have suggested?[3] Or were his discomforts
the consequence of his notorious opium habit? – opium having a profoundly debilitating effect on the gut.

Any attempt at a posthumous diagnosis is perilous, particularly one as
diagnostically and determinably slippery as hypochondriasis, which has
long had a reputation as a non-disease, or at least a condition so problematic in its ambiguity and protean transformations, or at least so heavily conjoined to genius, that it is incapable of definition.
Hypochondriasis was also the complaint of malingerers. As early as 1766
the commentator John Hill wrote, 'To call the Hypochondriasis a fanciful malady, is ignorant and cruel. It is a real, and a sad disease.'[4]
Historically, the *morbus hypochondriacus* first spoken of by Galen was a
severe disorder seated in the organs of the hypochondria or upper
abdomen (the spleen, liver, gall-bladder, and so on, the word deriving
from *hypo*, under, and *chondros*, cartilage), and was related to melancholia ('black bile') and emotional disorders such as the 'spleen' and
'vapours'.[5] Other more ancient commentators than Hill had pronounced
on the hypochrondria diagnosis and the difficulties involved in understanding it (for example, Galen, *On Prognosis*). By the eighteenth century
it was principally gendered as a male malady, a counterpart to female
'hysteria'.[6] Along with other 'nervous disorders', hypochondriasis was
increasingly being written upon by (male) physicians of eighteenth-century Britain, when it was seen as threatening the well-being of the whole
nation.[7] In 1733 in *The English Malady: Or, A Treatise of Nervous Diseases
of all Kinds, As Spleen, Vapours, Lowness of Spirits, Hypochondriacal, and
Hysterical Distempers, &c.* George Cheyne famously recorded that these
'nervous Disorders' were 'computed to make almost one third of the
Complaints of the People of Condition in England'.[8] It is unclear where
he derived his statistics but Cheyne was probably not far off the mark.
Two generations later, Thomas Trotter in his *A View of the Nervous
Temperament* (1806), doubled the number: he believed that 'nervous

diseases' now made up 'two-thirds of the whole with which civilized society is infested, and are tending fast to abridge the physical strength and mental capacities of the human race'.[9] Hence society – the culture into which Coleridge was born into in 1772 and then raised – was growing increasingly nervous. The ill, languorous, hypersensitive body thus quickly became a principal characteristic of the Romantic sensibility. In March 1801 Coleridge – still a young man of 29 – apologized to his friend Thomas Poole for having sent him a letter 'written in "a wildly-wailing strain"', confessing that he had been 'horribly hypochondriacal' when he wrote it.[10] Two years later, in October 1803, he even described his friend and poetic collaborator William Wordsworth as 'a brooder over his painful hypochondriacal Sensations',[11] a man becoming 'more & more benetted in hypochondriacal Fancies, living wholly among *Devotees*'.[12] The young Coleridge saw the world through hypochondriacal eyes: his culture was preoccupied with it by then so preponderantly that it had filtered down to household knowledge of educated people.

Roy and Dorothy Porter have identified the 'coming-out' (the phrase is ours rather than theirs and is intentionally chosen) of the hypochondriac as a human type in late eighteenth-century England as designating an important moment in the cultural history of medicine. As modern western society increasingly put a mark on the special, the interesting individual, especially the genius, they suggest that the ensuing social tensions 'between individual brilliance and polite conformity bred anxieties' which were 'somatized into physical complaints, which could be partly owned and partly disowned. Sickliness provided social alibis while suffering purchased the right to be different, to be oneself. Pain commanded a certain social bargaining power.'[13] The Romantic *sickly* poet thus became a type, one with legitimate medical credentials. Trotter wrote that 'it is to be supposed, that all men who possess genius, and those mental qualifications which prompt them to literary attainments and pursuits, are endued by nature with more than usual sensibility of nervous system'. In Trotter's opinion, the power and focus of the mind on higher subjects sapped the 'powers of digestion' and reacted upon 'the nervous part of the frame'. The 'literary character' was thus likely to suffer 'numerous instances of dyspepsia, hypochondriasis and melancholia'.[14] Digestion in its various forms – whether successfully completed or as indigestion and dyspepsia – was crucial to the developing hypochondriac. Our point in brief is that if illness was a necessary hallmark of all Romantic writers, hypochondria was the cornerstone of that individual talent because it was, ultimately, an exclusionary strategy.

The idea that the sedentary and studious type hovered in particular danger of illness had been a commonplace in Judaeo-Christian tradition since biblical times.[15] John Hill was only one in a long line of medical commentators, ancient and early modern, when he wrote how 'The finer spirits are wasted by the labour of the brain: the Philosopher rises from his study more exhausted than the Peasant leaves his drudgery'.[16] The sickly writer thus included almost all the prominent British writers in Coleridge's formative mindset: William Cowper, Thomas Gray, James Boswell, Samuel Johnson, Percy Shelley and John Keats. Yet despite Coleridge's own self-fashioning as an incurable hypochondriac (despite his protestations), his incessant ailments, his constant, endless references to his poor health, as well as the further features of the hypochondriacal subject we shall examine below, all combine to suggest an authentic case in its modern sense. Hence Coleridge both suffered the symptoms of which he endlessly complained, as well as sought to ensure that he could be a *malade*: he was thus both *malade vraiment* as well as *malade imaginaire*. In Coleridge we appear then to have the genuine article.

I

Coleridge's first physical illness occurred in 1779, when he was only seven and in his first year at school, which was hit by an epidemic of 'putrid fever'. But more telling than this early encounter with illness was his experience with his immediate family. As the precociously gifted youngest of ten children, with a father of 53 and a mother of 45, Coleridge was either bullied by or distanced from his eight brothers and spoilt by his parents. He recalled that as a child he 'became fretful, & timorous, & a tell-tale – & the School-boys drove me from play, & were always tormenting me'. He sought consolation in books, 'and I used to lie by the wall, and *mope* – and my spirits used to come upon me suddenly, & in a flood'.[17] A significant incident occurred when he was seven, when after an argument with one of his brothers he ran away from home to escape a scolding from his mother. He spent the night out of doors whilst family and friends searched for him. He later recalled that on being found, 'I was put to bed – & recovered in a day or so – but I was certainly injured – For I was weakly, & subject to the ague [fever] for many years after'.[18] He also recalled 'the tears stealing down his [father's] face' when he was brought home, and his mother's 'outrageous ... joy'. This event sets a pattern for Coleridge's adult life, of escape and blame, mixed with illness that is not of his own making.

As Holmes points out, the importance of this episode is shown by the number of times Coleridge referred to it in later life, and its recurrence in his notebooks.[19] The final traumatic event of early childhood was the sudden death of his beloved father after a heart attack in 1781, shortly before Coleridge's ninth birthday. Soon afterwards he was sent away to school at Christ's Hospital in London, from which date he virtually considered himself an 'orphan'. The deaths of a brother and sister in 1791 were also particularly emotional blows, provoking the lines:

> Pain after pain, and woe succeeding woe –
> Is my heart destin'd for another blow?
> O my sweet sister! and must thou too die?[20]

Our impression is thus of a sensitive, intelligent, highly imaginative youth, but a lonely one too, deeply affected by these early experiences. This is the type of character one might expect to develop into a hypochondriacal adult.

It was in the winter of his final year at Christ's Hospital school, 1790–91, that Coleridge came down with what he described as 'jaundice and rheumatic fever'.[21] He spent long periods of time in the school's sick-ward, and was given opium to help him sleep. He recorded his experience in the early poem, 'Pain: Composed in Sickness'. After this, rheumatism would frequently be referred to as a principal source of pain. An inflammatory disease, rheumatic fever has been described as 'an illness of skin, brain, heart, connective tissue, blood and serum, tonsils, and joints'.[22] It can make recurrent attacks, and involves such symptoms as joint pains, muscle and abdominal pain, skin nodules and vomiting. Coleridge's friend and host for the last 18 years of his life, Dr James Gillman, attributed 'all his bodily sufferings' to rheumatism,[23] and this would certainly explain some of the aspects of Coleridge's adult ill health. But it goes no way to explaining the recurrent problems of the gut we noted in our introduction, nor the sudden appearance and disappearance of his symptoms, nor his obsessive attitude to his condition, aspects of his case which we will consider in more detail below. Indeed, Walter Jackson Bate suggests that Coleridge's autopsy 'establishes that he had never had anything like "rheumatic fever"... nor in all probability anything else that would *organically* explain protracted physical sufferings as a boy or young man.'[24] It has, however, been suggested that the biological character of rheumatic fever changed in the very late eighteenth and nineteenth centuries, and that heart damage – as well as damage to the brain – is a feature only of this later incarnation of the disease.[25] Nonetheless, whilst rheumatic fever may explain *some* of Coleridge's physical pain, it by no means explains *all* his symptoms.

Coleridge began to point to anxiety as the source of his ailment. In 1794 he informed a friend that he had been 'seriously unwell' and 'heavy of head & turbulent of Bowels'.[26] But at this time Coleridge was also suffering from nervous anxiety associated with his relationship with his future wife, Sara Fricker, a disastrous match encouraged by his friend Robert Southey. When Southey admonished Coleridge for not writing to Sara, Coleridge claimed he had been 'taken ill – very ill . . . Languid, sick at heart', and could not write to her then (though he managed to pen an article of 'Nonsense' for the booksellers).[27] In 1796 a doctor informed him that his condition was 'altogether nervous', originating 'either in severe application, or excessive anxiety'. Coleridge seized upon this diagnosis: 'in excessive anxiety, I believe, it might originate!'[28] This became one point of focus, with, following his move to Cumbria in 1800, the weather and his diet becoming further key ingredients in the confused recipe of his disease.

It was in the Lake District that Coleridge discovered the potent opium-based medicine known as Kendal black drop, the effects of which were ruinous on his digestion. The effects of Coleridge's drug-use offer the strongest counter to the argument that he was truly hypochondriacal in the modern sense. Indeed, two of his worst periods of illness, in the early 1800s and the early 1830s, coincide with periods of heavy drug-use or attempts to reduce that use. Coleridge appears to have taken opium intermittently during the 1790s, and it appears that his problems with his gut developed at this time. In 1791 he claimed that 'Opium never used to have any disagreeable effects on me – but it has upon many.'[29] This is a stance that he would maintain at least until the later 1800s.[30] When in 1814 Coleridge suggested to Joseph Cottle that it would be best if he were incarcerated in 'a private madhouse' for a few months in order to overcome his opium habit,[31] Robert Southey told Cottle that the most 'mournful thing' about Coleridge's case 'is that while acknowledging the guilt of the habit, he imputes it still to morbid bodily causes, whereas after every possible allowance is made for these, every person who has witnessed his habits, knows that for the greater part . . . inclination and indulgence are the motives'.[32] Thus, as opposed to Gillman's claim for rheumatism, Cottle in his *Reminicences* [sic] declared that Coleridge's 'unhappy use of narcotics' was the 'true cause of all his maladies, his languor, his acute and chronic pains, his indigestion, his swellings, the disturbances of his general corporeal system'.[33] However, like rheumatism, opium use does not preclude a broader diagnosis of hypochondriasis, as contemporary doctors realized. In his account of the nervous temperament, Trotter made particular note of the effects the drug had in exacerbating such disorders:

> Opium alone gives relief, though it must feed the disease. Such persons seem to compound with their physician for sound nights, and days of ease; and if he does not comply he must be changed. Hard is the task imposed on the medical attendant; he must obey, or starve.[34]

In his 1817 *Essay on Hypochondriasis* the physician John Reid similarly noted the danger of the long-term prescription of opium, considering it 'a drug which is so likely to become a part of the daily regimen of an hypochondriacal invalid, and which often renders him incurably such'. But in Reid's opinion, the malady *antedated* the drug use, 'which is often begun to relieve bodily pain', and was a feature of the hypochondriac's intemperate character.[35] Usually it was, and another chapter on the body of melancholics would be needed to disentangle cause and effect here. Suffice it to say that Coleridge was persuaded beyond a shadow of doubt that he had drugged himself to relieve these symptoms.[36]

Intestinal disorders had been troubling Coleridge for some time when in the summer of 1803 he identified his condition as 'a compleat & almost heartless Case of Atonic Gout'.[37] He drew this self-diagnosis from an article in *Encyclopedia Britannica* (1797), which described 'atonic' gout as one affecting not the joints, but appearing as 'affections of the stomach, such as loss of appetite, indigestion, and its various attendants of sickness, nausea, vomiting, flatulency, and eructations, and pains in the region of the stomach'.[38] He complained at this time of 'this truly poisonous, & body-&-soul-benumming Flatulence & Inflation'.[39] He stuck to this diagnosis for some months, but his attempts 'to throw the Disease into the Extremities' by gout medicines and rigorous exercise failed to shift it.[40] By January 1804 he had firmly decided that his delicate constitution could stand the damp climate of England no longer. His illness had not been helped by making his home in the wet countryside of the Lake District, and as rain fell inexorably on the roof of the Wordsworths' Grasmere home, he complained to Robert Southey that his health was 'pitiable! . . . I must go into a hot climate'. Significantly, he had now reached the conclusion that his disease was not 'genuine gout, but primarily a Disease of the Skin, & affecting the Digestive organs by the diseased Action of the Skin'. He complained that physicians were 'utterly ignorant of the Skin . . . I have no doubt, that a violent Eruption which perhaps a hot Climate might bring on, would cure me'.[41] Two days later he added that it was 'hardly possible to give even a plausible conjecture' for his illness 'while we remain ignorant of the secret means & subtle passages of that sympathy that exist in so remarkable a degree between the Skin & Stomach.' He only expected to be able to 'find words & a theory to explain my own Disease by' when some medical philosopher had fully worked out this relationship.[42] He then had the idea of writing a book about his own disorder. He told Thomas Poole, 'Of it's Contents the Title will in part inform you – Consolations and Comforts from the exercise and right application of the Reason, the Imagination, and the moral Feelings, addressed especially to those in Sickness, Adversity, or Distress of mind, *from speculative Gloom*, &c.'[43] Soon after, in London, he was attacked by what he thought was cholera morbus, a dangerous diarrhoeal disease then relatively common in England.[44] But on reaching Portsmouth he told the Wordsworths that he believed his ongoing 'Hauntings and Self-desertions are, no doubt, connected with the irritable state of my Bowels & the feebleness of my Stomach; but both they & these, their bodily causes, are exasperated by the rapid Changes, I have undergone' – especially in his various travels and escapades since leaving Cumbria.[45] But over and again it is his gut which is the culprit, an area of the body still little understood in the mindset of the Enlightenment and nineteenth century.[46]

Though Coleridge never wrote a book on 'distress of the mind', as his letter to the Wordsworths reveals, this was nevertheless a period of mental as well as physical distress, alongside his increasing enslavement to opium. He was unable to work, was suffering nightmares, was financially embarrassed, and despairing in, and endlessly fretting about, his failed love for Sara Hutchinson. At odds with his 'cold' wife, he was clearly depressed. A year's residence in a hot climate, such as Madeira or Sicily, was the answer not just to his problems of health, but to most of his other problems as well. After quitting the Lakes early in 1804, he would not see his wife or children again until late 1806, informing the Wordsworths in November of that year that they had '*determined* to part absolutely and finally'.[47] In London his condition improved a little, though he wrote to the Wordsworths from Essex that throughout the realms of health he was still 'as faithful a Barometer' as he had been in Keswick, '& during all falling Weather am as asthmatic & stomach-twisted as when with you'.[48] Over and again, we encounter his interminable preoccupation with his digestive tract as the specific site of his daily condition as well as the inception of his nocturnal (as distinct from daytime waking) dreams. From the convoluted descriptions of his nightmares, it seems likely that Coleridge was regularly indulging in laudanum, though he continued to ascribe his illness to the weather mixed with his own brooding nature. He explained to Sir George Beaumont in February, in no equivocal terms, that 'Whatever affects my Stomach, diseases me; & my Stomach is affected either immediately – by disagreeing Food, or distressing Thoughts, which make all food disagree with me – or indirectly by any ungenial action upon *the Skin*, that terra incognita to Physicians and Metaphysicians.'[49] Dermis was a runner-up in this hierarchy of offending body parts: but comb through the thousands of pages of Coleridgeana and its appearances form only a fraction of the sub-hypochondriacal domain. And he told Southey in March, 'It is not *Cold* that hurts me . . . It is Damp without & anxiety, or Agitation, within that cause my Disease / and the former is often quite as predominant in our Summers as our winters'.[50] We are thus establishing the picture of a man with obsessive awareness of his health, seeking in external events and diagnoses potential explanations for his supersensitive maladies. That his soul, spirit, or unconscious self were essential components of his health, as he perceived them to be, we are the first to admit.

II

Even so, to what extent can we rely on Coleridge's attempts to find an *organic* explanation for his illness, and to what exact extent can we blame it wholly on his drug taking? If Coleridge's ailment was not wholly linked to his opium taking, the suggestion of his most recent biographer, Richard Holmes, that Coleridge suffered perhaps from irritable bowel syndrome (IBS), is a promising one, and one that links to Coleridge's own focus on anxiety. IBS is a chronic, relapsing functional disorder focused on the small and large intestine, whose 'cause and mechanism are unknown'.[51] In *Gut Reactions: Understanding Symptoms of the Digestive Tract* (1989), W. Grant Thompson explains that though the 'effects of *chronic* emotion or stress on gastric motility and secretion are not precisely known . . . there can be little doubt that they are important in the genesis of symptoms'. Certain emotions may be capable of precipitating gastric dysfunctions such as non-ulcer dyspepsia, and it is possible that 'a certain personality type with certain previous experiences and associations may undergo changes in gastric function or in awareness of gastric function in response to emotion'.[52] As Coleridge declared, it was 'Damp without & anxiety, or Agitation, within that cause my Disease'. Furthermore, the relationship between the gut and the brain is two-way traffic: one influences the other. The gut can thus 'learn' responses from the brain, and a Pavlovian reaction to certain stimuli particular to the individual is possible, though this is as yet unproved. Certain drugs, including opiates and alcohol, 'may also cause dyspepsia through unknown mechanisms', and Thompson adds that although hard scientific data is rare, 'it is generally accepted that emotion is important in the genesis of dyspepsia'.[53] Thompson also explains that nocturnal pain 'or spring and fall exacerbations of the pain all tilt the diagnosis toward peptic ulcer',[54] which would have the potential to explain some of Coleridge's symptoms. Medical research appears to show that IBS sufferers 'are more prone to chronic illness behavior and that this behavior is learned . . . Such illness behavior may be engendered not only by early life experiences but also by . . . psychological and personality abnormalities'.[55] Again, this appears to fit the pattern of Coleridge's complaint. Many of his attacks coincided with periods of personal emotional anxiety or stressful situations, and would undoubtedly have been exacerbated by his laudanum use, a dangerous mix of opium *and* alcohol. Dyspepsia or IBS would also explain Coleridge's recurrent claim that his bowel problems *preceded* his drug habit.

However, like rheumatic fever, IBS does not provide a full explanation for all of the features of Coleridge's case. Hypochondriasis, though, offers an alternative, if quite possibly linked, diagnosis. Unfortunately, like IBS hypochondriasis is an especially problematical condition to pin down, and medical opinion on the exact nature of the disorder remains divided: it is agreed 'that the diagnosis of hypochondriasis is not easy'.[56] In the eighteenth century, hypochondriasis was closely connected with the operation of the gut. In his *Medicinal Dictionary* (1743–5), Robert James defined 'Hypochondriacus Morbis' as

> a spasmodic-flatulent Disorder of the *Primae Viae*, that is, of the Stomach and Intestines, arising from an Inversion or Perversion of their peristaltic Motion, and, by the mutual consent of the Parts, throwing the whole nervous System into irregular Motions, and disturbing the whole Oeconomy of the Functions.[57]

In 1827 the former naval physician James Johnson would also focus his discussion of these nervous distempers on the gut, entitling his rapidly-selling study *An Essay on Morbid Sensibility of the Stomach and Bowels, As the Proximate Cause, or Characteristic Condition of Indigestion, Nervous Irritability, Mental Despondency, Hypochondriasis, &c. &c.* Johnson wrote that

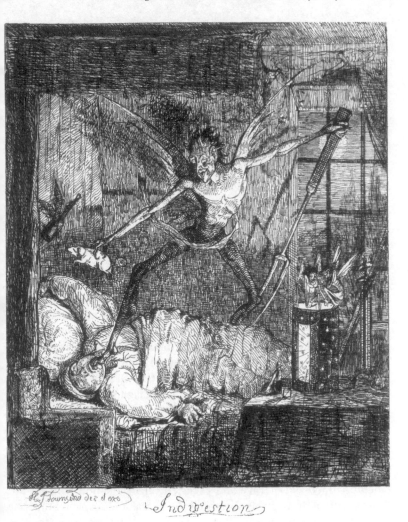

Illustration 11.1 Etching by H. J. Townsend of 'A monster, representing indigestion, torturing a man trying to sleep'. No date, approximately 1820

a *morbid sensibility* of the nerves of the stomach and the bowels, with or without the usual symptoms of disordered digestion, was the leading feature of the disease, and the cause of the varied and endless train of symptoms which develop themselves in the mind and in distant parts of the body.[58]

This focus on the guts is clearly useful for a contemporary explication of Coleridge's case. In his *A View of the Nervous Temperament*, Thomas Trotter, whom we cited above, also observed that these increasingly prevalent disorders included those diseases 'commonly called Nervous, Bilious, Stomach, and Liver Complaints; Indigestion; Low Spirits; Gout, &c'. All of these Trotter bracketed together collectively as 'nervous disorders', and they were 'to be referred in general, to debility, increased sensibility, or torpor of the alimentary canal'.[59] As Trotter rightly saw things, the

> human stomach is an organ endued by nature, with the most complex properties of any in the body; and forming a *centre* of sympathy between our corporeal and mental parts, of more exquisite qualifications than even the brain itself . . . In all those disorders whose seat is the nervous system, it particularly suffers.[60]

All forms of gout, for example, were 'preceded by stomach affection' and attended by dyspeptic symptoms.[61] Hypochondriasis was thus firmly linked by Trotter and other contemporary doctors with the operation of the digestive organs, and was often grouped alongisde dyspepsia and indigestion.[62] Individually, these 'nervous disorders' were, perhaps, more akin to what would now be identified as IBS, chronic fatigue syndrome, and anxiety disorders rather than hypochondriasis, though they all also feature as frequent diagnoses of the modern hypochondriacal patient.[63]

But what exactly is to be understood as hypochondriasis today – a necessary question, it would seem, in a discussion about the framing of disease? In the recent study *Hypochondriasis: Modern Perspective on an Ancient Malady* (2001), Dr Vladan Starcevic writes that it 'can be succinctly defined as excessive and persistent preoccupation with health, disease, and body, which is associated with a fear and suspicion that one is a victim of serious disease.'[64] Another characteristic feature, Starcevic claims, is its persistence over many months and years, though with fluctuating intensity. So chronicity is fundamental to the condition. Even when subjects (are they all patients?) possess an organic medical condition, 'the symptoms are experienced as far more intense than what could be expected on the basis of the objectively existing, organic pathology'.[65] Starcevic observes that whilst there are no symptoms *typical* of hypochondriasis, some symptoms – such as gastrointestinal and dermatological ones, or those affecting the central nervous system – are 'found more frequently among patients with hypochondriasis'.[66] This

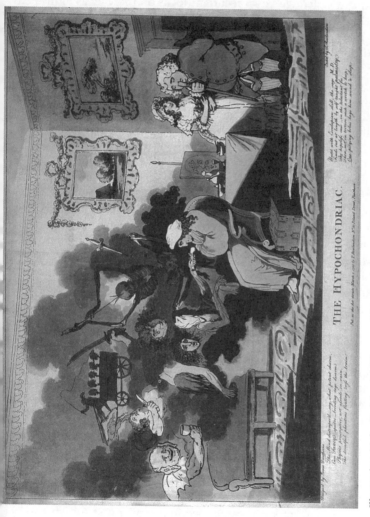

Illustration 11.2 Etching by Thomas Atkinson of a seated hypochondriac shivering in front of a fire surrounded by pills and, not so fortuitously, picture frames. Coloured aquatint, 1819.

may be so but how (again within the context of framing) are we to understand the victim – are these *all* patients without recourse to class and identity? And how are the fear and suspicion to be culturally contextualized? Even this modern transhistorical approach goes some way to explain Coleridge's own recurrent focus on these areas of his body, but this diagnosis also appears to cover aspects of Coleridge's condition that are not covered by IBS. Trotter noted the sensitivity of the hypochondriacal patient in a different work on naval medicine, writing how sailors suffering from scurvy recounted to each other their dreams of 'green fields, and streams of pure water'. These conversations were 'as earnestly conducted, as we sometimes observe hypochondriacs in relating their feelings, from any ruffle of temper occasioned by changeable weather, or other slight causes'.[67] Other defining features of hypochondriasis include the bodily preoccupation we have already seen in Coleridge, and a constant recourse to medical practitioners. Coleridge dismissed many of the physicians he consulted as failures, and wrote significantly in 1796, 'I know a *great many* Physicians. They are *shallow* Animals: having always employed their minds about Body and Gut, they imagine that in the whole system of things there is nothing but Gut and Body.'[68] Though Coleridge would come to praise some physicians, such as Thomas Beddoes and James Gillman, highly, when he decided that a warm climate was the best solution to his condition it is notable that he had been advised by no less than '*four* medical men' that his only hope for a cure was a 'regulated Diet, Tranquillity, and an even & dry climate'.[69] Perhaps it is no surprise that in 1823 he wrote that he considered it 'the chance of my life, that I have counted an unusually large number of medical men (several of them Men of great celebrity & eminence) among my friends'.[70]

A fascination with medical texts in an attempt to identify their disorder is another feature of the hypochondriacal personality shared by Coleridge.[71] On a number of occasions he described his ailment according to the symptoms in recently read books.[72] We have already seen how in 1803 the *Encyclopedia Britannica* provided him with a definition of 'atonic gout', which he at first accepted before then rejecting it in favour of an undefined 'disease of the skin'. Significantly, he blamed his first taking of opium on 'a medical Journal [where] I unhappily met with an account of a cure performed in a similar case (or what to me appeared so) by rubbing in of Laudanum, at the same time taking a given dose internally – It acted like a charm, like a miracle!'[73] In 1814, after reading Everard Home's *Practical Observations on the Treatment of Strictures in the Urethra* (1797), he declared that 'a mass of Evidence has crowded on me', and he prepared to have a physical examination made of his bladder. Yet the very thought of this operation engendered such 'distressful feelings . . . they now agitate me so as almost to overwhelm the Dread of having the Worst, I suspect, ascertained'.[74] Though the examination was permanently postponed, Coleridge was convinced that 'Since I have read on the Subject, I myself have no doubt of the melancholy fact. I am *quite certain*, that I have not deceived myself as to 9 Symptoms'.[75] And again in October 1824 he declared to Dr Gillman 'I have more than suspected Diabetes, ever since I first read Dr Prout's Work' on diseases of the urinary organs.[76] This feature of the hypochondriac personality appears to exceed what one might expect as Coleridge's undoubtedly considerable interest in medical texts per se: he recalled that as a boy he had been 'wild to be apprenticed to a surgeon. English, Latin, yea, Greek books of medicine read I incessantly'.[77] An ill man with a keen interest in reading, it might seem unsurprising that he sought in books a clue to his disease: but could he not have deceived himself to *nine* symptoms? Does this not seem an extreme diagnosis, especially as these diagnoses are often quite quickly discarded? Vickers observes that 'medicine was the empirical science against which Coleridge, repeatedly, judged the claims of metaphysics',[78] but it sometimes appears that his reading of medical texts, and his response to them, was more than simply objective interest. The text appears on more than one occasion to *inspire* the diagnosis, and this should be noted when we consider his interest in medicine. It might be suggested that Coleridge 'borrowed' symptoms in the same way that he 'borrowed' words in his now-famous acts of so-called plagiarism. Despite his extensive reading of medical and philosophical texts, therefore, it is hard always to portray him as a wholly objective reader.[79]

This 'borrowing' of symptoms is witnessed in Coleridge's manifest experience of a distemper new to eighteenth-century England: homesickness. When in January 1796 he wrote to a friend, 'to tell you the truth I am quite home-sick – aweary of this long absence from Bristol', he was using a word that does not have an earlier recorded appearance in England and that was destined to describe his prevailing geographical destiny: fated, like his mariner, to wander, always far from the places he loved, a front-runner in the ranks of the homeless.[80] 'Homesick' is a partial translation of the German *heimweh*, from which is derived the Latin 'nostalgia', a neologism coined by a French doctor, Johannes Hofer, in the late seventeenth century and derived from the Greek *nostos* (home) and *algia* (malady). Hofer's *Dissertation de Nostalgia* was published in Basel in 1678, and described a medical condition he had identified amongst Swiss mercenaries, who were sickening and even dying from this yearning to return home. Nostalgia would become established as a genuine disease in England by the early nineteenth century. In a prize-winning essay presented to the University of Edinburgh, the former president of the Hunterian Medical Society, Hector Gavin, dismissed the idea that nostalgia was an easily feignable complaint:

> It is almost impossible to imitate the alteration and expression of countenance, the languid appearance, and sadness, so impressed on all the features, which are always present in the real disease; the simulator is wanting in the involuntary abandonment, and the apathetic indifference for every thing, which is foreign to the cherished idea of the true nostalgic; as also in the sudden extravagance of joy, which the sight of some object connected with home produces: moreover, pretenders generally express a great desire to revisit their native country, whilst those who are really diseased are taciturn, express themselves obscurely on the subject of their malady, dare not to make an open avowal, and are little affected by the consolations which hope or promise affords them.[81]

When Coleridge left his wife and two young sons, Hartley and Berkeley, in 1798 in order to travel to Germany with his friends John Chester and William and Dorothy Wordsworth, he would have been more closely exposed to medical thought on this new malady. For example, at the University of Göttingen in 1799 he attended lectures by the professor of medicine, Johann Friedrich Blumenbach, Europe's foremost writer on comparative anatomy, who built on a long tradition of medical anthropology from the mid-eighteenth century days of figures such as Ernst Platner (1744–1818) who himself had contextualized *heimweh* in neurophysiological terms. Here, in Germany, Coleridge had likely heard the symptoms of medical nostalgia catalogued and discussed.[82] Did they, almost by sympathy we wonder, induce in him the hypochondriacal symptoms he was to endure for the rest of his life? In Germany Coleridge also experienced increasingly severe bouts of the new distemper, and his letters through the late winter and spring of 1798–99 contain frequent, if also shrill, cries for home, accompanied by the symptomatic feelings of lethargy, distraction and melancholy. For example, on 14 January, in a letter to Sara Coleridge, he wrote:

> My dearest Love – Since the wind changed & it became possible for me to have Letters, I lost all my tranquillity. Last evening I was

absent in company, & when I returned to Solitude, [was] restless in every fibre. A novel, which I attempted to read, seemed to interest me so extravagantly, that I threw it down – & when it was out of my hands, I knew nothing of what I had been reading. This morning I awoke long before Light, feverish & unquiet – I was certain in my mind, that I should have a Letter from you; but before it arrived my restlessness & the irregular pulsation of my Heart had quite wearied me down – & I held the letter in my hand like as if I was stupid, without attempting to open it. – 'Why don't you read the Letter?' said Chester – & I read it. – Ah little Berkley [*sic*] – I have misgivings – but my duty is rather to comfort you, me dear dear Sara! – I am so exhausted that I could sleep. – I am well; but my spirits have left me – I am completely home-sick. I must walk half an hour – for my mind is too scattered to continue writing . . . O God! I do languish to be at home![83]

These disjointed fragments contain the symptoms of nostalgia, but are they not also, and concomitantly, hypochondriacal? Was his a true nostalgia, a nostalgically loaded hypochondriasis, or a self-feigning excuse not to return to familial responsibilities, the excuse for the failings of a man who has told himself that his nostalgia has made him 'ill'? (According to Hector Gavin's medical criteria, Coleridge, with his 'open avowal' of homesickness, would be considered a feigner.) Coleridge returned to this *leitmotif* in April, by which time he had been in Germany almost seven months – much longer than the '3 or 4 months sojourn' he had originally intended.[84] 'My dear Sara,' he lamented, 'Surely it is unnecessary for me to say, how infinitely I languish to be in my native Country & with how many struggles I have remained even so long in Germany!'[85] But remain he did, if pathetically so. Even after hearing the news that 'little Berkley' had died, he did not return to his family for another six months. What are we to make of both symptoms and Coleridge's own accounts of them?

HOME-SICK. Written in GERMANY.

Tis sweet to him, who all the week
Thro' city crowds must push his way,
To stroll alone thro' fields and woods
And hallow thus the Sabbath day.

And sweet it is, in summer bower
Sincere, affectionate, and gay,

One's own dear Children feasting round,
To celebrate one's marriage day.

But what is all to *his* delight,
Who having long been doom'd to roam
Throws off the Bundle from his Back
Before the Door of his own Home?

Home sickness is a wasting pang
That feel I hourly more and more:
There's healing only in thy wings,
Thou Breeze, that play'st on Albion's shore!

Coleridge wrote this poem in May 1799 in Germany and introduced it to his friend Thomas Poole with the words 'O Poole! I am homesick. – Yesterday, or rather, yesternight, I dittied the following hobbling Ditty.' The full title is 'Homesick: Written in Germany, Adapted from Bürde.' By 1799 Samuel Gottlieb Bürde had translated Milton's *Paradise Lost* into German and published an account of his Grand Tour over the Alps and descent into Italy where he, like so many Germans before him, first experienced the pangs of *heimweh*. Bürde later versified these affective emotions in many of his poems. They are imbued with the spirit of 1790s nostalgia, vivifying how these attacks of longing grew so acute that they produced the onset of sickness, as they also do here. Coleridge frames nostalgia's daggers as 'no baby pangs' – i.e., not the homesickness experienced by children when they first leave, home but that of adults who can reflect on the reasons for their cravings for the hearth. The symptoms are alleviated only when the wanderer can 'throw off his Bundle from his Back' at his own door; hence Coleridge's 'healing Breeze' which will waft him back home. Coleridge's images crescendo into the joy he encounters in line 11. But he no sooner imagines the return home than he coins his most intriguing image in the poem: nostalgia's 'wasting'. The nostalgic's wasting away was the dominant image of the 1790s: *heimweh* framed as bodily wasting. Physicians then prolifically delineated how the 'wasting' occurs. For example, Leopold Auggenbrugger, discoverer of the percussion test which tapped the breast cavity, claimed it was caused by lesions in the heart which sapped up fluids in the wanderer's body and reduced him to a quasi-consumptive creature. The 'hourly' acceleration of time experienced by the narrator in Coleridge's poem dramatizes how this 'wasting' was psychologically perceived as an attack of anxiety, even panic.

Coleridge's biographical nostalgia, especially whilst in Germany, is a larger topic than can be adequately dealt with here. However, its relation to, and even imprecation in, the large configuration of hypochondriacal maladies is salient. There can be little doubt, that is, that Coleridge was combining these conditions in his own mind to produce a type of hypochondria diagnosis that was entirely idiopathic to himself and which, he thought, he could document. He is, of course, famous for his poor treatment of his family, and at one point in his notebooks in January 1804, shortly before he left England and his wife again, this time for the Mediterranean, he reflects unhappily on his feelings for Sara Coleridge, writing of 'the advantage to have had some remembered Instance . . . of some <heavy> Frailities & Hypochondriacal Selfishness'.[86] Tellingly, Coleridge did not complain of homesickness during his even longer sojourn in Malta and Italy. By this time, relations with his wife were irreparable.

In summary we are suggesting that if hypochondriasis was a vital word, and category, permeated with layers of meaning, however contradictory, for Coleridge and his contemporaries, it was also a concept that permitted him to explain to himself diverse strands of his life experience impossible otherwise to comprehend or reconcile. These certainly extended to his creative, imaginative life; the imagination – as he had been persuaded in Germany – so heavily dependent on neuroanatomical processes. Coleridge's hypochondriacal characteristics of impairment thus extended to his many unrealized ambitions and projects, a failure he ascribed to his ill health, exacerbated by opium use taken, he claimed, in his attempts to overcome bad health. This debilitation accounts in part for his contradictory behaviour whilst in Germany, especially since the hypochondriac's preoccupation with illness (to put the matter in modern DMS terminology that strengthens the larger point we are making about the modernity of Coleridge's hypochondria) 'causes clinically significant distress or impairment in social, occupational, or other important areas of functioning'.[87] But even this amalgamation of his hypochondria and nostalgia does not constitute the totality of a story he was telling himself about his almost Jobean decline.

For his dire bodily symptoms and turn for the worse constituted a persuasive excuse for unfulfilled projects. As he told Southey in 1803, 'No one who lived a month with me could have the least doubt as to the barometrical nature of my Health', adding immediately that he was 'weary & ashamed of talking about my intended works'.[88] The biographical record confirms the point, and the pattern of 'intended works' (endless projects he began and never finished) recurs throughout his letters. It was indeed his creative *work* that caused him the greatest anxieties: in 1828, for example (and it is merely one of many), he described himself as the now Jobean 'sick, anxious, embarrassed Man, constantly forced off either by ill-health or the necessity of the To Day, from completing the Works, to which the studies and Aspirations of more than half his Life had been devoted'.[89] To pain and illness and opium he blamed these failings, and he even went so far as to implicate divine providence in his imminent tragedy. Because he laboured in such agonies, he had been driven to medicate himself. He heard in 1814 God's accusation: ' "I gave thee so many Talents. What hast thou done with them"?'[90] He would continue to hear the indictment in his profuse nocturnal dream life, whether as Death-in-Life or its reverse.

As his letters, notebooks and poems reveal, Coleridge was also a man of incredible sensitivity and eloquence, and he constantly worried that people did not take his medical condition(s) seriously. He bombarded friends, acquaintances and virtual strangers with detailed snippets of information – itself, predictably, an almost universal feature of hypochondriasis that surfaces in all epochs without consideration of local context and situation.[91] In 1811 he told Daniel Stuart that 'The quickness, with which I pass from Illness into my best state of Health, is astonishing, & makes many think it impossible, that I should have been so ill, the day or two before'.[92] Coleridge's description indicates an ailment existing beyond the effects of his opium use. Like Southey, the Wordsworths also encountered Coleridge's ever-changing health. In June 1811, Dorothy wrote of their old friend:

> How absurd, how uncalculating of the feelings and opinions of others, to talk to your Father and Sister of dying in a fortnight, when his dress and everything proved that his thoughts were of other matters ... Poor William went off to London ... in consequence of his [STC] having assured Mrs. Coleridge that he *could* not live three months; and, when William arrived, he ... saw no appearance of disease which could not have been cured, or at least prevented by himself.[93]

William believed that 'The disease of [Coleridge's] mind is that he perpetually looks out of himself for those obstacles to his utility which exist only in himself.'[94]

Yet Coleridge continuously acknowledged his hypochondriacal nature and was hardly a stranger to it. If his nostalgia appeared more surprisingly and remotely to him, his hypochondriasis did not: it was a permanent pillar, daily intensifying, of his psychological and psychosomatic being. In describing his repertoire of symptoms and their rapid change from ill to well to another friend in September 1821, he worried that 'I should leave the impression of hypochondriasis rather than of any determinable malady.'[95] And in 1815 he had enquired sombrely of a Dr Sainsbury (of whom nothing else is heard in his correspondence) if he had 'ever heard of a man whose Hypochondriasis consisted in a constant craving to have himself [i.e., his entrails or abdominal cavity] opened before his own eyes?'[96] The 'constant craving' is another curious feature of his psyche and leads us directly to the interior chambers of his mind. As he told William Sotheby in 1828, it was 'a not unfrequent tragico-whimsical fancy with me' to imagine himself as 'an Assessor' at his own post-mortem, and giving 'this and that thought into the Mind of the Anatomist':

> Be so good as to give a cut just *there*, right across the umbilicar [sic] region – there lurks the fellow that for so many years tormented me on my first waking! – Or – a Stab *there*, I beseech you – it was the seat & source of that dreaded Subsultus [under the Hypochondrium], which so often threw my Book out of my hand, or drove my pen in blur over the paper on which I was writing!

Only then, thought Coleridge, when his bodily insides as signs of ailments were finally revealed to the world on the autopsy table, would he have 'justifying reason' for the actions of his life, and his 'only offences against others, viz. Sins of Omission'.[97] The actual biographical report of Coleridge's autopsy a decade later found extensive deformation in the hypochondria – an 'immensely enlarged' heart, an 'enormously distended' gall bladder, as well as over six pints of 'bloody serum' in cyst-like membranes in the chest cavity.[98] His friend and quondam patron in the 1820s, Dr Gillman, who could not bring himself to attend the dissection, told Cottle that these morbid features 'will account sufficiently for his bodily sufferings, which were almost without intermission during the progress of the disease, and will explain to you the necessity of subduing these sufferings by narcotics, and of driving on a most feeble circulation by stimulants'.[99] Coleridge had entered into correspondence with him about his symptoms, as well as revealing his troubled dreams and seeking the good doctor's signification. Coleridge's daughter Sara, however, wrote to her brother Hartley after the autopsy that their father's 'internal pain & uneasiness' was ascribed to 'some sympathetic nervous affection'[100] – everywhere the hint, by Coleridge and others, that all his complaints had ultimately been nervous. The cyst may well have been a pleural effusion occurring late in life, but the inflammation of the heart was probably the result of pericarditis, which can be caused by a viral infection such as the rheumatic fever from which Coleridge first suffered at Christ's Hospital. All these symptoms were grounded in fact and realism: Coleridge was not merely imagining himself in pain. Hypochondriasis was a felt, experienced disease, no less than gout or dropsy. That he was grasping, however and in addition, for a language of hypochondriasis – that is, trying to frame his malady – is our rationale of his presentation in this volume.

III

The foregoing evidence suggests that a diagnosis of hypochondriasis fits comfortably the pattern of Coleridge's ailments. Even so the psychological causes of hypochondriasis are notoriously difficult to establish and it may be worth the remaining space to attempt to eliminate some other possibilities before moving to our conclusion about framing Coleridge's hypochondriasis. We therefore return to some of the best modern studies as aids: as Arthur J. Barsky writes in Starcevic and Lipsitt's collected study, 'The prominent disease fears, beliefs, and preoccupations of hypochondriacal patients are thought to stem from a misattribution of benign bodily symptoms and normal sensations to serious disease.'[101] Hypochondriasis has thus been conceptualized

> as a disorder of bodily amplification, in which a wide range of somatic and visceral sensations are experienced as unusually intense, noxious and disturbing. Thus, hypochondriacal individuals may be thought of as especially sensitive to, and intolerant of, bodily sensation in general ... Hypochondriacal people, because their symptoms are so intense and uncomfortable, conclude that these sensations must be abnormal and pathological, rather than normalizing them by attributing them to a benign cause such as overwork, insufficient rest, inadequate exercise, or dietary indiscretion.[102]

Unfortunately, whilst all four of these latter possible attributions apply amply to Coleridge, modern empirical investigation of this thesis has been 'relatively sparse'. That which has been undertaken, however, does appear to suggest 'that hypochondriacal subjects are more sensitive to physiological sensations'.[103] Generalized as the characteristics are to all hypochondriacs, this assessment would nevertheless appear to fit with the picture we have of Coleridge as a supersensitive observer. The possible examples of this sensibility are many and well documented; they would fill many pages if culled from his letters and marginalia. As he described his restless self in 1797, 'Frequently have I, half-awake & half-asleep, my body diseased & fevered by my imagination, seen armies of ugly Things bursting in upon me'.[104] The symbolism of these ugly objects can be interrupted according to the corpus of pre-1800 dream symbolism, but it is equally significant that Coleridge pauses first to comment on his diseased body. Then there were the observations about his hypersensitivity by those who knew Coleridge, especially the strange way his body had predisposed him. Humphry Davy was only one of several to remark on his friend's 'excessive sensibility'.[105] Barsky, using modern categories but aiming to account for the same phenomena, notes that anxiety, depression and dysphoric mood states all help to amplify bodily distress. We have already noted Coleridge's ascription of his disease to anxiety, and Barsky explains that anxiety 'increases self-consciousness, and this apprehensive self-scrutiny amplifies pre-existing symptoms and brings previously unnoticed sensations to conscious awareness'.[106] Coleridge's anxiety also includes another characteristic of the hypochondriac personality: a vivid fear of death. As Porter and Porter have written, 'Coleridge feared sleep, since his nightmares were intolerable. Above all, a paralysing dread of death seized him.'[107] Erasmus Darwin believed that 'the cause of what is term'd hypochondriasis in men' derived from a 'general debility' in the stomach and bowels, 'which is always attended with so much fear, *or expectation*, of dying, as to induce them to think of nothing but their own health'.[108] In *Zoonomia* Darwin classified hypochondriasis as a disease of the mind, if not a form of actual madness, though modern studies suggest that 'in the majority (62%–88%) of hypochondriacal patients, there is at least one comorbid mental disorder', with depressive and anxiety disorders being the most common.[109] Coleridge clearly suffered from both depression and anxiety, and considered his inability to control his opium habit to be 'a species of madness'.[110]

IV

We have launched a case for Coleridge's hypochondriasis as the *main* feature of our framing. In this sense we extend Richard Holmes's biographical quest to understand 'what the idea of "health" meant to the Romantics; and what place – if any – it had in the New Sensibility of Feeling'.[111] It may be claimed that these are but footnotes on Coleridge's medical case history; a position we would endorse and even amplify by affirming that it could be rigorously shown, if sufficient medical history were imported to philosophical and literary sources, that Coleridge was suffering almost textbook hypochondriasis compounded by the opium and other drugs he imbibed. However, our aim here is not to compile medical case histories but to reflect on these conclusions for framing disease. In our methodology Coleridge's own vocabulary of hypochondriasis has led us to his gut, and the gut – more specifically, his dreaming gut – to his dream theory. As evidence that our framing has not been fanciful, we have also performed the sequence backwards: from his dream theory (as recorded in the vast jungle of commentary he compiled over the course of his lifetime) back to his gut and from the gut to his hypochondriasis as a sign of his genius. Perhaps it will be useful to consider each block separately as another route to this version of framing.

Coleridge's hypochondriasis has yet to be reconstructed, block by block, as it were, discussed and pondered. So canonical a figure as Coleridge, in whom so much is at stake in the development of Romanticism, cannot lightly be classified, or diagnosed, as imbued with any malady unless it has been derived independently by different assessors working towards a common goal. Coleridge could have been suffering other illnesses; his malady need not have been hypochondriasis. Yet we have tried to demonstrate the decades of his concern for his ailments: not merely a particular fleeting disquietude or momentary flirtations with (for example) cholera, but with the larger picture adding up to hypochondriasis. We especially think his troubled domestic life and homelessness, even the nature of his love for Sara Hutchinson and his paranoid fantasies about his infidelity, were part and parcel of a fundamentally hypochondriacal personality using sickness to shield the victim from a hard world and chronically medicating himself in a clearly vicious circle of malady leading to further malady. His obsession was with the gut rather than any other part of the human body – from the almost daily bouts of intestinal trouble to his perceived sense that he had cholera – and the preoccupation fortified him against the possibility that he was a lesser talent after all. As Roy Porter has claimed, and as we agree: 'the gut was the cradle of genius'.[112]

We might have taken an alternative route by framing his main malady through his troubled sleep and nocturnal rituals. Had we done so we would have recreated his contexts of night thoughts and graveyard sensibility. Starting in the kingdom of sleep we might have derived his concerns for the gut and self-diagnosis from netherly and dark realms in the land of sleep – or sleeplessness. This would have been taking a different route to the same place. In the end what counts is a malady framed and context developed that are both commensurate with the subject of the attention.

This route would have indeed captured the sleepless Coleridge better than we have, and highlighted what it was like to sleep as little and as poorly as he often did – troubled as he was by one or another concern – but would also have falsified the specificity of his hypochondriasis. Many hypochondriacs and male hysterics warred with themselves at night, experienced one hell after another as they tossed 'alone, all alone on a wide, wide sea', but who were not preoccupied with their gut as he was. Read the Coleridge of the letters, the Coleridge of the notebooks and marginalia, and you soon realize that this is a man possessed by the devil of his entrails. He has demonized the gut to the point that it must forever let him down; in doing so it also, through contradiction and paradox, proves to be the site of his greatest imagination, genius, and talent. Whatever he was as a man and whether philosophical dualist or monist – now proponent of one, now the other, always sparring with the two without coming to any conclusion – he was the possessor of a defective gut that was both his virtue and his defect. And he had no embarrassment divulging this to anyone, not even his patrons, as in his numerous letters to his friend and sponsor James Gillman.

Yet another alternative route was through Coleridge the dreamer. This avenue was the one taken by Jennifer Ford in *Coleridge on Dreaming*, discussed above, and we think it paid handsome dividends; not merely in explaining why Milton and Swedenborg were so crucial for Coleridge's understanding of his own dreams but also in heralding the trumpet call that anatomical and physiological processes could not be omitted. In view of Coleridge's chronic illnesses, the announcement pertained to his medicine, especially his variety of maladies, as well as understanding of the complex processes underpinning them.

There is no need to summarize Ford's important work here or to repeat its findings. Suffice it to invite our own readers to consult her pages on Swedenborg (pp. 147–52), since they form the heart of the post-Cartesian matter about mind–body interaction in the gut, and also her last chapter – the eighth – entitled 'the dreaming medical imagination' (pp. 183–202). We think this eighth chapter likely to be omitted by students of Coleridge's dreaming, yet it represents the conclusions of Ford's own long voyage with the subject and points to the future direction of research in this area. If there is any gap in her conclusions they lie in gauging Coleridge's tone in his ephemeral notes and marginalia, especially in relation to the theorists he was reading about materialism, dualism and dreaming, from Milton and Swedenborg through Andrew Baxter and the post-Baxterian dualists right up to his own time.

Coleridge, we believe, was often ironic and contradictory in these writings. Many of the Coleridgean passages cited by Ford in her book cannot be construed literally. This is especially true of the comments on Swedenborg, which embody a particular hurdle in Coleridgean exegesis about the understanding of dreams because Coleridge annotated the Swede so prolifically. We do not engage here in close textual analysis but invite the reader to do so. Select any of the passages Ford cites on pp. 147–52, for example, even the long letter dated November 1824 to James Gillman about 'feculent metempsychosis' and the way 'certain foul Spirits of the lowest order are attracted by the precious Ex-viands', and you have a narrator with tongue in cheek only half of whose voice means what he literally says. This ambivalence does indeed pose a problem for all of Coleridge's framing of dreams and – furthermore – understanding of illness. But it is not one that can be discounted or altogether overlooked.

This small caveat notwithstanding, Ford's contribution to the progress of Coleridge scholarship is significant. When she writes (p. 185) that it is 'the medical imagination' in all its complexity that has been overlooked in Coleridge studies she puts her finger on a lacuna that could fill not one, but several books. When you consider the role the imagination plays in Coleridge's aesthetics and literary criticism (especially in the *Biographia Literaria*), Coleridge is often said to be the Father of theories about the role of imagination in poetry[113] – yet Ford claims that we have overlooked essential features of his notion of that same imagination. When Ford recounts, page after page, how that same imagination could become 'diseased' in the parlance of the late eighteenth and early nineteenth centuries, she treads on the border of just the sort of framing disease we are proposing here. When she argues for a unity of 'medical, physiological and poetic imagination' (p. 194) she comes close to the hypochondriacal Coleridge who required just this sort of 'diseased imagination' to persuade himself that his pain was real. When she expends energy trying to demonstrate that 'the imagination's power as a translational organ of the body . . . also creates a poetic world' (p. 200) she connects realms medical and literary in just the sense we have been prescribing. And it is – finally – impossible to avoid the conclusion that in his dreams and dream processes Coleridge unified all these views.

You could make these claims without framing Coleridge's hypochondriasis, but you could not see how it had coloured much in his life and work and especially informed the great poetry which he conceived as so many dreams translated by the imagination. If Coleridge represented the end of a long tradition summing up melancholy, hypochondriasis, and their central activity in the gut, he also anticipated the future: not merely in Thomas De Quincey and the other Romantic opium prophets, but in towering European hypochondriacs such as Henri Amiel, Dostoevsky and Marcel Proust who also had nocturnal lives that revelled in the gut. We would go so far as to claim that this mystical system-builder whose imagination has so haunted us was not so far in his new sensibility from that other visionary, Dostoevsky. Susan Sontag has captured an essential feature of what is at stake when she described the summer in Baden-Baden of the latter:

> Perhaps only an obsessive, death-haunted hypochondriac, such as Tsypkin seems to have been, could have devised a sentence form that is free in so original a way. His prose is an ideal vehicle for the emotional intensity and abundance of his subject. In a relatively short book, the long sentence bespeaks inclusiveness and associativeness, the passionate agility of a temperament steeped, in most respects, in adamancy.[114]

Appendix A

DSM-IV diagnostic criteria for hypochondriasis, reproduced from the *Diagnostic and Statistical Manual of Mental Disorders* (4th edn, American Psychiatric Association, 1994).[115]
A. Preoccupation with fears of having, or the idea that one has, a serious disease based on the person's misinterpretation of bodily symptoms.
B. The preoccupation persists despite appropriate medical evaluation and reassurance.
C. The belief in Criterion A is not of delusional intensity (as in Delusional Disorder, Somatic Type) and is not restricted to a circumscribed concern about appearance (as in Body Dismorphic Disorder).
D. The preoccupation causes clinically significant distress or impairment in social, occupational, or other important areas of functioning.
E. The duration of the disturbance is at least 6 months.
F. The preoccupation is not better accounted for by a Generalized Anxiety Disorder, Obsessive-Compulsive Disorder, Panic Disorder, a Major Depressive Episode, Separation Anxiety, or another Somatoform Disorder.

Appendix B

Representative sample of the types of medical dissertations being written while Coleridge was annotating his own hypochondria and commentaries:

Berthelen, C. A. 'De hypochondriasis origine.' Leipzig, 1846.

Birotheau, A. L. 'Sur l'hypochondrie.' Paris, 1830.

Bourrelly, E. J. F. 'Sur l'hypochondrie.' Paris, 1819.

Bouteiller, F. 'Essai sur l'hypochondrie.' Paris, 1820.

Brequin, H. L. J. 'Sur l'hypochondrie.' Paris, 1831.

Calestroupat, J. H. 'Sur l'hypochondrie.' Paris, 1823.

Carilian, A. F. V. 'Sur l'hystérie et l'hypochondrie.' Paris, 1818.

Champagne, J. P. 'Sur l'hypochondric.' Paris, 1827.

Chauvin, A. E. C. A. 'Paralléle de l'hypochondrie avec la mélancholie.' Strasbourg, 1824.

Dubois d'Amiens, E. F. *Histoire philosophique de l'hypochondrie et de l'hysterie.* Paris, 1837.

Falret, J. P. 'Del'hypochondrie et du suicide. Considérations sur les causes, sur le siége et la traitement de ces maladies, sur les moyens d'en arréter les progrés et d'en prévenir le développement.' Paris, Croullebois, 1822.

Flemyng, Malcolm. *Neuropathia; sive de morbis hypochondriacis et hystericis, etc.* 1746.

Gillespie, R. D. 'Hypochondria: Its Definition, Nosology and Psychopathology.' *Guy's Hospital Rep.* 78 (1928): 408–60.

Goullin, P. M. B. 'Sur l'hypochondrie.' Paris, 1821.

Hall, M. *On the mimoses: or, A descriptive, diagnostic and practical essay on the affections usually denominated dyspeptic, hypochondriac, bilious, nervous, chlorotic, hysteric, spasmodic , etc.* London: Longman [& others], 1818.

Haro, A. 'Considérations générales sur l'hypochondrie.' Strasbourg, 1834.

Ladee, G. A. *Hypochondriacal Syndromes.* Amsterdam: Elsevier, 1966.

Lecadre, A. A. 'Sur le siége et la nature de l'hypochondrie.' Paris, 1827.

Louyer-Villemary. 'Sur l'hypochondrie.' Paris, 1802.

Private, F. 'Coup-d'oeil sur l'hypochondrie.' Paris, 1827.

Reid, J. 'Essays on hypochondriacal and other nervous affections.' Philadelphia, M. Carey & Son, 1817.

Rowley, Wm. *A treatise on female, nervous, hysterical, hypochondriacial, bilious, convulsive disease; apoplexy & palsy with thoughts on madness & suicide, etc.* C. Nourse, 1788.

Schiller, E. 'De hypochondria.' Prague, 1841.

Venables, P. *De hypochondriasi.* Edinburgh, 1803.

Wirtz, J. M. 'De sede et causa proxima hypochondriae.' Bonn, 1830.

Notes

1. Samuel Taylor Coleridge (hereafter STC) to Sir George Beaumont, 6 April 1804, in *The Collected Letters of Samuel Taylor Coleridge* (hereafter *CL*), ed. Earl Leslie Griggs, 6 vols (London: Oxford University Press, 1956–1971) 2: 1122. We have written with one secondary work constantly before us: Jennifer Ford's *Coleridge on Dreaming: Romanticism, Dreams and the Medical Imagination* (Cambridge: Cambridge University Press, 1998), which George Rousseau reviewed when it first appeared; see *Medical History* (January 2000): 139–41 and which he esteems with this caveat developed below: Ford relies rather too much on Swedenborg and the sense of Coleridge's approbation of some of that mystic's explanation of the physiology of dreams and nightmares. We

think instead that Coleridge tried hard, over many years, and in prolific annotations that would amount to a book on Swedenborg in itself to concur with the Swedish mystic but – in the end – could not. Close textual analysis of the evidence suggests that Coleridge was typically ironic or sardonic or dismissive but, in the end, unable to find himself in agreement with Swedenborg's theosophical solutions. George Rousseau is also grateful to Dr Matthew Gibson, astute student of the visionary tradition from Coleridge down through Yeats, with whom he was privileged to discuss the former throughout the year 2001.

2. Griggs, *CL* 1: xxxv. Our essay builds on the authoritative biographical record of Coleridge as compiled by Walter Jackson Bate, *Coleridge* (London: Weidenfeld & Nicolson, 1969), Norman Fruman, *Coleridge: the Damaged Archangel* (New York: George Braziller, 1971), Molly Lefebure, *Samuel Taylor Coleridge: a Bondage of Opium* (London: Quartet Books, 1977) and especially Richard Holmes's two-volume study, *Coleridge: Early Visions* (London: Hodder & Stoughton, 1989) and *Coleridge: Darker Reflections* (London: HarperCollins, 1998), as well as the various Bollingen editions.

3. For previous references to Coleridge's possible hypochondriasis, see Holmes, *Early Visions*, 15, and Holmes, *Darker Reflections*, 110; Thomas McFarland, 'Coleridge's Anxiety', in John Beer (ed.), *Coleridge's Variety: Bicentenary Studies* (London and Basingstoke: Macmillan Press, 1974) 134–65; Bate, *Coleridge*, 102; Neil Vickers, 'Coleridge, Thomas Beddoes and Brunonian Medicine', *European Romantic Review* 8 (1997) 47–94, 59; Roy Porter and G. S. Rousseau, *Gout: the Patrician Malady* (New Haven and London: Yale University Press, 1998) 156. Despite all these previous references, to our knowledge no diagnosis has previously been attempted in any depth. This contrasts with the considerable interest that has been taken in other early-nineteenth-century English patients, for example Byron, Keats ('Ah, what ails thee knight at arms/alone and palely loitering?'), Shelley, and, most notably, Charles Darwin about whom a library of books exists. See, for example, Ralph Colp, *To Be an Invalid: the Illness of Charles Darwin* (Chicago and London: The University of Chicago Press, 1977) and 'To Be an Invalid, Redux', *Journal of the History of Biology* 31 (1998) 211–40.

4. John Hill, *Hypochondriasis. A Practical Treatise on the Nature and Cure of that Disorder; Commonly Called the Hyp or Hypo* (London, 1766) 3. By 'real' Hill meant that it had an organic origin, the 'obstruction of the spleen by thickened and distempered blood' (ibid.). Our study has been assisted by a recently published collection of essays written by leading contemporary psychologists, *Hypochondriasis: Modern Perspective on an Ancient Malady* (Oxford: Oxford University Press, 2001). Edited by scientists Dr Vladan Starcevic and Dr Don R. Lipsitt, it aims 'to produce a text on this ancient disorder that will provide "state of the art" knowledge on hypochondriasis for years to come'; see Vladan Starcevic and Don R. Lipsitt, 'Introduction', in Starcevic and Lipsitt (eds), *Hypochondriasis*, xiii. Especially useful here is German E. Berios, 'Hypochondriasis: History of the Concept', 3–20. Also valuable are: Susan Baur, *Hypochondria: Woeful Imaginings* (Berkeley and Los Angeles: University of California Press, 1988); G. A. Ladee, *Hypochondriacal Syndromes* (Amsterdam and New York: Elsevier, 1966); Gernöt Böhme, 'Hypochondria as an illness caused by civilisation in the eighteenth-century', talk delivered at the

Conference on Nature and the Body convened by Gianna Pommata in Bologna, Italy, Summer 1997; Alan Ingram, *Boswell's Gloom* (London: Macmillan, 1984); R. D. Gillespie, 'Hypochondria: Its Definition, Nosology and Psychopathology', *Guy's Hospital Report* 78 (1928) 408–60. For historicized pre-twentieth-century conceptualizations of hypochondriasis, see Esther Fischer-Homberger, 'Hypochondriasis of the Eighteenth Century – Neurosis of the Present Century', *Bulletin of the History of Medicine* 46 (1972) 391–401. We agree with the assessment of hypochondria in the role of genius made by Roy Porter and Dorothy Porter, *In Sickness and in Health: the British Experience, 1650–1850* (London: Fourth Estate, 1988) 203–10, and Roy Porter, *Bodies Politic: Disease, Death and Doctors in Britain, 1650–1900* (London: Reaktion Books, 2001) 154–64. For a modern statement about the role of the condition in our world see Adam Sage, 'Hypochondria threatens France's economic health', *Times*, 24 June 1997.

5. See Fischer-Homberger, 'Hypochondriasis of the Eighteenth Century', 391–401.

6. Ladee, *Hypochondriacal Syndromes*, 8.

7. See Porter and Porter, *In Sickness and in Health*, 203–10.

8. George Cheyne, *The English Malady: Or, A Treatise of Nervous Diseases of all Kinds, As Spleen, Vapours, Lowness of Spirits, Hypochondriacal, and Hysterical Distempers, &c.* (London, 1733) i–ii. Other major works on the subject from this period include Richard Blackmore, *A Treatise of the Spleen and Vapours: Or, Hypochondriacal and Hysterical Affections* (London, 1725), Nicholas Robinson, *A New System of the Spleen, Vapours, and Hypochondriack Melancholy: Wherein all the Decays of the Nerves, and Lowness of the Spirits, are Mechanically Accounted For* (London, 1729), and Robert Whytt, *Observations on the Nature, Causes, and Cure of those Disorders which have been Commonly Called Nervous, Hypochondriac, or Hysteric; to which are Prefixed some Remarks on the Sympathy of the Nerves* (Edinburgh, 1765).

9. Thomas Trotter, *A View of the Nervous Temperament; Being a Practical Enquiry into the Increasing Prevalence, Prevention, and Treatment of Those Diseases Commonly Called Nervous, Bilious, Stomach, and Liver Complaints; Indigestion; Low Spirits; Gout, &c.* (2nd edition, London, 1807) viii.

10. STC to Poole, 24 March 1801, *CL* 2: 710. (The quote is from one of his own fragmentary poems.)

11. STC to Poole, 3 October 1803, *CL* 2: 1010.

12. STC to Poole, 14 October 1803, *CL* 2: 1013. See also Holmes, *Coleridge: Early Visions*, 357.

13. Porter and Porter, *In Sickness and in Health*, 209. Detailed texts on hypochondriasis appeared later on the Continent than they did in Britain (and hence, of course, Cheyne's description of this as 'the English malady'), but their dates reflect the intense medical attention given to the condition in Coleridge's lifetime: see for example Louyer-Villemary, *Dissertation sur l'hypochondrie* (Paris, 1802), E. J. F. Bourrelly, *Dissertation sur l'hypochondrie* (Paris, 1819), J. P. Falret, *De l'hypochondrie et du suicide. Considérations sur les causes, sur le siége et la traitement de ces maladies, sur les moyens d'en arréter les progrés et d'en prévenir le développement* (Paris, 1822); A. E. C. A. Chauvin, *Paralléle de l'hypochondrie avec la mélancholie* (Strasbourg, 1824); J. M. Wirtz, 'De sede et causa proxima hypochondriae' (Bonn, 1830); E. Schiller, *De hypochondria* (Prague, 1841) and Appendix B.

14. Trotter, *A View of the Nervous Treatment*, 39.
15. See Roy Porter, 'Reading: A Health Warning', in Robin Myers and Michael Harris (eds), *Medicine, Mortality and the Book Trade* (Folkestone: St Paul's Bibliographies, 1998) 131–52.
16. Hill, *Hypochondriasis*, 6. See also James Boswell, *Boswell's Column: Being his Seventy Contributions to the London Magazine Under the Pseudonym the Hypochondriack from 1777 to 1783, Here First Printed in Book Form in England* (London: W. Kimber, 1951). For the line of commentators and their proliferation in the eighteenth century see Anne C. Vila, 'The Scholar's Body: Health, Sexuality and the Ambiguous Pleasures of Thinking in Eighteenth-Century France', in Angelica Goodden (ed.), *The Eighteenth-Century Body: Art, History, Literature, Medicine* (Oxford and Bern: Peter Lang, 2002) 115–34; for the thriving debate about hypochondria during Coleridge's lifetime see our Appendix A providing a sample of the range of works. Elsewhere we have assembled an archive of almost one hundred dissertations.
17. STC to Poole, 9 October 1797, *CL* 1: 347.
18. STC to Poole, 16 October 1797, *CL* 1: 353–4.
19. Holmes, *Coleridge: Early Visions*, 17.
20. Quoted in ibid., 38.
21. James Gillman, *The Life of Samuel Taylor Coleridge* (London: William Pickering, 1838) 33.
22. Peter C. English, *Rheumatic Fever in America and Britain: A Biological, Epidemiological, and Medical History* (New Brunswick, New Jersey, and London: Rutgers University Press, 1999) xvii.
23. Gillman, *Life of Samuel Taylor Coleridge*, 33.
24. Bate, *Coleridge*, 103–4.
25. See English, *Rheumatic Fever*, chapter 1, 'The New Face of Rheumatism, 1798–1840', 17–31.
26. STC to George Dyer, 11 September 1794, *CL* 1: 101.
27. STC to Southey, 19 September 1794, *CL* 1: 105.
28. STC to Poole, 5 November 1796, *CL* 1: 250. See Giovanni A. Fava and Lara Mangelli, 'Hypochondriasis and Anxiety Disorders', in Starcevic and Lipsitt (eds), *Hypochondriasis*, 89–102.
29. STC to George Coleridge, November 1791, *CL* 1: 18.
30. Porter and Porter (1988) 223.
31. STC to Cottle, 26 April 1814, *CL* 3: 477.
32. Footnote to Letter 921, Southey to Cottle, no date given, *CL* 3: 479.
33. Joseph Cottle, *Reminiscences of Samuel Taylor Coleridge and Robert Southey* (New York: Wiley and Putnam, 1847) 351.
34. Trotter, *A View of the Nervous Temperament*, 137. Coleridge eventually admitted this fact to himself, reflecting in 1814 that he had 'for many years . . . been attempting to beat off pain, by a constant recurrence to the vice that reproduces it'. STC to Josiah Wade, 26 June 1814, *CL* 3: 511.
35. John Reid, *Essays on Hypochondriasis, and Other Nervous Affections* (3rd edition, London, 1823) 178–9.
36. For further discussion of chicken and egg here see Raymond Aron, *The Opium of the Intellectuals with a new introduction by Harvey C. Mansfield; foreword by Daniel J. Mahoney and Brian C. Anderson* (London: Secker & Warburg, 1955); Martin Booth, *Opium: a History* (London: Simon & Schuster, 1996).

37. STC to Southey, 14 August 1803, *CL* 2: 974.
38. See *Encyclopedia Britannica* (1797), vol. 9, article on 'Medicine'. On Coleridge's condition as gout, see Porter and Rousseau, *Gout*, 155–9.
39. STC to Southey, 14 August 1803, *CL* 2: 974.
40. STC to Sir George and Lady Beaumont, 22 September 1803, *CL* 2: 993.
41. STC to Southey, 11 January 1804, *CL* 2: 1027.
42. STC to Southey, 13 January 1804, *CL* 2: 1028–31.
43. STC to Poole, 15 January 1804, *CL* 2: 1035–6.
44. See G. S. Rousseau and David Haycock, 'Coleridge's Choleras: Cholera Morbus, Asiatic Cholera, and Dysentery in Early in Nineteenth-Century England', *Bulletin of the History of Medicine*, 77 (2003), 298–331. In 1831–2 Coleridge would also suspect that he had been attacked by Asiatic cholera. It is interesting to note the belief that an attack of Asiatic cholera could be brought on by simple *fear* was strongly held, and persisted through the nineteenth century. Sir William James Moore, in an overview of the diseases of India published in 1890, observed that 'During epidemics of cholera nervous persons sometimes imagine they are attacked, a condition which has been called "choleraphobia", and which occasionally actually terminates in an illness which cannot be distinguished from cholera.' See *The Constitutional Requirements for Tropical Climates and Observations on the Sequel of Disease Contracted in India* (London 1890) 40.
45. STC to the Wordsworths, 4 April 1804, *CL* 2: 116.
46. We need large-scale treatment of it and nothing less than a study of the cultures of the gut from the Renaissance to the Romantics will do, especially as a prolegomenon to understand how the seat of genius continued to be lodged there. For contextual material that is ironic, see especially Sydney Whiting, *Memoirs of a Stomach, Written by Himself, That All Who Eat May Read. With Notes, Critical and Explanatory, by a Minister of the Interior* (London: W. E. Painter, 1853).
47. STC to the Wordsworths, *c.*19 November 1806, *CL* 2: 1200.
48. STC to the Wordsworths, 8 February 1804, *CL* 2: 1059.
49. STC to Beaumont, 2 February 1804, *CL* 2: 1052.
50. STC to Southey, 12 March 1804, *CL* 2: 1084. See Jennifer Ford, *Coleridge on Dreaming*, note 1.
51. W. Grant Thompson, *Gut Reactions: Understanding Symptoms of the Digestive Tract* (New York and London: Plenum Press, 1989) 210
52. Ibid., 82. Thompson points out that the complexity of the enteric nervous system that links the gut with the brain is exceeded in complexity only by the brain itself, and that the medical understanding of functional bowel disease remains 'rudimentary'. Thompson, *Gut Reactions*, 189, 184.
53. Ibid., 141.
54. Ibid., 144.
55. Ibid., 191. Thompson nevertheless notes that 'we remain uncertain of the extent to which the psychological phenomena observed in IBS patients are cause, effect, or coincidence'.
56. Issy Pilowsky, 'Hypochondriasis, Abnormal Illness Behavior, and Social Context', in Starcevic and Lipsitt (eds), *Hypochondriasis*, 249–62, 254.
57. Robert James, *Medicinal Dictionary* (London, 1743–5), article on 'Hypochondriacus Morbis', quoted in G. S. Rousseau's introduction to John

Hill's *Hypochondriasis: a Practical Treatise* (Los Angeles: William Andrews Clark Memorial Library, 1969).

58. James Johnson, *An Essay on Morbid Sensibility of the Stomach and Bowels, As the Proximate Cause, or Characteristic Condition of Indigestion, Nervous Irritability, Mental Despondency, Hypochondriasis, &c. &c.* (London: Thomas and George Underwood, 1827) 60.

59. Trotter, *A View of the Nervous Temperament*, xvi.

60. Ibid., 205–6. Trotter's work is not mentioned amongst Coleridge's letters or notebooks.

61. Ibid., 173–4.

62. See, for example, James Rymer, *A Tract Upon Indigestion and the Hypochondriac Disease: With the Method of Cure, and a New Remedy of Medicine Considered* (London: T. Evans, 1785); William Rowley, *A Treatise on Female, Nervous, Hysterical, Hypochondriacal, Bilious, Convulsive Diseases; Apoplexy and Palsy; With Thoughts on Madness, Suicide, etc.* (London, 1788); M. Hall, *On the Mimoses: Or, A Descriptive, Diagnostic and Practical Essay on the Affections Usually Denominated Dyspeptic, Hypochondriac, Bilious, Nervous, Chlorotic, Hysteric, Spasmodic , etc.* (London: Longman, Hurst, Rees, Orme, and Brown, 1818); James Woodforde, *A Treatise on Dyspepsia, or Indigestion: With Observations on Hypochondriasis and Hysteria* (2nd edn, London: Longman, Hurst, Rees, Orme and Brown, 1821); Stephen Waterman Avery, *The Dyspeptic's Monitor: Or, The Nature, Cuases, and Cure of the Diseases Called Dyspepsia, Indigestion, Liver Complaint, Hypochondriasis, Melancholy, etc* (New York: E. Bliss, 1830).

63. Vladan Starcevic, 'Clinical Features and Diagnosis of Hypochondriasis', in Starcevic and Lipsitt (eds), *Hypochondriasis*, 21–60, 38.

64. Ibid., 21–60, 21.

65. Ibid., 23.

66. Ibid., 23. According to Starcevic, 'Clinical Features and Diagnosis of Hypochondriasis', 45, 'a diagnosis of hypochondriasis is not incompatible with the presence of organic disease'. Keats is an example of a hypochondriacal personality whose relationship to illness was exacerbated by the effects of organic disease – in his case, consumption.

67. Thomas Trotter, *Observations on the Scurvy; with a Review of the Opinions Lately Advanced on that Disease, and a New Theory Defended*, (2nd edn, London, 1792) 44.

68. STC to Charles Lloyd, Senior, 14 November 1796, *CL* 1: 256.

69. STC to Beaumont, 2 February 1804, *CL* 2: 1053 (emphasis in original).

70. STC to Mrs Charles Aders, 30 December 1823, *CL*, 5: 319. On Coleridge's relationships with doctors, see R. Guest-Gornall, 'Samuel Taylor Coleridge and the Doctors', *Medical History* 17 (1973) 327–42. The relationship between doctor and patient in hypochondriasis is a complex one, and would need further exploration in Coleridge's case than we can give here. Pilowsky observes that the diagnosis of hypochondriasis itself 'emerges from a development at some point in the doctor–patient relationship'. Pilowsky, 'Hypochondriasis', 254. There is, oddly, no record that any of Coleridge's doctors diagnosed him as hypochondriacal in their casebooks.

71. See Starcevic, 'Clinical Features and Diagnosis of Hypochondriasis', 30.

72. Coleridge's medical reading was wide-ranging, in several languages, and included (in English) such works as George Berkeley, *Siris: a Chain of Philosophical Reflexions and Inquiries Concerning the Virtues of Tar Water* (1744); Sir John Pringle, *Observations on the Diseases of the Army* (1765); Erasmus Darwin, *Zoonomia; or, The Laws of Organic Life* (1794–6); James Hamilton, *Observations on the Utility and Administration of Purgative Medicines in Several Diseases* (1805); Thomas Bateman, *A Practical Synopsis of Cutaneous Disease* (1813); *The Quarterly Journal of Foreign Medicine and Surgery* (1818–19); *Transactions of the Medico-Chirurgical Society of Edinburgh* (1826). Furthermore, his awareness of German medical anthropology, which touched on hypochondriasis and its nervous origins, should not be minimized.

73. STC to Cottle, 26 April 1814, *CL* 3: 476, 489.

74. STC to the Morgans, 30 June 1814, *CL* 3: 515.

75. Ibid. *CL* 3: 516, emphasis in original.

76. STC to James Gillman, 6 October 1824, *CL* 5: 376. See William Prout, *Inquiry into . . . Gravel, Calculus, and Other Diseases of the Urinary Organs* (1821).

77. Gillman, *The Life of Samuel Taylor Coleridge*, 23.

78. Vickers, 'Coleridge, Thomas Beddoes and Brunonian Medicine', 59.

79. See, for example, Coleridge's *Theory of Life,* published posthumously in 1848 and reproduced in *The Collected Works of Samuel Taylor Coleridge: Shorter Works and Fragments, Volume I,* ed. H. J. Jackson and J. R. de J. Jackson (Princeton: Princeton University Press, 1995) 481–557. For Coleridge's plagiarisms in this work see Fruman, *Coleridge,* chapter 12, '*Theory of Life* and Coleridge's Writings on Science', 121–34. Fruman writes (126), 'Coleridge's reputation as a profound thinker has profited by a process in which his absurdities are either reinterpreted so as to seem insightful, or simply ignored.'

80. STC to Revd John Edwards, 29 January 1796, *CL* 1: 179. See 'home-sick', *Oxford English Dictionary,* 2nd edn. Further on we discuss Coleridge's homelessness briefly; it needs, in particular, to be compared with Wordsworth's lack of it or, at least, the latter's sense of lack. Poems such as Coleridge's 'The Delinquent Travellers' (1824) indicate how profoundly the condition moved him. For the medical and cultural formulation of nostalgia, see G. S. Rousseau, *Nostalgia: The History of an Idea* (forthcoming).

81. Hector Gavin, *On Feigned and Factitious [sic] Diseases, Chiefly of Soldiers and Seamen, On the Means Used to Simulate or Produce Them, and on the Best Modes of Discovering Impostors: Being the Prize Essay in the Class of Military Surgery, in the University of Edinburgh, Session, 1835–6, with Additions* (London: John Churchill, 1843) 176.

82. He may have read about Ernst Platner's theories in Christian Friedrich Ludwig's (1751–1823) recently published four-volume collection, *Scriptores neurologici minores selecti . . .* (1791–95), widely available in German libraries and handsomely illustrated. Ludwig's anthology was just the sort of work, with its vivid descriptions of the hypochondrium's nervous sensibility and consequently the susceptibility of sedentary genius to its derangements, to appeal to Coleridge. Platner also wrote about memory as a neuroanatomical process, a theory that influenced Blumenbach who discussed Platner in the lectures Coleridge heard him give.

83. STC to Sara Coleridge, 14 January 1799, *CL* 1: 459–60.

84. STC to Poole, 3 August 1798, *CL* 1: 414.
85. STC to Sara Coleridge, 23 April 1799, *CL* 1: 484. See also Coleridge's poem, 'Home-Sick. Written in Germany', in Samuel Taylor Coleridge, *The Complete Poems* (London: Penguin, 1997) 260–1.
86. *The Notebooks of Samuel Taylor Coleridge, Volume 1: 1794–1804*, ed. Kathleen Coburn (London: Routledge & Kegan Paul, 1957) 1816.
87. See Appendix A, DSM-IV, point D.
88. STC to Southey, 17 May 1803, *CL* 2: 943.
89. STC to Gioacchino de' Prati, 14 October 1828, *CL* 6: 767.
90. STC to Cottle, 26 April 1814, *CL* 3: 476.
91. See Starcevic, 'Clinical Features of Diagnosis of Hypochondriasis', 23.
92. STC to Daniel Stuart, 28 April 1811, *CL* 3: 319.
93. Dorothy Wordsworth to Catherine Clarkson, 16 June 1811, in *The Letters of William and Dorothy Wordsworth, 1806–1811*, ed. E. de Selincourt, 2nd edn, revised M. Moorman (Oxford: Clarendon Press, 1969) 495.
94. William Wordsworth to Thomas Poole, 30 May 1809, ibid., 353.
95. STC to C. A. Tulk, 21 September 1821, *CL* 5: 174.
96. STC to Dr Sainsbury, July 1815, *CL* 4: 578.
97. STC to William Sotheby, 9 November 1828, *CL* 6: 769–70.
98. 'Report of Examination of the body of S. T. Coleridge', in *CL* 6: 992.
99. Gillman to Cottle, 2 November 1825, *CL* 6: 992–3, footnote.
100. Sara Coleridge to Hartley Coleridge, 5 August 1834, *CL* 6: 992.
101. Arthur J. Barsky, 'Somatosensory Amplification and Hypochondriasis', in Starcevic and Lipsitt (eds), *Hypochondriasis*, 223–48, 223.
102. Ibid., 224.
103. Ibid., 225.
104. STC to Poole, 9 October 1797, *CL* 1: 348.
105. Cottle, *Reminiscences*, 293.
106. Barsky, 'Somatosensory Amplification', 229.
107. Porter and Porter, *In Sickness and in Health*, 222.
108. Ersasmus Darwin to Elizabeth, Lady Harrowby, 21 May 1796, in *The Letters of Erasmus Darwin*, ed. Desmond King-Hele (Cambridge: Cambridge University Press, 1981) 295. On fear of death in hypochondriasis, see Starcevic and Lipsitt (eds), *Hypochondriasis*, 28, 34, 38, 47, 50, 68, 79, 109–10, 112, 297.
109. Starcevic, 'Clinical Features and Diagnosis of Hypochondriasis', 34. See also Russell Noyes, 'Epidemiology of Hypochondriasis', in Starceiv and Lipsitt (eds), *Hypochondriasis*, 127–54, esp. 139–41.
110. STC to Cottle, 26 April 1814, *CL* 3: 477.
111. Holmes, *Early Visions*, 15. Hitherto most discussions of Coleridge and the new sensibility have omitted his medicine, Ford being the exception.
112. Roy Porter, *Bodies Politic* (London: Reaktion Books, 2001) 162, a crucial statement about the role of the gut in the development of theories of genius.
113. I. A. Richards continued to make this point about the importance of Coleridge's contribution to English aesthetics throughout his (Richards') writing career.
114. Susan Sontag, 'Loving Dostoyevsky', *The New Yorker* 2001: 98–105.
115. Starcevic and Lipsitt (eds), *Hypochondria*, 35.

Part IV

Towards a Poetics and Metaphorics of Disease

12
Paradoxical Diseases in the Late Renaissance: the Cases of Syphilis and Plague

Agnieszka Steczowicz

In their study of plague and syphilis, the authors of *The Great Pox* argue that the 'experience of the two diseases jointly altered European medicine'.[1] It is not uncommon for these two diseases to be discussed together, whether in contemporary medical treatises or in studies of Renaissance medicine. *Medicine from the Black Death to the French Disease*, a collection of essays spanning the 'long fifteenth century', which begins with the pan-epidemic of bubonic plague, around 1348, and ends in the 1490s when syphilis first appeared, is a case in point.[2] In the century following the outbreak of the 'French disease', plague provided a ready-made pattern of interpretation for the more recent epidemic. This is partly due to the popularity of medieval plague tracts, which served as a model for treatises dealing with syphilis.[3] But syphilis in turn changed the nature of debates about plague, perhaps as a result of the influential new theories prompted by its emergence. In the late Renaissance, similar kinds of explanations were put forward to account for both plague and syphilis, frequently by the same physicians.[4] Both were seen as virulent, intractable, and contagious. Traditional medicine, centred on the individual's receptiveness to particular diseases, failed to explain the rapid spread of these diseases or to come up with a successful cure. This gave some the justification for promoting alternative accounts of disease, challenging ancient authorities and received medical opinions. In the words of Petrus Severinus, 'paradoxical diseases produce[d] paradoxical doctors'.[5]

Syphilis and plague have attracted a great deal of interest on the part of historians of medicine, and the literature devoted to them is extensive.[6] This essay is specifically concerned with the relation between these two diseases and paradox; it is both limited in its scope and highly selective in the writers discussed. Its aim is to explore the ways in which paradox, both as a concept and as a genre, provided ways of framing and imagining disease in the late Renaissance. My understanding of paradox, by contrast with that of most critics who have written about Renaissance paradoxes,[7] rests entirely on contemporary definitions of the term, rather than on what we today take to be paradoxical. By paradox we nowadays understand a 'statement or proposition which on the face of it seems self-contradictory, absurd, or at variance with common sense, though, on investigation or when explained, it may prove to be well-founded' (*OED*, 2.a.). Yet the sixteenth-century author or reader of paradoxes had a very different understanding of the notion, much closer than ours to the etymology of the word. 'Paradox' was taken to mean what is 'besides' and 'contrary to' (*para*) common or received opinion (*doxa*), and it was synonymous of 'new' and 'strange'. Surprisingly from a modern-day perspective, paradoxes were also a genre of serious scholarly disputation, loosely modelled on Cicero's *Paradoxa Stoicorum*, and most prevalent in medical, legal, theological and philosophical writings.[8]

In the first part of this essay, I explore the semantic field of 'paradox', and particularly its associations with novelty and wonder, in relation to new diseases. To call a disease paradoxical, I argue, may be seen as an attempt to imagine and categorize it so as to come to grips with its inexplicable nature. Syphilis, the most emblematic of these diseases, and the one that gave rise to the most vigorous debates, will be the focus of this section, but plague and other new diseases will also be considered alongside it. I then turn to paradoxes as a genre dealing with diseases such as syphilis and plague. This subject has up until now received fairly little scholarly attention, although recent studies have drawn attention to this new genre of medical writing and its popularity in the sixteenth century.[9] Far from being mere rhetorical and literary devices, paradoxes were used as polemical tools in various medical debates. I shall briefly outline some of the characteristic features of this genre, before examining how it was used for framing discussions about disease. This section will be centred on two vernacular paradoxes devoted to plague: Claude Fabri's *Paradoxes de la cure de peste* (1568) and Silvestro Facio's *Paradossi della pestilenza* (1584). In these works, plague is likened to syphilis, and the explanatory schemes devised for the more recent disease are used in discussions of the older one.

Imagining disease: the notion of disease as paradoxical

Traditional Galenic medicine, a synthesis of Hippocratic writings and Aristotelian natural philosophy, proved largely ineffective in dealing with a number of epidemics which plagued Europe from the late Middle Ages onwards. Faced with contagious diseases for which there were no obvious precedents in ancient or medieval literature, university-trained physicians were at pains to account for them in terms of temperamental imbalance or humoural disorder. Underlying such explanatory categories was the notion that disease affects the individual interacting with a specific environment. Galen's method and his account of disease come under attack in Petrus Severinus' *Idea medicinae philosophicae* of 1571 precisely for being unable to cure new illnesses:

> The host of new diseases in our age, and the fact that the remedies of the ancients proved ineffectual and vain in dealing with these diseases, gave rise to great medical controversies; meanwhile every one of Galen's principles and his method, preserved and handed down for centuries, were tried in search of causes and remedies to such unusual symptoms and unyielding diseases. Thus *paradoxical diseases give rise to paradoxical doctors* (my own emphasis).[10]

Playing on different senses of the adjective 'paradoxical', Severinus makes a causal connection between the so-called new diseases ('paradoxi morbi') and unorthodox medical thinkers ('paradoxi medici'). In the sixteenth century, the word 'paradox' had the meaning of 'unheard of' and it was closely associated with novelty and wonder.[11] It could thus be used as an image for the recent epidemic outbreaks of syphilis, whooping cough, the 'English Sweats', rickets, smallpox, and even plague which, if not strictly speaking new, is often counted among them.[12] Plague, not unlike the more recent epidemics, was perceived to be a novel phenomenon at the time of the Black Death. Although it continued to be identified with pestilential fever, its contagiousness, the role of poisonous vapours in its propagation, and the presence of buboes made it unlike any of the diseases previously described by either Greek or Arabic authorities.[13] The notion of a 'paradoxical' disease aptly reflects the disarray into which university-based medicine was thrown by the emergence of new diseases, which did not fit neatly into existing classificatory schemes or respond to traditional therapeutic methods. The most prominent of the new diseases and the one that gave rise to the largest number of medical controversies is the great pox, named 'syphilis' after the hero of Girolamo Fracastoro's poem of 1530,[14] and often referred to by its vulgar name, *morbus gallicus*, in Renaissance treatises. The disease is presented as unusual ('morbum insuetum') in the first lines of Fracastoro's *Syphilis*, and it is frequently portrayed as new and marvellous in the rest of the poem.[15] Interestingly, these are also qualities attributed to plague in the first book of the poem, where Fracastoro compares the appearance of plague two centuries before to the more recent outbreak of syphilis.[16] Of disputed origin, the French disease spread across Europe in the 1490s, after the French army had been contaminated with it at Naples, and it was thought to have been initially contracted by Columbus' crew in the New World. Both the supposed provenance of this strange new disease and the recourse to indigenous remedies, such as the bark of guaiac wood imported from the Indies,[17] justify Laurent Joubert's calling it an 'exoticus affectus' by association with other 'morbi peregrini', in a tract entitled *De vairola magna*.[18] Joubert considers it to be a 'new disease' not so much because its appearance can be dated to 1494, but because he deems it just as strange and inexplicable as the plague, very difficult to treat, spectacular in its symptoms, and contagious. Galenic categories do not seem to apply to this singular disease: 'an illness which is not common, merely hot or cold, humid or dry, or composed of these [qualities], but of the total (as they call it) substance'.[19] Far from original, Joubert's characterization of the new disease makes use of notions developed by 'paradoxical doctors', chief amongst them Fracastoro and Fernel.

By the time Joubert's short treatise was first published, in 1571, the notion of a 'new disease' had ceased to be paradoxical. But in the decade following the first outbreak of syphilis, the very idea that an illness could appear *de novo* was highly controversial and stimulated much discussion both in courtly and in academic circles. The first in a long line of treatises dealing with this issue, Nicolò Leoniceno's *Libellus de epidemia quam vulgo morbum gallicum vocant* of 1497, stems from a dispute which took place at the court of Ferrara.[20] While he does not see any reason for identifying the recent outbreak with any of a number of well-known diseases displaying similar symptoms (*elephantiasis, asaphati, pruna, ignis persicus,* or *lichenas*), he refuses to think of it as an entirely new disease. Since neither human nature nor the causes of disease are subject to change, he argues, this disease must have been known to ancient authorities by a different name, which we are yet to discover.[21] To a Hellenist like Leoniceno, this view had the advantage of preserving the authority of *prisca medicina* intact. Sebastian Montuus invokes this precise argument in his refutation of Fuchs's paradox dealing with the French Disease.[22] Fuchs follows Leoniceno, *contra* Symphorien Champier whose view Montuus defends, in distinguishing between syphilis and the disease called *lichen* in Greek and *impetigo* in Latin. But he departs from Leoniceno's opinion by calling the disease new and unknown to the ancients: 'The illness which is generally called "French disease", is not that which the Greeks call *lichen,* and the Latins *impetigo,* but rather a new disease unknown to the ancients.'[23] To most physicians in Fuchs' day this assertion was nothing short of paradoxical.

Having looked at the controversial nature of 'new diseases' and the sense in which they may be described as paradoxical, we may now turn to the 'paradoxi medici' in the above-mentioned statement. Severinus has in mind physicians such as Jean Fernel, to whose concept of 'diseases of the total substance' operating through occult properties he briefly alludes, and perhaps Girolamo Fracastoro, whose theory of contagion and 'seeds of disease' could be applied to syphilis as well as to other intractable diseases, plague amongst them.[24] Other physicians, such as Argenterius, also used the notion of 'disease of the total substance', affecting the total substance or form of the body rather than the balance of its qualities, to account for the spread of plague and syphilis.[25] These new theories were elaborated from ancient doctrine and used to classify specific illnesses that did not fit into habitual categories of disease, based on the theory of temperaments. But Severinus, an exponent of Paracelsian medicine, thinks that Fernel and other such doctors did not go far enough in their rejection of traditional concepts. In his eyes, they have kept the principles, the method and the cures set out by Galen virtually intact. He sees Paracelsus, who 'entirely transformed the medicine of our times' (4), as far more radical. Paracelsus may be seen as an unorthodox thinker on several counts: he rejected the authority of ancient and medieval doctors, professed a contempt for learned medicine, advocated the use of empirical remedies, waged battle against humours and qualities, and introduced in their place a new cosmology, which combined mystical, alchemical and astrological elements. Not surprisingly, he had a large following among empirics, apothecaries and surgeons, all of whom were less concerned with establishing the nature of a disease than with finding effective remedies for it.

Severinus is not the only one to have drawn a parallel between new diseases and unorthodox medical views. In a work entitled *De morbis novis interpola, cum aliquot paradoxis,* published in Poitiers in 1541, Baptista ex Cavigolis considers whether there are such things as new illnesses, what they are, and lists some possible causes. He gives the usual examples of the English sweating sickness, whooping cough, typhus, and smallpox, but also lists a variety of less-known local epidemics.[26] Unlike Fuchs, who saw no real need to prove that new diseases existed, since the 'French disease' was known to have appeared in 1494, Baptista ex Cavigiolis appeals to reason and experience in arguing for the theoretical possibility of new diseases. In a manner directly opposed to Leoniceno's way of thinking, he argues that neither Greek nor Arabic doctors can have known the same diseases as his contemporaries, since they lived in very different geographical areas, had different habits and practices, and ate different foods. He claims to have observed new diseases peculiar to the region of Poitiers, which called for new treatments. Cavigioli goes on to discuss the causes of new diseases (divine wrath, the influence of stars, elements, individual constitutions, winds, regions, alimentary regimes), the study of which occasions many almost discrete paradoxical developments. He argues, for instance, that three rather than four elements enter into the composition of simples, an opinion which ran counter to that of most contemporary philosophers.[27] Paradoxes are, to use his own expression, woven into the study of new diseases, and they appear naturally to grow out of it. This is true of paradoxes at large, a genre whose appearance may be directly linked to the spread of new diseases and the vigorous debate about the nature and the transmission of disease that it occasioned.

Framing disease: the genre of paradox dealing with disease

From the third decade of the sixteenth century onwards, various medical works calling themselves 'paradoxes' were printed both in Latin and in the vernacular. These ranged from individual paradoxes dealing with a specific disease (the plague, catarrh) or medical field (anatomy, surgery),[28] to entire collections of paradoxes in the works of Leonhart Fuchs, Laurent Joubert and Felix Platter.[29] Medical paradoxes were above all attacks on authorities, whether these be Arabic and medieval, ancient or 'neoteric'. Like the cognate genre of *errata*, paradoxes were devoted to exposing and rectifying erroneous medical opinions. Judging by the works of Fuchs and of Joubert, where these two notions are closely allied, paradoxes may in fact be seen as an outgrowth of error literature.[30] Whether or not the appearance of this new kind of writing was in any way linked to the invention of printing,[31] its novelty was not without appeal to an audience used to more traditional forms of medical debate such as the commentary and the *quaestio*. Placed at the head of a tract or a collection, the word 'paradox' promised controversy and departure from accepted norms and habitual ways of thinking at a time when these were frequently challenged by innovative physicians and surgeons. Although the genre of paradox continued to be used as a polemical tool well into the eighteenth century, in medicine, its rise to prominence coincided with various trends associated with the 'medical

Renaissance':[32] the humanist rejection of scholastic and Arabic authorities, the challenge to traditional Galenic medicine posed by discoveries in botany and anatomy, the appearance of new diseases and the radical alternatives to Greek medical thought propounded by men like Paracelsus.

While paradoxes were not confined to any specific part of medicine, they were particularly prominent in the fields of anatomy, botany, and pathology which were the theatre of some of the most radical depatures from established theory and practice in the late Renaissance. Fuchs's *Paradoxorum medicinae libri tres* of 1535, the earliest extant collection of medical paradoxes, is exemplary in this respect and sets the trend for later paradoxists. The three books of paradoxes, devoted respectively to 'medical matter' or botany (book I), diseases and their cure (book II) and anatomy (book III), closely parallel Leoniceno's interests and those of the school of Ferrara.[33] Leoniceno's *De Plinii ac plurimum aliorum in medicina erroribus*, on which Fuchs's errors and paradoxes are modelled, deals with botany and anatomy, and his *Libellus de epidemia quam vulgo morbum gallicum vocant*, although chiefly concerned with syphilis, describes and attempts to identify several other diseases. In the preface to the second book, Fuchs directs his criticism specifically at the erroneous opinions of vulgar doctors regarding the causes of various diseases and their cures.[34] Like Leoniceno, and other prominent members of the school of Ferrara, Fuchs is especially concerned with nomenclature and giving the correct name to a disease. In paradox XVIII of the second book, for instance, he accuses his contemporaries of giving four different names to the same disease, an error largely resulting from their ignorance of Greek and the fact that they follow the lessons of the Arabs.[35] The sense that a lack of equation between *res* and *verba* in medical matters can pose a serious threat to human health lies behind his efforts at stabilizing medical terminology.[36]

Of the paradoxes dealing with disease a great number are dedicated to putrid or pestilential fever and to plague, topics that were frequently confused with one another.[37] I shall consider two roughly contemporary works written by less well known figures, specifically devoted to plague: Claude Fabri's *Paradoxes de la cure de peste* (1568) and Silvestro Facio's *Paradossi della pestilenza* (1584).[38] By contrast with most paradoxes which were composed in Latin, the *lingua franca* of the learned community of physicians, these works are written respectively in French and Italian. This is not, however, highly unusual given their subject-matter. For charitable reasons, paradoxes dealing with diseases, particularly the epidemic ones, tended to be composed in the vernacular so that the less educated might benefit from them. Writers of such paradoxes often felt obliged to justify their use of the vernacular. In a Latin epistle addressed to fellow physicians, which follows one in the vernacular, Claude Fabri explains that he opted for the French tongue so as to make his paradox accessible to those surgeons and apothecaries not versed in Latin.[39] His insistence on method and the need to seek out the true causes of the disease rather than simply prescribing remedies reaffirms his credentials as a university-trained physician. Fuchs himself, in the preface to the second book of his paradoxes, dismisses practical medicine and favours a rational approach which begins by methodically investigating the causes of a disease and only then turns to remedies.[40] The methodical approach which Fabri sees as a mark of his originality sets his treatise apart from the majority of plague tracts, which often amounted to little more than a list of prophylactic treatments and cures, where the author would advertise his own remedies.[41]

However, Fabri's approach is far from what we would consider today as rational and scientific. He describes himself on the title page as a 'medecin et astrophile'. This last qualification accounts for his use of an astrological figure with the help of which he predicts an onslaught of the plague throughout Christian Europe for the year 1568. Insisting that the plague is unlike most diseases, Fabri likens it to the *grosse verolle* which arrived in Europe some sixty years before, sent by God as a punishment for our sins. He goes on to explain that the cause of pestilential fever has long been 'hidden, occult and doubtful', partly as a result of plague being (like syphilis) a 'contagious disease'.[42] Physicians and empirics, both ancient and modern, have greatly erred in prescribing phlebotomy and purgation as if they were effective remedies for pestilential fever. For Fabri, the root of their error lies in ignoring the true cause of the event:

> We had more concern for the putrefaction of humours than for the occult, secret, specific and celestial cause, coming from above, and not having its origin in the elements and their qualities, or in the humours, as in the case of other illnesses. It is necessary to seek essential and proven remedies other than phlebotomy and purgation to withstand such a poisonous quality.[43]

Implicit in this statement is a criticism of the classical Galenic account of disease based on such notions as 'temperamental imbalance', and the 'putrefaction' of humours in the case of pestilential fever. In his

51202

PARADOXES

DE LA CVRE DE PESTE,

PAR VNE METHODE SVCCIN-
cte, contre l'opinion de ceux qui en
ont escrit & pratiqué au passé.

PAR

CLAVDE FABRI, MEDECIN

& Astrophile, natif de Prelz en Ar-
gonne, demeurant à Dijon.

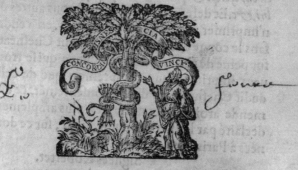

Ἀρχὼ ἰᾶθαι πολὺ λώϊον ἤε τελευτὼ.

A PARIS,

Chez Nicolas Chesneau, rue S. Iaques, à l'ensei-
gne de l'escu de Froben, & du chesne verd.

M. D. LXVIII.

AVEC PRIVILEGE DV ROY.

Illustration 12.1   Title page of Claude Fabri, *Paradoxes de la Cure de Peste*, 1568

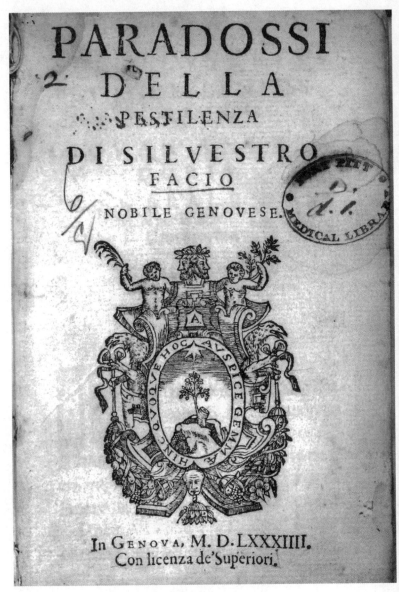

Illustration 12.2   Title page of Silvestro Facio, *Paradossi della Pestilenza*, 1584

eyes, a new disease calls not only for new remedies but also for rethinking the very foundations of traditional medicine in which elements, qualities and humours take the place of all other explanations. Not unlike Paracelsus, with whom he shares an enthusiasm for astrological and religious causes, Fabri claims that God made remedies readily available to all, and in the name of Christian charity he urges the reader to dispense them to all those in need of cure. The 'unorthodox' elements of Fabri's thought can thus easily be traced to Fernel, Fracastoro and Paracelsus, even though none of these authorities is directly invoked.

By contrast, Silvestro Facio's *Paradossi della pestilenza*, published in Genoa two decades later, are explicitly a criticism of Fracastoro's theory of contagion in favour of the traditional aetiology of miasma or bad air as an explanation of the spread of plague. Facio's paradoxes take the form of a dialogue between three characters who are all described as physicians ('Medici') at the outset of the dialogue, and one of whom is the author himself: Steffano Mari, Giuseppe Ratto and Silvestro Facio. The three characters and the functions that they fulfil within the paradoxical dialogue call to mind Philiatros, Brutus and Eudoxus in Fernel's *De abditis rerum causis*.[44] Ratto, much like Brutus, is committed to defending the *doxa* against the more paradoxically-minded Eudoxus, in this case Facio himself, and Mari convenes the speakers in the first place and weighs the relative merits of the arguments as Philiatros did in Fernel's dialogue. The courtly and literary qualities of the dialogue are further enhanced by the fact that the dialogue spans over a period of seven days, described as *Giornata Prima, Seconda, Terza*, and so on, in a manner evocative of Boccaccio's *Decameron*. Such a literary allusion, unusual in an otherwise serious medical work, is pleasing and appropriate since Boccaccio's work opens with one of the most celebrated accounts of plague-stricken Florence. The dedication to the prince, which begins by alluding to the recent outbreak of plague from which Facio's countrymen are suffering, contains the initial formulation of the paradox, which is then fully exposed and borne out by arguments in the course of the seven *giornate*:

> The mortality which of late has filled this country with such dread
> . . . made me long to find out whether it came from the outside and
> was carried over in infected things from Lombardy, *as is the common
> cry*, or whether it was spread by means of pestilential air in this coun-
> try. But prompted by two *vivid reasons and palpable experiences* to
> think that it did not come from outside the city, but was born out of

bad air, I went even further, and judged that the belief that any pestilence can be kindled by means of a few infected objects brought into
cities or provinces is based on weak foundations. *This opinion, though
contrary to the opinion of all men, is I believe not far removed from truth*
(my own emphasis).[45]

Most paradoxes begin with a justification of their title; Facio's dedication is exemplary in this respect. According to Facio, the opinion of the
vulgar ('as is the common cry') has it that the current outbreak of plague
had spread from Lombardy by means of infected objects carrying disease, rather than having been caused by pestilential air. Facio rules out
the first theory, which he sees as based on weak foundations, and considers that only the latter may be taken into consideration. In a manner
typical of a paradoxist, he claims that his own opinion is consonant
with reason and experience ('vivid reasons and palpable experiences')
and, though it runs counter to the views commonly held ('the opinion
of all men'), it is nevertheless close to the truth.[46]

Translated into medical terms this amounts to a partial rejection of
Fracastoro's theory of contagion, namely of the *fomites* or intermediaries
such as food or clothes, which were thought to carry within them 'seeds
of disease' able to generate putrefaction in a healthy host. Although the
theory of contagion was initially devised to account for the spread of
syphilis, it was usually invoked in contemporary discussions about
plague.[47] Ratto, in his exposition of the general belief that plague is contagious, alludes to the similarly contagious *mal Francese*:

I will not fail to recall in this regard the French disease, similar in its
mode of contagion, which as everyone knows was brought over from
the New World, and first broke out in Italy in the year 1494, while
the French were conquering the kingdom of Naples, and which by
means of pure contagion spread throughout the Old World.[48]

By contrast with Fabri, the author of the Italian work has a much firmer
grasp of the vocabulary and the theories in question. In the course of
the dialogue, plague is precisely defined and distinguished from pestilential air, contagion and its three different modes (direct contact, by
means of intermediaries, at a distance) are discussed at length, as are
Fracastoro's other views before they are rejected. Facio denies that contagiousness is an essential quality of plague, basing his claims on the
authority of doctors who have witnessed recent and past pestilences (to
his mind the disease has always existed), reason which forbids him to

summon a particular cause such as the *fomites* for what he defines as a 'common disease', and the experience of the most recent outbreak of plague in Genoa.[49] The formal sophistication of the arguments deployed is worthy of note, even if, with hindsight, his conclusions appear to be false.

In this essay, I have considered paradox both as a metaphor and an image for strange and new diseases, and as a genre framing debates about diseases such as syphilis and plague. To call a disease 'paradoxical', in the sixteenth-century meaning of the term, is another way of saying that it is new and strange, and that it runs counter to common medical opinion regarding disease. Many puzzled over new diseases in the wake of the outbreak of syphilis, deeming them difficult to categorize, to name, and therefore to treat. But Petrus Severinus was among the first to draw a causal connection between the new diseases and the unorthodox medical thought that they engendered. His claim that 'paradoxical diseases produce paradoxical doctors' is highly pertinent for the study of 'framing and imagining disease': new diseases are metaphorically designated as 'paradoxical' so as to emphasize their heuristic value and the role that they played in subsequent medical discoveries and innovations.

Notes

1. Jon Arrizabalaga, Roger French and John Henderson, *The Great Pox: the French Disease in Renaissance Europe* (New Haven and London: Yale University Press, 1997) 235.
2. See Roger French, Jon Arrizabalaga, Andrew Cunningham and Luis García Ballester (eds), *Medicine from the Black Death to the French Disease* (Aldershot: Ashgate, 1998).
3. On the influence of medieval plague tracts in discussions of the French disease, see Anthony Grafton, April Shelford and Nancy Siraisi, *New Worlds, Ancient Texts: the Power of Tradition and the Shock of Discovery* (Cambridge, MA and London: Belknap Press of Harvard University Press, 1992) 180.
4. Vivian Nutton, 'The reception of Fracastoro's theory of contagion: the seed that fell among thorns?', *Osiris*, 2nd series, 6 (1990): 226–7.
5. Petrus Severinus, *Idea medicinae philosophicae, fundamenta continens totius doctrinae Paracelsicae, Hippocraticae et Galenicae* (Basle, 1570) 3. For an interpretation of this quote, see Ian Maclean, *Logic, Signs and Nature in the Renaissance: the Case of Learned Medicine* (Cambridge: Cambridge University Press, 2002) 23.

6. For an overview of plague and syphilis scholarship, see Ann G. Carmichael, *Plague and the Poor in Renaissance Florence* (Cambridge: Cambridge University Press, 1986) 166–75 and Arrizabalaga et al., *The Great Pox*, 3–10.

7. The most influential interdisciplinary study on the subject is Rosalie Colie's *Paradoxia Epidemica: the Renaissance Tradition of Paradox* (Princeton: Princeton University Press, 1966). Colie, however, operates with a loose understanding of 'paradox', which enables her to include in her study oxymorons, self-contradictions, statements of self-reference, negations and mock-encomia. For a criticism of this approach, see Frances Yates's review in the *New York Review of Books*, 23 February 1967: 27–8.

8. See Brian Vickers's *'King Lear* and Renaissance Paradoxes', *The Modern Language Review* April 1968: 305–8.

9. See in particular Iain M. Lonie's 'Fever pathology in the sixteenth century: tradition and innovation', in *Theories of Fever from Antiquity to the Enlightenment*, eds W. F. Bynum and V. Nutton, *Medical History*, Supplement no. 1 (1981): 20; and Maclean, *Logic, Signs and Nature in the Renaissance*, 193.

10. 'Nostra ætate nova morborum cohors, & antiquorum remedia in morbis nostris irrita & vana, magnas in arte medica peperere controversias: dum unusquisque ex Galenicis Principiis & tot seculis custodita ac quasi per manus tradita Methodo, tam insolentium Symptomatum, & cedere non volentium morborum, causas & curationes eruere conatur. Itaque paradoxi morbi, paradoxos medicos peperere' (Severinus, *Idea medicinae philosophicae*, 3; all translations are my own). See Maclean, *Logic, Signs and Nature in the Renaissance*, 22.

11. Cicero famously defined paradoxes as 'admirabilia contraque opinionem' (*Paradoxa Stoicorum, Prooemium*, 4). Contemporary dictionaries retained and elaborated upon this definition. Randle Cotgrave, for instance, defines 'paradox' as 'a strange, and odd conceit, or assertion, which differs from the common-received opinion' in *A dictionarie of the French and English tongues* of 1611. For a study of the notion, see Letizia Panizza's 'The semantic field of "paradox" in 16th and 17th century Italy: from truth in appearance false to falsehood in appearance true: a preliminary investigation', in *Il Vocabolario della République des lettres: terminologia filosofica e storia della filosofia. Problemi di Metodo* (Florence: Leo S. Olschki editore, 1997) 197–220.

12. On new diseases, see Laurence Brockliss and Colin Jones, *The Medical World of Early Modern France* (Oxford: Clarendon Press, 1997) 45, and Andrew Wear, 'Medicine in early modern Europe, 1500–1700', in Laurence I. Conrad, Michael Neve, Vivian Nutton, Roy Porter and Andrew Wear (eds), *The Western Medical Tradition 800 BC to AD 1800* (Cambridge: Cambridge University Press, 1995) 218–20.

13. See Melissa P. Chase, 'Fevers, Poisons, and Apostemes: Authority and Experience in Montpellier Plague Treatises', in Pamela O. Long (ed.), *Science and Technology in Medieval Society* (New York: NYAS, 1985) 153–8.

14. *Hieronymi Fracastorii Syphilidis, sive morbi gallici, libri tres, ad Petrum Bembum* (Verona, 1530).

15. See, for instance, book I, 12, 14, 243, 261 and book II, 4–5 and 16.

16. See book I, 189, where Fracastoro speaks of 'insolita . . . febris'.

17. A treatment popularized by Ulrich von Hutten in a famous treatise entitled *De guaiaci medicina et morbo gallico*, published in Mainz in 1519.

18. Laurent Joubert, *De vairola magna*, in *Opera omnia* (Lyons, 1582), vol. 2, 225–34.

19. '[I]ntemperies non . . . vulgaris, calida tantum, vel frigida, humida aut sicca, vel ex suis composita, sed totius (ut vocant) substantiæ (Joubert, *De variola magna*, 226).

20. For the exact circumstances of the dispute and its participants, see chap. 4 of *The Great Pox*.

21. *Liber de morbo gallico* (Venice, 1535) a3.

22. See Sebastianus Montuus, *Dialexeon medicinalium libri duo* (Lyon, 1537) 87.

23. 'Morbum quem vulgo Gallicum vocant, non esse eum quem Graeci Lichenem, Latini vero Impetiginem appellant, sed novum potius et veteribus incognitum'. See Leonhart Fuchs, *Paradoxorum medicinae libri tres* (Paris, 1546) 157r.

24. For a detailed account of these theories, see Vivian Nutton's 'The reception of Fracastoro's theory of contagion: the seed that fell among thorns?', *Osiris*, 2nd series, 6 (1990): 196–234; and Linda Deer Richardson's 'The generation of disease: occult causes and diseases of the total substance', in Andrew Wear, R. K. French and Iain M. Lonie (eds), *The Medical Renaissance of the Sixteenth Century* (Cambridge: Cambridge University Press, 1985) 175–94.

25. See Wear 'Medicine in early modern Europe', 262.

26. Baptista ex Cavigiolis, *De morbis novis interpola*, 3 and 7. Less typical is his inclusion of some local diseases, or heartache (*cordis dolore*) and anxiety.

27. Ibid., 65.

28. See, for instance, Claude Fabri's *Paradoxes de la cure de peste par une méthode succinte contre l'opinion de ceux qui ont en escrit . . . au passé* (Paris, 1568); Nicolas Habicot's *Paradoxe myologiste, par lequel est demontré que le diaphragme n'est un seul muscle* (Paris, 1610); and Jacques Fontaine's *Deux paradoxes appartenant à la chirurgie: le premier contient la façon de tirer les enfans du ventre de leur mère par la violence extraordinaire . . . l'autre est de l'usage des ventricules du cerveau, contre l'opinion la plus commune* (Paris, 1611).

29. Leonhard Fuchs, *Paradoxorum medicinae libri tres* (Paris, 1546); Laurent Joubert, *Paradoxorum decas prima atque altera* (Lyons, 1566); Felix Platter, *Quaestiones medicae paradoxae et endoxae* (Basle, 1625).

30. Fuchs's *Paradoxorum medicinae libri tres* of 1535 is an amended and closely expanded version of the author's *Errata recentiorum medicorum* published in 1530. Joubert's reputation as a controversial writer rests chiefly on his vernacular *Erreurs populaires au fait de la medecine et regime de santé* (1578) and the *Paradoxorum decas prima atque altera* (1566).

31. As I. M. Lonie argues in 'Fever Pathology in the Sixteenth Century: Tradition and Innovation', claiming that printing created an 'indeterminate audience' for genres such as paradox (Lonie, 'Fever pathology in the sixteenth century', 20).

32. On this notion, see the introduction to *The Medical Renaissance of the Sixteenth Century*, ix–xi.

33. For an account of Leoniceno's and other members' of the School of Ferrara influence on Fuchs, see Luigi Samosa's 'Le ripercussioni in Germania dell'indirizzo filologico-medico leoniciano della Scuola Ferrarese per opera di Leonardo Fuchs', *Quaderni di Storia della Scienza e della Medicina*, 4 (1964): 7–41.

34. Fuchs, *Paradoxorum medicinae*, 103.
35. '*Pruna* or *ignis persicus, carbunculus* and *anthrax* are not different kinds of diseases, as many doctors think today, but rather it is one and the same disease that is designated by these different names' (Fuchs, *Paradoxorum medicinae*, 160–1).
36. On the different categories of 'error' in Leoniceno and Fuchs, see Maclean 214.
37. Joubert devoted three of his paradoxes to putrid fevers: paradoxes 2–4 of the second decade. On the controversy surrounding these paradoxes, see Lonie 36–9. Platter's *Quaestiones paradoxae et endoxae* includes questions such as 'Whether air is the cause of pestilential venom' and 'Whether the internal cause of pestilential fever resides in the corruption of humours or not' (Platter 75–8).
38. Claude Fabri, *Paradoxes de la cure de peste, par une methode succinte, contre l'opinion de ceux qui en ont escrit et pratiqué au passé* (Paris, 1568); Silvestro Facio, *Paradossi della pestilenza di Silvestro Facio nobile genovese* (Genova, 1584).
39. Fabri, *Paradoxes de la cure de peste*, 5.
40. Fuchs, *Paradoxorum medicinae*, 103.
41. Chase, 'Fevers, Poisons and Apostemes', 153.
42. Fabri, *Paradoxes de la cure de peste*, 2.
43. '[O]n a eu plus d'égard à la putrefaction des humeurs, qu'à la cause occulte, secrette, specifique & celeste, venant d'enhaut, & n'ayant origine premiere des elemens ny de leurs qualitez, ny des humeurs comme les autres maladies. Dont convient chercher autres remedes premiers & certains que phleubotomie & purgation, pour obvier à une telle qualité veneneuse' (Fabri, *Paradoxes de la cure de peste*, 3).
44. On this distribution of roles, see Linda Deer Richardson, 'The generation of disease', 179.
45. 'La mortalità che ultimamente con tanto spavento ha tormentato questa patria ... ha desto nell'animo mio uno ardente desiderio di sapere se stata sia forestiera venuta col mezo di robe appestate di Lombardia, come suona il publico grido, overo paesana tratta dall'aria pestifera. Ma da vive ragioni e palpabili esperienze invitato a non istimarla forestiera, ma partorita dalla malvagità dell'aria, sono entrato tanto oltre col pensiere, che ho giudicato haver deboli fondamenti lo stimare che alcuna pestilenza per l'introduttione di poche robe di appestati nelle città, o provincie si accenda giamai. Laqual oppenione, come che contraria all'oppenione di tutti gli huomini: credo nondimeno che non si lontani del vero' (Facio, *Paradossi della pestilenza*, a2–a3).
46. On the equation of truth and paradox, see Panizza, 'The "semantic" field of paradox', passim.
47. See Nutton, 'The reception of Fracastoro's theory of contagion', 201–3 and 225ff.
48. 'Ne mancherò di ricordare a questo proposito il mal Francese nel contagio simile alla peste, il qual si sa che fu recato dal mondo nuovo, e si scoperse in Italia l'anno 1494, mentre i Francesi vincevano il regno di Napoli, e con forza poi del puro contagio si diffuse per tutto il mondo vecchio' (Facio, *Paradossi della pestilenza*, 28).
49. Ibid., 104.

13

'Proved on the Pulses': Heart Disease in Victorian Culture, 1830–1860

Kirstie Blair

In 1841, *The Times* reported an inquest on Honoria Brien, a young woman who died unexpectedly in a state of poverty and starvation. The cause of her death was recorded as heart disease: largely, it seems, due to a witness who reported that Honoria told her 'my heart is so compressed, and I am sure it is breaking'.[1] A sense of 'compression' in the chest does have some authority as a symptom of cardiac illness, but the chief weight of the statement lies in the theory of heartbreak. The inquest could interpret a figurative expression as a physical event, and was supported in this by medical authority. 'Violent feelings not only agitate, but may kill the heart in a moment; in short, broken hearts are medical facts', wrote the medical and philosophical writer James Wilkinson in 1851.[2] In the same decade, but in a different discourse, William Gladstone argued, in a review of Tennyson's poems, that passion and feeling were vital aspects of contemporary life, concluding, 'Does any one believe that ever at any time there was a greater number of deaths referable to that comprehensive cause a broken heart?'[3] Honoria's death from a broken heart, it seems, was a peculiarly Victorian cause, one supported by both literature and medicine.

'Heartbreak' is one example of a figure of speech (the physical heart cannot literally break) which is imagined as a medical possibility, if not a probability. The heart, this essay argues, lends itself to such transformations, constantly blurring the boundaries between cultural supposition and apparent medical fact. Although the late eighteenth and early nineteenth century saw the gradual establishment of physiology and medicine as separate, professionalized discourses, the language of the heart in medical texts before 1870 rarely discusses this organ in purely physical terms. The decades between 1830 and 1860 are perhaps the last moment when the heart maintains the level of cultural importance it had accrued in earlier periods, and indeed, particular factors current in the nineteenth century – including the rise of physiology – highlighted this importance. The focus on sensibility in late-eighteenth-century culture and literature, for example, meant that the feeling heart became a symbol of moral worth as well as passionate susceptibility to emotion. Evangelicalism, a form of Christianity which stressed individual, heartfelt response, also rose to prominence in the Anglican Church, meaning that the traditional religious symbolism of the heart gained a new currency. And both romantic love and family affections (heart and hearth) were glorified in Victorian ideology. Such a priori involvement of the heart in a wider network of cultural and literary reference meant that physiologists and medical writers inevitably found in the heart the qualities which metaphorical uses had taught them to look for.

Yet this kind of influence runs both ways. References to medical and physiological texts and debates should be read in conjunction with later examples from literature, not necessarily as a gloss on them, nor as evidence that poets were reading physiology (though in many cases this was true), but as examples of how the imagination of the heart in Victorian Britain worked simultaneously through and in these different discourses. The sick heart comes to be a focus of interest across disciplines, as increasing suspicion of sensibility from the early nineteenth century onwards, and doubts about the validity of feeling and faith in a mechanistic and materialistic society, meant that the heart came to seem an untrustworthy prop. In *Aids to Reflection*, for example, Coleridge wrote that his contemporaries feared to examine their feelings, for:

> There is an aching hollowness in the bosom, a dark cold speck at the heart, an obscure and boding sense of a somewhat, that must be kept *out of sight* of the conscience; some secret lodger, whom they can neither resolve to eject or retain.[4]

The terms used recall the language of pathology, with the heart concealing a cancerous growth or a secret, undermining sickness. Coleridge's use of 'at' (rather than 'in' or 'on') gives a vaguer sense of something near or around the heart, and also hints at the phrase 'at heart', meaning inwardly or secretly ('he was sick at heart'). If medical concentration on the pathological heart may in part have stemmed, as we shall see, from sources such as Coleridge's account, Coleridge and his contemporaries were simultaneously engaging with the new medical vocabulary of the heart, as it meshed with general cultural disquiet about 'heartsickness', and insinuated itself into the textual corpus and, effectively into the bodies of poets themselves.

In recent years scientific and medical historians and literary critics have argued for the existence of 'one culture' in Victorian Britain, a shared discourse in which 'not only *ideas* but metaphors, myths, and narrative patterns could move rapidly and freely to and fro between scientists and non-scientists'.[5] Perhaps surprisingly, however, the discourse of heart disease has rarely been examined in this context. In her influential study of illness and metaphor, Susan Sontag argues that heart disease has been 'hitherto little culpabilized' because it is seen as purely mechanical failure.[6] But it cannot be assumed that the organ which has traditionally been perceived as the innermost and most sensitive part of the self was (or is) purely seen as 'mechanical' in its actions – for nineteenth-century writers coming to terms with mechanistic physiological explanations, this concept was terrifying and alienating. Moreover, in the early to mid-Victorian period, as we shall see, heart disease tended to be seen as highly culpable, and was blamed for a variety of other physical and emotional ailments.

Recent studies of pathology in nineteenth-century Britain have concentrated almost exclusively on the brain and nervous system, and on the interconnected narratives of madness, hysteria and nervousness; illnesses in which psychology and physiology meet. Unlike the heart, which has been a continuous topic in medical (and cultural) discourse since antiquity, the nervous system was a relatively new discovery in the nineteenth century, and so it appears peculiarly representative of Victorian attitudes and theories. But its sudden rise to prominence, around the mid-century, has tended to obscure the significance of earlier, stubbornly resistant, theories of disease. In a recent discussion of Victorian pathology and literature, Jane Wood writes:

> To the lay mind, it seemed logical that the nervous system formed the vital bridge between the body's sensations and the mind's consciousness of them. Neurophysiologists, moreover, were confident that it was the mediating properties of the nervous system which explained how invisible impulses translated into human action and behaviour.[7]

However, neurophysiologists would naturally wish to claim the importance of their chosen field of study, the nervous system. To the 'lay mind' of the 1830s, a period in which nerve action was only just beginning to be explained, it seemed more reasonable, I argue, to assume that the 'vital bridge' was provided by the heart, whose ambiguous position between body and mind was already well established. The older humoural theory, which gave primary importance to the blood and circulation, still had a grip over the practice of physicians and the imagination of their patients.

By the 1830s, moreover, the heart was already well established as a leading topic of investigation and research. Christopher Lawrence writes that:

> Interest in the morbid anatomy of the heart and its clinical manifestations can be said to form a continuous tradition in British medicine, beginning at the end of the eighteenth-century ... Increasingly, physicians wrote books on the disorders of anatomically defined organs, including the heart.[8]

In 1846, the Pathological Society was formed as a new forum for discussion, and 31 heart cases were discussed in the opening season; not surprisingly, given that the first president (Charles Williams) was an expert on the pulse.[9] At the newly established University College Hospital in London, several of the professors were researching the heart.[10] The first hospital specifically for the treatment of heart disease opened in London in this period, and in 1857 the National Hospital for Diseases of the Heart was founded.[11] Advances in classification were extremely rapid: the early nineteenth century was the era in which most major types of heart disease were identified and named, including angina, endocarditis, pericarditis, hypertrophy and fatty degeneration. An awareness of these diseases gradually spread into wider Victorian culture. 'Fatty degeneration', for instance, was described as a 'fashionable complaint' in 1852,[12] and the medical historian A. D. Morgan notes that around this period: 'fatty degeneration became a popular diagnosis, so much so that it infiltrated everyday speech and even mid-Victorian literature'.[13] He is doubtless thinking of George Eliot's Casaubon in *Middlemarch* (1872), who suffers from this degenerative disease, Eliot implies, from an inability to love as much as from organic causes.[14]

Many of these discoveries were enabled by the invention of new clinical instruments and diagnostic techniques. By the 1860s the sphygmograph, which produces a diagram of the wave patterns of the pulse, and various experimental apparatuses for measuring blood pressure, were gradually coming into use. But the most revolutionary new instrument of the period was, of course, the stethoscope, first used by Laennec in

1819. *The Times* reported in 1824: 'A wonderful instrument called the stethoscope . . . is now in complete vogue in Paris . . . It is quite a fashion . . . to have recourse to the miraculous tube'.[15] It was widely used in Britain from the 1830s onwards. 'Auscultation' (first discussed by Leopold Auenbrugger in the mid-eighteenth century), the practice of identifying heart and lung problems by tapping on the chest and listening intently to the reverberations beneath, was another important diagnostic tool. Along with the stethoscope, it introduced a greatly increased sensitivity to the movements and sounds of the heart, and a clinical method of precise investigation rather than general surmise. Kenneth Keele argues that in the 1830s, 'the nature and causes of the heart sounds and murmurs were to be sufficiently rationally elucidated as to satisfy most clinicians' demands ever since'.[16] Not without dissension, however. There was a heated technical debate on the subject in the *Lancet* between 1832 and 1835, which was also the year when the British Association for the Advancement of Science appointed a committee to enquire into 'the heart's sounds and movements'.[17] James Hope and Charles Williams, leaders in the field, were rival investigators into the cause of the heartbeat, and their dispute remained unresolved.

The new vocabulary of murmurs, thrills and whistles which resulted from listening to the heart could be said to give it 'eloquence', a voice and a language. Suddenly it was theoretically possible for anyone in possession of a stethoscope and a guide to auscultation to describe accurately an anomaly in the heart's sound, and to proceed to diagnose the disease. In their attempts to describe sounds, doctors and other investigators resorted to a range of striking and inventive similes. Laennec, for instance, heard sounds like a whip, and like a dog lapping water.[18] John Elliotson remarked a noise 'exactly like the cooing of a dove', and J. J. Furnivall heard a 'creaking, or new leather sound' and 'the rumpling of silk or parchment'.[19] In 1836, Peter Mere Latham, one of the most famous doctors and lecturers of the period, familiarly nicknamed 'Heart Latham', wrote on the praecordial region:

> Within this space we cannot see. But at this space we can listen, and feel, and knock, and so put it to question, whether all be right beneath. And there is no spot of it which does not in its turn make answer to the ear, to the touch, or to the tapping of the finger, and tell something of the organ that lies herein.[20]

He envisages a responsive heart, although his phrasing suggests that it is not the heart itself, but the echoes from the dark space in which it lies, that allow a process of deduction as to the mysterious organ within. The attempt to enter into dialogue with the heart, to persuade or force it to reveal its secrets, is a common literary trope. But the revelations here are of the heart's illness. Asking 'whether all be right beneath' raises the likelihood that in that obscure and dark region, something might be wrong.

Nineteenth-century medical research into the heart unquestionably concentrated on its pathology. In a later treatise on heart disease, J. Milner Fothergill remarks:

[C]uriously, both the public who furnish the patients and the medical men who give advice, have to a great extent neglected the normal working of the heart; both, however, feeling keenly the fascination which the diseases of this organ unquestionably possess for all.[21]

It is impossible to say whether heart disease proved of such interest because it was perceived as one of the most common diseases of the time, or whether it owes this status as a common disease to earlier popular fascination. The well-known biblical quotation describing the heart as the organ 'out of which are the issues of life' (Proverbs 4.23), a phrase cited by many writers in different discourses, lent a religious colour to the heart's accepted cultural status as the most vital part of the body. Such apparent biblical proof, in an era when Christianity was still the dominant mode of thought, seemed to guarantee the heart's centrality even as it also implied the dangers inherent in heartsickness. In medicine, this centrality meant that unidentifiable diseases or unknown causes of death tended to be ascribed to underlying cardiac problems. One medical writer notes that, in 1845, a third of all deaths in London were caused by 'diseases of the chest'.[22] The leading doctor James Paget wrote to his fiancée in 1839, when he was in the early stages of his career:

I have found out something . . . by which I hope I shall gain a little more reputation: for I shall be able to prove that nearly half the adult population have had a disease of the heart at some time of their lives – not indeed an important, not perhaps an injurious one, but still one that is discernible.[23]

The breadth of his claim makes 'a little more' seem like understatement. In an atmosphere where the sick heart was 'fascinating', Paget might well think that his discovery could cause a sensation. One year later, *The Times* reported this summing up of a case of sudden death by the chief coroner, who was also the influential editor of the *Lancet*: 'Mr Wakley said he had no doubt that deceased's death was occasioned by disease of the heart, which was now fearfully prevalent; and which an eminent physician had told him recently was the cause of 95 sudden deaths out of 100.'[24] Reports on the frequency and unpredictability of heart disease clearly carried a frisson of interest, and the statistics circulating in popular and medical reports about the likelihood of contracting it were high enough to be definitely alarming.

While it is unlikely that specialized treatises on heart disease were widely read by a lay public, the explosion of theory did have an impact on popular culture, and was reported in newspapers, journals and, apparently, at dinner-table conversations. John Ruskin, for instance, wrote to his father in 1861, after attending a party: 'Miss Cooke thought I must be threatened with disease of the heart, and spoke almost with tears in her eyes to me about minding what I was about in time – she is herself a sufferer from heart disease.' In the same letter he adds, 'It's very tiresome the way people notice my face now. A lady . . . was dining here to-day, and I had no sooner gone out of the room than she asked Miss Bell if I had heart disease.'[25] If we believe Ruskin's report, it does suggest informed knowledge, as at least one popular medical writer warns that a 'violet or red tint to the face' can be a sign of hypertrophy.[26] It is not necessary to have read medical textbooks, moreover, to be aware of the cultural status of a particular disease. Mark Pattison, a leading Oxford reformer, writes in his *Memoirs* that when he and his fellow dons began discussions about revising the Oxford syllabus in 1845, 'The great discoveries of the last half-century in chemistry, physiology, etc, were not even known by report to any of us.' But two years later, when he was suffering from 'palpitation of the heart' due to overwork, fasting and emotional involvement with Tractarianism, Pattison tells the reader that he went to London 'to take the advice of Dr Williams, or Dr Latham, I forget which'.[27] Williams (possibly John Williams, author of a treatise on palpitation) and Latham were experts on nervous diseases of the heart. Not only did Pattison clearly know of them at the time: his casual reference also implies that he expects readers in 1885 to recognize the names.

The rapid advances in diagnosis and classification thus made heart disease more visible, and more commonly recognized, yet not therefore more explicable. The author of one of the most important early treatises on the subject, Allan Burns, warns:

The heart, from the intricacy of its structure, and from its incessant action, is liable to many diseases, and these from the importance of the function of this organ, are at all times highly alarming. Some of them are extremely insidious in their commencement, are attended with obscure and perplexing symptoms, and in their result are almost uniformly and speedily fatal.[28]

Burns presents the heart as a delicate organism subjected to deliberate attack by disease. His repeated use of intensifying adverbs ('highly', 'extremely', 'uniformly', 'speedily') heightens the rhetorical urgency of his warning. Rather than reassuring his readers (whether they are a doctor hoping to diagnose heart disease or a patient), Burns plays on their fears, painting an exaggerated and foreboding picture. 'Observation has traced back, with fearful fidelity', writes Latham, 'a long line of formidable and fatal diseases to their pathological parentage in the heart.'[29] The heart becomes a parent, or a womb, generating diseases as its offspring, an image which taps into contemporary fears about heart disease and heredity. The relish in Latham's alliteration deliberately adds a dramatic flourish, portraying the physiologist as an intrepid investigator, fearing what he will encounter – the sensational hidden source of all disease, the sick heart.

If the source of sickness is evident, however, the cause is less so. Medical writers often resorted to speculation in arguing why individuals contracted heart disease. The heart's symbolic and metaphorical status in other discourses lent credibility to various hypotheses, fostering beliefs that organic heart disease could be caused both by internal emotions, such as grief or love, and by external events, such as the decline of religious belief or the economic uncertainty of the period. It was generally accepted that the heart responded directly to feelings, whether mental or physical, registering how they impinged on the individual. In the early to mid-nineteenth century, however, it was perceived as more likely to register emotions and events which had a negative effect on bodily health. The expansive term 'sympathy', which is defined as the influence of one organ on another, but also as emotional identification and empathy, becomes an index of disease. 'By its all-pervading sympathy, it feels all that is hurtful throughout the body;' writes Latham on the heart, 'and by its own peculiar mode of action it tells all that it feels, and telegraphs intelligence of it through every artery that can be felt.'[30] He describes a physical action of the heart in language which, again, extends into the figurative, introducing a productive uncertainty as to how far concepts like 'sympathy' can be taken.

'Intelligence' conveys a sense that the heart is the thinking operator of this system: in a metaphor borrowed from contemporary technology, it is simultaneously the telegraph operator and the mechanism itself, as the pulse beats out the messages. If sympathy is vital, because it implies beneficial affective responses, it is also dangerous because it transmits threatening feelings of hurt and passion.

'Sympathetic' heart disease was the subject of a wealth of medical textbooks and advice manuals throughout these decades. Associated with emotion and feeling, it encompassed any symptoms which apparently lacked a clear organic origin, and mimicked the symptoms of organic disease with such success that diagnosis was extremely difficult. In his book on palpitation, John Williams writes:

> From the intimate connection that exists through the medium of the nervous system, between the heart and other organs ... symptoms may arise 'par sympathie', so similar, in every respect, to those which proceed from absolute disease of the heart itself, as to baffle the closest inquiry.[31]

Of course, this allows any organic disease to be diagnosed as sympathetic in origin, as well as vice versa. Williams's treatise is devoted to the theory that the increasing importance of the nervous system in medicine highlights new causes of heart disease, because the nerves sympathetically communicate with the heart. He and other writers point out that whereas those actually suffering from cardiac disease are relatively unlikely to realize it, those undergoing nervous heart disorders experience symptoms so alarming that they insist they have organic disease. As James Hope, author of one of the most influential accounts of cardiac disease, remarks:

> There are few affections which excite more alarm and anxiety in the mind of the patient than this. He fancies himself doomed to become a martyr to organic disease of the heart, of the horrors of which he has an exaggerated idea; and it is the more difficult to divest him of this impression, because the nervous state which gives rise to his complaint, imparts a fanciful, gloomy and desponding tone to his imagination.[32]

In imitating the symptoms of 'real' disorders, sympathetic disease could induce such apprehension in the sufferer that organic disease would eventually be produced. Hope's language – 'fancies', 'idea', 'impression', 'imagination' – stresses that disease is acting on or in the mind as much as the body. The patient is trapped, because the nervous state associated with inorganic, sympathetic disease, in itself, by manifesting the symptoms of heart disease (a disordered pulse, an unbalanced circulation) is likely to cause these symptoms to become permanent and thus lead to organic disease. This theory of a causal link between sympathetic and 'real' heart disease was very tempting, not least because it indicated the need for mental and moral regulation and control over impulsive emotions. In addition, it suggested that belief in the sick heart was itself enough to make the heart sick. Hence the prevalence of heart disease in society could literally stem from discussions – whether medical or not – of its prevalence, creating a nervous apprehension.

In a relatively late study, Robert Semple repeats the common claim that heart disease is associated with 'mental emotion and excitement, a very common cause, especially in this active and enterprising age; the influence of the passions, especially that of love; the pursuit of study to an excessive degree', combining public events and private emotions in his list of causes.[33] Sympathetic disorders of the heart, and related organic diseases, were assumed to be more common among those who were unduly sensitive or over-emotional: young men, women and artists. To take a literary example, in Elizabeth Gaskell's *Wives and Daughters* (1865), Osborne Hamley, a sensitive, poetic young man who marries unwisely for love, dies from 'Something wrong about the heart.' Technically, his complaint is defined as 'aneurism of the aorta', but it seems logical when his father blames his death on anxiety about his hidden marriage: 'care killed him. They may call it heart disease –'.[34] Osborne's emotional and familial problems, besides his character, would have been presumed to be important factors.

The combination of causes listed by Semple made it particularly likely that writers would suffer from heart disease, given that reading and writing were commonly linked to illness, and that poetry, and to a lesser extent novels, were traditionally expected to be written 'from the heart', discussing the author's heartfelt emotions and conveying them to the reader's heart. For this reason, Victorian poets were particularly anxious about the state of their own hearts, and their poems and letters provide some of the most vivid imaginings of cardiac disease. In Elizabeth Barrett Browning's 1838 poem, 'The Student', for example, a young over-ambitious student dies at his desk with his 'breast and brow' pressed to his book:

> Words which had often caused that heart to throb,
> That cheek to burn; though silent lay they now,

> Without a single beating in the pulse,
> And all the fever gone![35]

These lines shift so that the heartbeat and blush of the student, caused by the excitement of reading (or writing, if these words are his), are strangely transferred to the written page. The words themselves have a pulse, which came alive in the act of reading, when the student animated it with his own fever and desire. Barrett Browning does not need to explicitly state the cause of the student's death: the symptoms clearly allude to a rush of blood from the heart to the head, a well-documented complaint of writers and readers. She herself suffered from rapid circulation and a dangerously fast pulse:

> I had a doctor once who thought he had done everything because he had carried the inkstand out of the room – 'Now', he said, 'you will not have such a pulse tomorrow.' He gravely thought poetry a sort of disease . . . and held as a serious opinion, that nobody could be properly well who exercised it as an art – which was true, he maintained, even of men – he had studied the physiology of poets.[36]

The 'physiology of poets', although Barrett Browning mocks it, was taken seriously by her doctor. Robert Browning, likewise, was urged by a friend to give up writing for the state of his health, and to plunge his head regularly into cold water, which 'will lower the circulation of the blood within and with it the *necessity* for thinking'.[37] Thought itself here resembles a physiological function, the irresistible impulse to think caused directly by the rapid circulation of the blood.

Symptoms which came to be considered characteristic of the 'physiology of poets' also mark the bodies of poetic characters and leave their traces in form, rhythm and language. Alfred Tennyson, for example, continually writes of sensitive young men who suffer unbalancing shocks to the heart due to love or grief, leaving them incapable of manly action and decision and with hearts which either beat too fast or too slow. The hero of *Maud* (1855), for instance, is overcome by realization of his father's death:

> And my pulses closed their gates with a shock on my heart as I heard
> The shrill-edged shriek of a mother divide the shuddering night.[38]

This shock is insistently physical due to Tennyson's placing of the phrase 'on my heart'. Although 'shock' probably refers back to the pulses it appears to act *on* the physical organ, as the gates, the valves of the heart, shut upon it. A shock 'in' the heart would not carry the same implication of a blow falling, a physical jolt to the passive heart. The 'beat' of the verse is speeded up by the driving anapaests of line 14 ('with a shóck on my héart'). Such moments can leave the heart per- manently weakened: 'In *grief*, or long protracted and severe affliction, such is the influence of the mind on the heart, that the circulation of the blood becomes extremely languid, and sometimes to such a degree as to produce syncope.'[39] The morbidly susceptible lover Julian, in Tennyson's *The Lover's Tale*, suffers these effects after losing his beloved to his rival:

> [M]y blood
> Crept like marsh drains through all my languid limbs;
> The motions of my heart seemed far within me,
> Unfrequent, low, as though it told its pulses.[40]

This imagery recalls Percival Barton Lord's *Popular Physiology* (significant because Tennyson was given a copy for Christmas in 1838) where two pages are devoted to the comparison of the circulatory system with the drainage system of a city. The blood circulating through Julian's veins is not purified blood, 'bright and lively' through exposure to the air in the lungs, but the 'black and impure' blood, compared to sewage, that has been moving sluggishly around the body.[41] The 'sunken' heart, another common image, shows his isolation from human feeling – the heart has withdrawn into the depths, the void of the body, so that its movements are scarcely perceptible.

These Tennysonian sufferers are the more remarkable because Tennyson himself also had cause to worry about his heart. Besides his fears that the 'black blood' of the Tennysons might be hereditary, his father suffered from 'spasms of the chest', and he himself wrote in 1829: 'For the last quarter of a year I have been most distressed by a determin- ation of blood to the Head.'[42] Most significantly, Arthur Hallam, also a poet and writer, whose early death inspired Tennyson's *In Memoriam* (1850), had allegedly died of a heart-related illness. His father ascribed his death to 'a sudden rush of blood to the head' (in fact cerebral haemorrhage) and 'the symptoms of deranged circulation'.[43] John Brown, doctor, popular author and friend of Ruskin, Thackeray and other writers, alleged in a memoir that Hallam's diseased heart made him sympathetic in the wider sense of the word, more 'easily moved for others – more alive to pain – more filled with fellow-feeling'.[44] But the demands of that sympathy seemed to prove too much – it was reported that a post-mortem examination showed 'a weakness of the cerebral vessels, and a want of sufficient energy in the heart'.[45]

In 'A Farewell', Matthew Arnold writes:

> I too have felt the load I bore
> In a too strong emotion's sway;
> I too have wished, no woman more,
> This starting, feverish heart away.[46]

'No woman more' (like Barrett Browning's '*Even* of men') emphasizes the fact that the weak, intermittent heart was perceived as a feminine ailment – women were expected to be more liable to heart disease because of their particular emotional sensitivity, and because of the strong medical belief in the relation between heart and womb. The speaker here stresses his connection to the feminine heart even as 'wishing' it away. Arnold too feared for his own heart: his father had died of angina pectoris (Latham's case history of his death became the standard textbook account of the disease), and Arnold had been warned that his own pulse was irregular. Yet there is more pride in this stanza than is apparent, because Arnold's weakness, like that of other poets, can also be read as proof positive of his poetic destiny. Given the connections between heart disease, poetic sensitivity and intellectual activity – which might outweigh its associations with effeminacy and over-emotion – suffering from it could potentially be read as a mark of distinction. Certainly none of these poets attempt to hide these symptoms – rather, both they and their poems call attention to them.

In eighteenth-century and early Romantic literature, the heart is a common image, yet one that tends to be relatively unproblematically associated with sympathy, affection, romantic love and religion.[47] Only in early-nineteenth-century poetry does the heart start to be personified as a dangerously conscious organ, an active agent in the spread of disease throughout body and mind. There are few specific references to heart disease in the letters and other writings of Wordsworth, Keats, Shelley and Byron (Coleridge is the exception), while virtually every Victorian poet explicitly worried about his or her heart. Yet poets are only particularly evident examples of a general cultural imagination of heartsickness. Writers in all fields claimed that heart disease, in the widest sense, was particularly endemic in Victorian society, a contemporary evil. The 'sympathetically' diseased heart was commonly linked by many writers to politics, and indeed to the state of the nation itself. National traumas or upsets, doctors warned, could seriously damage the hearts of the population. Jean-Nicholas Corvisart, one of the pioneers in the study of cardiac pathology, claimed at the start of the century, in an oft-quoted passage, that heart disease rose as a direct consequence of the French Revolution.[48] William Newnham, another philosophical medical writer, refers to his work in claiming that,

> [D]isease of the heart has been of much more common occurrence of late years, especially after any season of commercial distress, or political excitement. This was very remarkably exemplified after the revolution in France, and in our own country after seasons of great and unfortunate speculation.[49]

He suggests the importance of economic factors: disturbances in the smooth circulation of capital (common in this period of booms, speculative mania, panics and slumps) might alter the circulation of those affected. Newnham in fact published his book at the lowest point of a period of pronounced economic depression, in 1842. He does suggest that the apparent rise in heart disease might be due to the attention paid to it by medical writers, but he emphasizes that this does not entirely explain the sudden rise in cases. Forbes Winslow, in a popular book on avoiding insanity, notes on the heart:

> Diseases of this organ are, I regret to say, alarmingly on the increase, and I much question whether the circumstance is not to be attributed to the unnatural political excitement in which the people of this country have been kept for the last few years.[50]

This was also written in 1842, and Winslow stresses economic anxiety as well as apprehension about the possibility of revolutionary disturbances. He neatly lays the blame for heart disease on the politicians, not on the weak hearts of the people.

Whereas the hearts of British people are expected to beat as one under pressure, this discourse suggests that they are instead prone to collapse and to develop nervous heart disorders. Whether it was organic (as some writers argued) or psychosomatic in origin, the nervous heart seemed a particularly damning comment on the state of Britain, given the extent to which political and nationalistic rhetoric used the language of the heart to bolster its claims. The minor poet Henry Ellison nicely demonstrates this when he describes how the State's interests should be infused with 'One same Lifespirit from the mighty Heart, / Pulsing unwearied thro' every Vein'; a circulation which will keep the body politic in health. The state will act by:

> Blending tenmillion [*sic*] Hearts into one Pulse,
> One mighty Pulse of universal Love,
> Of Tolerance, and Truth and Liberty,
> Whose Beatings should be those of *God's own Heart!*[51]

The title of this poem implies that the need to make all hearts beat together is once more a response to economic panic, as well as to political ills. This metaphorical 'blending' of hearts into one religious ideal (shown by Ellison's blending of two words in 'tenmillion'), where individual pulses are subsumed both to the nation's and to God's, is a deeply conservative goal, because it denies a hearing to any dissenting impulses of the individual heart and brings its beatings into line with established opinion.

Heart disease, by forcing the individual to focus on their own emotions and to shun sympathetic communication with others, which might worsen the sickness, might then be read as a disruptive, even a revolutionary force. It upsets the natural and divinely ordained order of the body and, implicitly, of society. At the start of the century, Wordsworth's famous phrase from 'The Old Cumberland Beggar', 'For we have all of us one human heart', is designed to create a sense of community, the hearts of his readers beating as one in their sympathy for the character.[52] But when this is reworked by Arnold in the 1850s as 'The same heart beats in every human breast', it is placed in the middle of a poem filled with doubt and uncertainty, and immediately succeeded by 'But'.[53] For Wordsworth, everyone participates in a general humanity, a unified heart, and this is undeniably positive. Arnold is not so sure. His line is much more specific about the heart's location and its action, meaning that it is pinned down to the physical 'human' organ, rather than being a diffusive spiritual presence. Since one theme of 'The Buried Life' is the inaccessibility of the heart, stating that everyone has a similar heart becomes an image of isolation rather than community. Arnold's heart is lodged in a morbid individual incapable of 'blending' with others, and its behaviour is unpredictable and potentially pathological.

In all this, it is particularly characteristic of its age, and representative of a shift in the ideology of the heart in its period. The heart as 'wonderful machine' designed by God, as William Paley described it at the start of the nineteenth century, in his textbook *Natural Theology*,[54] is frequently replaced in later writings by the heart as a wayward, passionate force, dark and alienated, mysterious in its workings. 'What can be said of palpitations of the heart, and intermissions, and irregularities of its beats which come and go during a man's whole existence', writes Latham: 'They must come from something, but we know not what.'[55] As in Tennyson's *The Princess* (1848), the heart is beyond – or above – comprehension:

> [S]omething wild within her breast,
> A greater than all knowledge, beat her down.[56]

The ambiguity of 'something' and 'A greater' position the heart as a separate, inhuman entity, capable of overcoming the will and intellect. Until the 1870s and 1880s, when the focus of medical debates started to change, and the paradigm of heart disease became gradually supplanted by new interest in the nerves and the brain, the sick heart was an object of fascination to commentators because of its unsettling powers. It stood at the intersection of several discourses, it evaded societal control and regulation, failing to beat in time. Heart disease, as imagined by both poets and physicians in these decades, was therefore disruptive but also productive and even creative, both something to be lamented and, perversely, a source of fascination and pride.

Notes

1. 'Inquest on Honoria Brien', *The Times*, 15 January 1841: 5.
2. James John Garth Wilkinson, *The Human Body and its Connexion with Man* (London: Chapman and Hall, 1851) 219.
3. William Gladstone, 'Tennyson's Poems – *Idylls of the King*', *Quarterly Review* 106 (1859): 485.
4. Samuel Taylor Coleridge, *Aids to Reflection*, ed. John Beer (London: Routledge, 1993) 24.
5. Gillian Beer, *Darwin's Plots* (London: Routledge, 1983) 7. See also George Levine (ed.), *One Culture: Essays in Science and Literature* (Madison: University of Wisconsin Press, 1987).
6. Susan Sontag, *AIDS and its Metaphors* (New York: Farrar, Strauss and Giroux, 1989) 25.
7. Jane Wood, *Passion and Pathology in Victorian Fiction* (Oxford: Oxford University Press, 2001) 3.
8. Christopher Lawrence, 'Moderns and Ancients: the "New Cardiology" in Britain 1880–1930', in W. F. Bynum, C. Lawrence and V. Nutton (eds), *The Emergence of Modern Cardiology* (London: Wellcome Institute for the History of Medicine, 1985) 5.
9. A. D. Morgan, 'Some Forms of Undiagnosed Coronary Disease in Nineteenth-Century England', *Medical History* 12 (1968): 346.

10. For example, John Elliotson helped establish University College Hospital and worked there until 1838. Richard Quain was Professor of Anatomy at the hospital in 1830, W. H. Walshe was Professor of Morbid Anatomy in 1841, and John Marshall was Professor of Surgery in 1866. All four published on heart disease. Information from the *DNB*.
11. Lawrence, 'Moderns and Ancients', 11.
12. Archibald Billing, *Practical Observations on Diseases of the Lungs and Heart* (London: S. Highley, 1852) 73.
13. Morgan, 'Some Forms of Undiagnosed Coronary Disease', 349.
14. George Eliot, *Middlemarch*, ed. W. H. Harvey (Harmondsworth: Penguin, 1965) 460–1.
15. Cited in P. E. Baldry, *The Battle Against Heart Disease* (Cambridge: Cambridge University Press, 1971) 63.
16. Kenneth D. Keele, 'The Application of the Physics of Sound to 19th-Century Cardiology: with Particular Reference to the Part Played by C. J. B. Williams and James Hope', *Clio Medica*, 8 (1973): 198.
17. E. L. Bryan, 'Letter to Editor on Committee's Report', *Lancet* (1835–6) I: 501–2.
18. René Laennec, *A Treatise on the Diseases of the Chest and on Mediate Auscultation*, trans. John Forbes, 3rd edn (London: Thomas and George Underwood, 1829) 555, 573.
19. John Elliotson, *On the Recent Improvements in the Art of Distinguishing the Various Diseases of the Heart* (London: Longman, Rees, Orme, Brown and Green, 1830) 15; J. J. Furnivall, *The Diagnosis, Prevention and Treatment of Diseases of the Heart* (London: John Churchill, 1845) 8, 36.
20. Peter Mere Latham, *Lectures on Subjects Connected with Clinical Medicine, Comprising Diseases of the Heart*, 2nd edn, 2 vols (London: Longman, 1846) 2.
21. J. Milner Fothergill, *The Heart and its Diseases, with their Treatment*, 2nd edn (London: H. K. Lewis, 1879) 2.
22. Herbert Davies, *Lectures on the Physical Diagnosis of the Diseases of the Lungs and Heart* (London: John Churchill, 1851) 1–2.
23. Stephen Paget, *Memoirs and Letters of Sir James Paget*, 3rd edn (London: Longmans, Green, 1901) 107–8.
24. 'Inquest on Sir W. H. Pringle', *The Times*, 29 December 1840: 7.
25. John Ruskin, *The Works of John Ruskin*, eds E. T. Cook and Alexander Wedderburn, 39 vols (London: George Allen, 1909) 36: 360.
26. Thomas J. Graham, *On the Diseases of Females; A Treatise . . . Containing also an Account of the Symptoms and Treatment of Diseases of the Heart*, 7th edn (London: Simpkin, Marshall, 1861) Appendix 10.
27. Mark Pattison, *Memoirs* (London: Macmillan, 1885) 237, 239.
28. Allan Burns, *Observations on Some of the Most Frequent and Important Diseases of the Heart* (Edinburgh: James Muirhead, 1809) 1.
29. Latham, *Lectures*, 1: x.
30. Latham, 'The Heart and its Affections, Not Organic', *The Collected Works of P. M. Latham*, ed. Robert Martin, 2 vols (London: New Sydenham Society, 1878) 2: 521.
31. John Williams, *Practical Observations on Nervous and Sympathetic Palpitation of the Heart*, 2nd edn (London: John Churchill, 1852) 3.
32. James Hope, *A Treatise on Diseases of the Heart and Great Vessels* (London: William Kidd, 1832) 488.

33. Robert Semple, *A Manual of the Diseases of the Heart: Their Pathology, Diagnosis, Prognosis and Treatment* (London: J. & A. Churchill, 1875) 265.
34. Elizabeth Gaskell, *Wives and Daughters*, ed. Pam Morris (Harmondsworth: Penguin, 1996) 554, 381, 567.
35. Elizabeth Barrett Browning, 'The Student', lines 41–4. *The Complete Works of Elizabeth Barrett Browning*, eds Charlotte Porter and Helen A. Clarke, 6 vols (New York: AMS Press, 1973).
36. 'Letter to Robert Browning', 11 August 1845. *The Brownings' Correspondence*, eds Philip Kelley and Scott Lewis, 13 vols (Winfield, KA: Wedgstone Press, 1992–) 11: 24.
37. Alfred Domett, 'Letter to Robert Browning', 30 January 1846. Kelley and Lewis, *Brownings' Correspondence*, 12: 31.
38. Alfred Tennyson, *Maud*, Part 1: 4, lines 14–15. *The Poems of Tennyson*, ed. Christopher Ricks, 2nd edn, 3 vols (Harlow: Longman, 1987).
39. James Wardrop, *On the Nature and Treatment of Diseases of the Heart, with some New Views on the Physiology of the Circulation* (London: John Churchill, 1837) 67.
40. *The Lover's Tale*, 2, lines 51–4.
41. Percival Barton Lord, *Popular Physiology* (London: John W. Parker, 1834) 206–10.
42. *The Letters of Alfred Lord Tennyson*, eds Cecil Y. Lang and Edgar Shannon, 3 vols (Oxford: Clarendon Press, 1982) 1: 23, 41.
43. Henry Hallam (ed.), *Remains, in Verse and Prose, of Arthur Henry Hallam* (London: W. Nichol, 1834) xxxiv.
44. Hallam Tennyson (ed.), *Tennyson and His Friends* (London: Macmillan, 1911) 455.
45. Hallam, *Remains*, xxxv.
46. Matthew Arnold, 'A Farewell', lines 29–32. *The Poems of Matthew Arnold*, ed. Kenneth Allott, 2nd edn, revised Miriam Allott (Harlow: Longman, 1979).
47. On eighteenth-century literature and the heart, see Robert Erickson, *The Language of the Heart 1600–1750* (Philadelphia: University of Pennsylvania Press, 1997). On Romantic poetry, see John Beer, *Wordsworth and the Human Heart* (London: Macmillan, 1978).
48. Jean-Nicholas Corvisart, *A Treatise on the Diseases and Organic Lesions of the Heart and Great Vessels*, trans. C. H. Hebb (London: Underwood and Blacks, 1813) 323.
49. William Newnham, *The Reciprocal Influence of Body and Mind Considered* (London: J. Hatchard, 1842) 258.
50. Forbes Winslow, *On the Preservation of the Health of Body and Mind* (London: Henry Renshaw, 1842) 92.
51. Henry Ellison, 'To England, on occasion of the moneypanic', *Madmoments: or First Verseattempts by a Bornnatural*, 2 vols (London: Painter, 1839) 1: 438.
52. Line 19. William Wordsworth and Samuel Taylor Coleridge, *Lyrical Ballads*, eds R. L. Brett and A. R. Jones, 2nd edn (London: Routledge, 1991).
53. Arnold, 'The Buried Life', line 23.
54. William Paley, *Natural Theology*, 3rd edn (London: R. Faulder, 1803) 170.
55. Latham, *Works*, 519.
56. Tennyson, *The Princess*, VII lines 222–3.

14
Tropenkoller: the Interdiscursive Career of a German Colonial Syndrome

Stephan Besser

The cover illustration of Henry Wenden's colonial novel *Tropenkoller* (1904) shows a remarkable combination of two pictorial elements. The image is framed by a stylized representation of the war flag of the German Empire, which divides the illustration into four equal-sized parts. From the right margin a white male hand, firmly holding a whip, projects into the picture. The lower part of the emblematic illustration is dominated by the some-what menacing *inscriptio* 'Tropenkoller'. The delicate ambiguity of the image results from the fact that it facilitates two readings without privileg-ing one of them: On the one hand, the whip-swinging hand can appear as a disturbing intruder in the square heraldic order of the flag and can there-fore be seen to highlight the incompatibility of German imperial authority and pathological forms of violence. On the other hand, it may also be regarded as a new heraldic element of the flag that is tentatively added to point to an intrinsic affinity between imperial power and sadistic violence.

In my exploration of the discursive history of Tropenkoller I shall attempt to show that the ambivalent conflation of the political and the pathological rather than being an accidental effect of this suggest-ive cover illustration is, in fact, an essential characteristic of the syn-drome to which Wenden's novel is devoted. Tropenkoller was an overdetermined cultural phenomenon: Circulating between politics, literature and sciences it was conceptualized according to a number of different cultural 'frames' that were neither intrinsically contradictory nor simply reducible to each other. In the first two parts of this chap-ter I will examine the conditions of Tropenkoller's overdetermination in political and medical discourse. The third part scrutinizes the emer-gence of the syndrome as a crucial juncture in colonial discourses on sexuality and race. I end with a concluding remark on the question of how far this nervous disorder was a specifically German phenomenon.

I

In contrast to the naming of many other nervous disease entities – for example, George M. Beard's 'Neurasthenia' – the term 'Tropenkoller' was not coined by professional physicians but on the street. According to a contemporary handbook of colloquial expressions, the buzzword 'Tropenkoller' – a compound of the German words for 'tropics' and 'choleric' – first appeared around 1895 in Berlin dialect as a mocking designation for the 'pathological irritability' (*krankhafte Reizbarkeit*)[1] of European officers and officials in tropical colonies. The notorious linguistic inventiveness of the Berlin vernacular was most probably stimulated by various reports which were reaching the German capital at this time, about individual acts of violence against African natives – the so-called 'colonial scandals'. The metropolitan public of Berlin became especially agitated about the violent crimes of Heinrich Leist, the chancellor and deputy governor of the Cameroons, who in 1893 had ordered the whipping of a group of naked Dahomeydian women in front of their husbands and who forced some native female prisoners into prostitution. The public's attention was also captured by the cases of Ernst Wehlan, an assistant judge in the Cameroons, who had let his troops burn down some native villages and slaughter their inhabitants, and the excessive cruelty of Carl Peters, a famous German colonial pioneer in East Africa, who in 1891 had ordered the execution of his native concubine and her supposed lover. In this historical context, the newly invented disease entity obviously fulfilled a contemporary need to categorize and name: Over the course of the following decade Tropenkoller became a widely discussed issue in political debates on colonial politics as well as in the discourses of tropical medicine and contemporary psychiatry. And within a few years two Tropenkoller-novels appeared, by Frieda von Bülow (1896) and Henry Wenden (1904).

The popular origin of the syndrome had a key influence on Tropenkoller's discursive history. Rather than being a clearly defined disease entity, the syndrome emerged as a polyvalent cultural topos that acquired a multitude of divergent meanings, definitions and discursive functions. In his theory of interdiscursivity, the literary critic Jürgen Link has termed this kind of semantically over-saturated cultural topoi 'collective symbols'. Drawing on Foucault's notion of 'interdiscursive configurations',[2] Link assumes that modern societies are characterized by a dialectics of discursive differentiation and interdiscursive reintegration of knowledge: On the one hand, the increasing societal division of labour leads to the emergence of specialized discourses, such as medicine and jurisprudence, which create their own language and grammar. On the other hand, these specialized discourses also tend toward a reintegration and coupling within the highly selective 'interdiscursive language games'[3] of popular knowledge and literature. Whereas the terminology of specialized discourses is typically characterized by a striving towards monosemantic clarity, the popular 'interdiscourse' connotatively charges its objects of knowledge with a multitude of divergent and often ambivalent meanings.

Being an 'interdiscursive' and thus highly polysemic syndrome from the beginning, Tropenkoller invited divergent ideological investments and therefore soon came to play a prominent role in public and parliamentary debates on the 'colonial scandals'. Significantly, both sides of the political spectrum embraced the newly invented phenomenon and relied on it in their argumentation. For apologists of the colonial project the notion of Tropenkoller provided a possibility to attach a suggestive term to the common imagery of the tropics as a zone of climatic dangers.[4] As such it could be used to excuse the brutalities which presented a flagrant inversion of the official ideology of colonialism as a civilizing mission. In a parliamentary debate in February 1894, for example, the conservative member of parliament, Ehni, explicitly resorted to Tropenkoller as a possible 'excuse' for the colonial brutalities. Citing a famous epigram from Goethe's *Wahlverwandtschaften*, 'one does not walk under palm trees with impunity', he stated that it was a well-known fact that the tropics had a 'devastating influence not only on the body, but also on the mind and to a certain extent on morality'.[5] Mitigating circumstances were also claimed by the perpetrators themselves. In an 1896 article for the political journal *Die Zukunft*, Heinrich Leist defended himself by pointing to the intensity of tropical sunlight as a cause for the 'increased irritability of the nervous system' in the tropics, which could easily lead to uncontrolled 'fits of anger' and 'sexual temptations'.[6] The more or less implicit assumption of these statements was that European standards of behaviour were not always applicable in the colonial situation. Beyond providing threadbare excuses for the deeds of individual criminals, however, Tropenkoller could also be deployed for the establishment of subtle differentiations between legitimate and illegitimate forms of colonial violence. In 1896, at a time when the German colonial army in Africa was engaged in several military operations against the native population, the director of the Colonial Office pointed to the cases of Leist and Wehlan as regrettable 'exceptions' that proved the rule that 'on the whole the officers and officials in our protectorates (*Schutzgebiete*) perform their hard duty in a faithful and honourable way'.[7]

Whereas the advocates of colonialism used the notion of Tropenkoller to exonerate the perpetrators, the liberal and especially the Social Democratic opposition tried to depict the syndrome as a characteristic symptom of the depravity of imperialist politics. Already in the spring of 1894, the Social Democratic newspaper *Vorwärts* noted in an ironic commentary, that the 'rampantly growing Tropenkoller'[8] of characters such as Wehlan and Leist had to be attributed to the immoderate consumption of alcohol and sexual excesses in the colonies. Suggesting a deep affinity between military violence and sadism, the social democrat von Vollmar interpreted the common habit among German officers and officials in Africa to wear whips, as a telling symptom of colonial 'megalomania'.[9] Following a similar line of argument, another article in *Vorwärts* stated in 1899 that Tropenkoller was not caused by the tropical climate but had to be traced to the moral degeneration of the ruling classes in Europe: 'These are the consequences of Europakoller, for which the defenders of colonial crimes try to blame the tropical climate, but which in reality is nothing else than the well-known European phenomenon of degeneration called dashingness (*Schneidigkeit*).'[10]

This cursory overview of the various invocations of the syndrome within the context of the 'colonial scandals' shows that, in political discourse, Tropenkoller was a highly ambiguous phenomenon. Participating in the ethical ambivalence of the pathological, the disease could be used to excuse as well as to accuse, could label patients as well as perpetrators. Paradoxically, it is especially the various rhetorical manoeuvres intended to determine what Tropenkoller 'really' was that most clearly point to the syndrome's rhetorical status as a highly connotative signifier that created the meaning it was supposed to denote: In a significant inversion of the conventional order of naming, most political invocations of the phenomenon started from the term Tropenkoller itself, and *then* tried to charge it with meaning and a suitable definition. The overdetermination of Tropenkoller as a polyvalent collective symbol, however, also implied that none of the speakers had complete control over its meaning. Since, as a contemporary neurologist noted, in colloquial language the term was often used to ironically hint to the fact that 'for all brutal acts in the tropics an excuse can be presented'[11] every exculpatory invocation of the Tropenkoller was at risk of deriding itself as a flimsy excuse. In the scandalizing propaganda of the Social Democrats, on the other hand, it was never quite clear whether the phenomenon had to be regarded as a mere pseudo-disease or whether it actually *did* exist, as its reading as a symptom of bourgeois degeneration suggested. Talking about Tropenkoller was thus a way of making political sense of colonial violence, in which the 'sense' itself remained essentially unsettled and ambiguous.

This polymorphous nature of the syndrome becomes especially apparent in Frieda von Bülow's *Tropenkoller* (1896). Published in the heyday of the 'colonial scandals', her text represents a distinctly polemic intervention into the ongoing political debate on colonial violence. Being a fervent supporter of German colonialism and a former lover of Carl Peters, von Bülow held radical nationalist views, which she tried to combine with feminist positions.[12] Set in an imaginary colonial village in German East Africa, her novel is designed to re-encode the notion of Tropenkoller from a colonial perspective. The concern about the devastating influence of African fever and climate on the psychosomatic condition of the German colonists, which runs through the text, is paradigmatically articulated by the novel's heroine Eva Biron, who worriedly remarks that 'everybody gets nervous here, even men, who in Germany have only unbelievingly laughed about the word "nerves" '.[13] Unfortunately, however, this anxiety does not seem to be shared by the metropolitan public back home in Germany. For Eva, this indifference becomes especially obvious in the recent invention of the mocking term 'Tropenkoller' in the German capital: 'The Berliners, never at a loss for funny words', she angrily complains, 'once they have found a name for a thing, they are done with it and no longer interested in the exploration of its nature.'[14] Her opposite, the seasoned colonial officer Ludwig von Rosen, takes this remark as a starting point for a lengthy talk about the aetiology of the syndrome. According to Rosen, one has to distinguish between two major types of tropical nervousness: a 'climatic' form, caused by the incompatibility of Nordic races with the heat of tropical climates, and a 'pernicious' form, resulting from the 'bad character' of the person affected.[15] In Bülow's narrative, these two types of tropical nervousness are epitomised in the forest assessor Udo Biron, Eva's blond and blue-eyed brother, and Ludwig Drahn, the brutal and megalomaniac director of a colonial railway construction company.

The medical history of the irascible but good-natured Teuton Udo is closely modelled after the phenotype of the 'colonial scandals': gradually losing his health and temper to fever and climate, Biron breaks up a noisy midnight party of local natives by whipping several of the participants and later hangs the evil leader of a group of Arab slave traders. Drahn's Tropenkoller, by contrast, is not exclusively directed towards the native population but also at his German fellow countrymen. The character of his disorder becomes suddenly apparent to Rosen when the selfish and boastful colonial entrepreneur denies him access to his business premises: ' "The glory of command in the land of the savages goes straight to the head of these servant types," he thought; "that's it! They are so unaccustomed to being masters that they lose their poor little bit of common sense and end up with a ridiculous form of megalomania." '[16] The tragic and accusatory turn that Bülow's novel takes consists in the fact that Drahn's colonial profiteering eventually triumphs over Biron's imperial enthusiasm. Annoyed about a derogatory remark by Udo, Drahn sends one-sided defamatory reports about his misdeeds to the Colonial Office in Berlin, which cause a public scandal and lead to Biron's recall to Germany. At the deathbed of the feverish Udo the other colonists are left with the distressed conclusion that the blind Moloch of public opinion in the capital needs, from time to time, an innocent 'scape-goat'[17] to cleanse itself from its own sins.

The fatal confrontation of Udo and Drahn highlights von Bülow's attempt to establish clear political and moral distinctions in the wide and ambiguous semantic field of colonial nervousness. Significantly, Rosen states that the deleterious effects of the climate for the nervous system are 'something very different'[18] from Drahn's Tropenkoller. This splitting up of tropical nervousness into a regrettable but understandable and a 'pernicious', egoistic form corresponds to von Bülow's nationalist critique of a wrong since too capitalist form of colonialism. From this perspective, Tropenkoller can indeed be seen to figure in Bülow's text 'as a metaphor for the psychological disorders produced by an inadequately democratic colonialism'[19] that becomes particularly obvious in the metropolitan public's hypocritical reaction. The distinction between idealistic and evil forms of colonial violence, whose effects on the native victims are not depicted in Bülow's book, may also be interpreted as a way for the author to come to terms with her own continuing fascination for Carl Peters.[20] In a letter written to Peters in 1897, Bülow declares: 'I know that you can be brutal, and I certainly don't love brutality. But I also know that this brutality is almost inseparable from certain qualities that are rare and of the highest value, and that it is necessary in some situations'.[21]

In her novel, Tropenkoller emerges as a central topos for the articulation of this ambivalent fascination with colonial violence. Significantly, von Bülow's attempt to narratively distinguish between two different forms of Tropenkoller makes a clear definition of the syndrome impossible. Instead, her double strategy of simultaneously deploying the disease for exculpatory and accusatory purposes results in a curious conflation of various forms of tropical nervousness. In fact, Eva's initial observation that '[e]verybody gets nervous here'[22] is true to such an extent that virtually every colonist in the novel to a certain degree seems to be affected by a combination of the two paradigmatic forms of tropical nervousness. Playing out the various associative possibilities of the syndrome, Bülow's novel points to the political overdetermination of the colonizers' nerves that characterized the entire debate about the colonial scandals.

II

Considering that Tropenkoller was an invention of 'laymen'[23] and first emerged as a politically framed disease, it is unsurprising that most professional doctors and experts in tropical medicine treated the syndrome with hesitation. Several physicians flatly doubted that one could speak of an 'actual disease' (*eigentliche Krankheit*)[24] at all. Although others were less reluctant and maintained that Tropenkoller was not just a 'delusion' (*leerer Wahn*)[25] because its symptoms could be frequently observed in tropical colonies, a general scepticism manifested itself most significantly by way of the quotation marks which usually accompanied the popular term in medical texts: These marks indicate exactly the discursive boundary Tropenkoller crossed when it became an issue in German tropical medicine around 1900.

Although the term 'Tropenkoller' was not unreservedly included into the medical lexicon, the phenomenon clearly left its mark in contemporary medical discourse. The idea that tropical climates had a weakening and exhausting influence on the European nervous system was in itself not new, but a commonplace in nineteenth-century tropical medicine.[26] Physicians had also speculated since the seventeenth century about the relationship between malaria and mental disorders.[27] It seems, however, that the invention of the term *Tropenneurasthenie* (tropical neurasthenia), which in German medical texts first appeared in the late 1890s, was at least partly stimulated by the pervasive Tropenkoller discourse. Many of the medical authors who explicitly doubted or rejected the existence of Tropenkoller as an actual disease, stated at the same time, that the unfavourable circumstances in the tropics could cause a number of neurasthenic symptoms ranging from nervous irritability, hallucinations and paranoia to psychosis.[28]

Although the deployment of tropical neurasthenia can be viewed as a strategy to evade the politically contaminated term Tropenkoller, the moral and forensic assessment of colonial crimes of violence still posed a major problem for tropical medicine. The question of whether climate and fever could actually affect the moral sense of Europeans in the tropics divided tropical medicine. In 1905 it became the object of a controversy between two of the leading protagonists of the discipline: the Dutch psychiatrist P. C. J. van Brero, and Albert Plehn, a German governmental doctor in Cameroon. In a chapter 'Nervous Disorders and Mental Diseases' that van Brero contributed to the canonical *Handbuch der Tropenkrankheiten*, he stated that the term 'Tropenkoller' was nothing more than 'a new word for an old thing'. Citing an ancient proverb from one of Horace's odes – 'Coelum non animum mutant, qui trans mare currunt' ('Those who travel over sea, change the sky but not the mind') – van Brero claimed that 'neither climate, nor unfavourable circumstances, nor both of them together' could explain the excesses. Rather, they should be traced to the ubiquitous 'bête humaine'. Having thus depicted Tropenkoller as an anthropological and philosophical rather than a medical issue, van Brero consequently denied any competence in judging the problem of criminal responsibility. That was a 'question for the judge'.[29]

In the same year, Albert Plehn vigorously criticized van Brero's position in a lecture on 'Tropical Brain Dysfunctions and Their Assessment' (*Tropische Hirnstörungen und ihre Beurteilung*) delivered to the medical section of the German Colonial Congress. Considering several aetiological factors contributing to the nervous irritability of Europeans in the tropics including sunlight, alcoholism, bad nutrition, and infection with malaria fever, Plehn maintained that the psychosomatic influences of the tropics could indeed affect a person's character: 'Man changes out there. Many of us might have experienced this themselves, if they, back at home after years abroad, reconsider their feelings and deeds out there.'[30] Plehn drew the conclusion that at least some of the criminal offences in tropical colonies should be judged more leniently than in Europe. In order to demonstrate the destructive influence of tropical fever on the cerebral cortex, he presented to his audience a number of slide preparations from the brains of malaria patients.

These two positions in the medical debate closely resemble the double aetiology of Tropenkoller in Bülow's novel. Plehn's explanation, that the tropics can deform a person's moral physiognomy beyond recognition, can be seen as an attempt to exterritorialize colonial violence – 'out there' – by putting it down to influences for which the patient

himself cannot be held responsible. Van Brero, on the other hand, formulates the far more pessimistic idea that the journey into the tropical
'heart of darkness' merely reveals a barbaric disposition in the traveller
himself. At this point, the highly ambiguous relationship between
pathology and violence, encoded in the name 'Tropenkoller', can be
seen to overdetermine the syndrome as a medical phenomenon: in the
discourse of tropical medicine, Tropenkoller either had to be translated
into the psychosomatic phenomenon of 'Tropenneurasthenie' (Plehn)
or to be rejected as a pseudo-disease (van Brero).

Since Tropenkoller's existence as an actual disease was ultimately a
question of moral perspective, it is significant that one of the rare texts
in which a physician unreservedly acknowledged the existence of the
syndrome was written as a first-person narrative. It is to be found in
Ludwig Külz's *Blätter und Briefe eines Arztes aus dem tropischen
Deutschafrika* (1906), a collection of thematically framed diary entries, in
which the author combines accounts of his experiences as a German
governmental doctor in Africa with reflections on political and medical
issues. In an entry from May 1905, Külz wonders why most of his medical colleagues rashly denied that Tropenkoller was a genuine disease.
Since the entire human organism was 'tuned to a different pitch'[31] in the
tropics, Külz regarded it as highly likely that this would also apply to the
nervous system. In order to verify his assertion, he reported his own
experience: suffering from a light attack of fever, he sat one night on his
veranda when he suddenly heard a whizzing noise at his right ear.
Although the local population was absolutely peaceful, the doctor was
convinced that the sound must have been caused be an arrow fired at
him. Suspecting an attack on his life, he alarmed his native servants and
patrolled the vicinity with a loaded rifle. Only half an hour later he realized that the ominous noise might well have been caused by a bat: 'But
I am sure', Külz concludes his story, 'that if on this ghost hunt I unfortunately had bumped into a black sitting in the grass I would have shot
him. And who would later have believed my explanation of the event?'[32]

Külz's question and his astonishment as to his own reaction point
exactly to the core of the medico-legal undecidability of Tropenkoller. It
is only because, in this case, the 'I' of the narrator brings together the
voice of the patient and the voice of the doctor – personal experience and
medical authority – that Tropenkoller can become a genuine disease. Külz
himself, however, admits that from the outside it was virtually impossible
to separate those 'pathological changes' of the nervous system from manifestations of the predatory character of human nature. In order to
describe this evil trait he ends his entry with a quote from Nietzsche's

Genealogy of Morals, thereby implicitly indicating that Tropenkoller raised questions that exceeded the competence of medical discourse: 'The same men who are so strongly bound by custom, honour, habit, thankfulness [. . .] once outside where the strange world, the foreign begins, [they] are not much better than beasts of prey turned loose.'[33]

III

Henry Wenden's *Tropenkoller* (1904) was the second novel on the topic to appear during the German colonial period. In contrast to von Bülow's novel, which contains no explicit descriptions of violence, Wenden's book blatantly exposes the sexual and pathological dimensions of the 'colonial scandals'. Significantly, the book starts with a psychologizing preface in which Wenden declares his intention to contribute to the 'clarification and perhaps also to the healing' of Tropenkoller.[34] Deploying an indirect but almost literal quote from psychiatrist Iwan Bloch's then recently published *Psychopathia Sexualis* (1903), Wenden asserts that Tropenkoller had to be regarded as a particular form of sadism. According to Wenden, it manifests itself in individuals disposed to sexual perversion due to the almost unlimited power enjoyed by Europeans in the colonies: 'Not only are they removed from their customary environment, not only are they cut off from the influence of civilisation, but they are also suddenly supplied with subordinates who belonged to a strange race, a race which appears to the proud, fastidious European even more inferior than in reality it is [. . .]'.[35] Legitimized by the popular scientific foreword, the narrative itself indulges in detailed depictions of violent crimes committed by Kurt Zangen, a young German colonial officer in East Africa. Initially Kurt participates only as an excited visitor in the secret whippings of African natives organized by the director of a local trading post. His later promotion to leader of a military expedition into the interior gives him ample opportunity to act out his sadistic perversions. In a key scene of violence Kurt satisfies his desire for the sight of 'pretty red blood on black skin'[36] by whipping a young native girl: 'A malicious, barbaric lash came down, a second, a third, a fourth followed, and pitilessly the whip cracked and hissed over the small bosom and young belly.'[37] The native woman Ataya, who initially resists him, acquiesces after Kurt threatens to whip her to death. Eventually apprehended and thrown in jail in Berlin, Kurt avoids legal proceedings and punishment by committing suicide.

The depiction of Tropenkoller as a specific form of sexual perversion in Bloch's and Wenden's novels points to a medico-political constellation that stimulated the enormous proliferation of the Tropenkoller discourse in general. In her recent attempt to bring the basic assumptions of Foucault's *History of Sexuality* to bear upon colonial texts, Ann Laura Stoler has argued that nineteenth-century discourses of tropical hygiene fulfilled an important role in the colonial 'education of desire': 'They reaffirmed that the "truth" of European sexuality was lodged in self-restraint, self-discipline, in a managed sexuality that was susceptible and not always under control.'[38] Challenging the common psychoanalytic assumption of many colonial studies that an – often implicitly essentialized – 'White desire' should be regarded as a driving force of European colonialism, Stoler shifts the focus from the repression and sublimation of desire and sexual perversion to their discursive production and cultural productivity. For her, as for Foucault, sex is not linked to power by repression and silence, but rather by the garrulous attention given to it.

The cultural significance of Wenden's novel resides in the fact that Kurt's perversion and the obscenely detailed descriptions thereof, unite and almost pornographically expose two prime motives of contemporary debates on Tropenkoller: the idea of an out-of-control and sadistically perverted male sexuality, and the fantasy of sexual race mixing. (In one scene Kurt becomes sexually aroused by the sight of 'blood streaming down the crotch and the thighs' a native being whipped and fantasises about tasting 'the delicious, stimulating liquid on his tongue'.)[39] In order to understand the regulatory function that Tropenkoller fulfilled in the colonial 'education of desire', it is important to note that the beating and whipping of natives as a means of punishment and their 'education' represented an essential – and for many colonizers indispensable – component of everyday colonial life. Elaborate, if often violated, rules existed for the correct method of whipping in which colonial authorities attempted to establish permissible forms of flogging, and imposed standards for those allowed to arrange and execute the punishment. Medical testimonies were concerned with forms of instrumentation – rope ends or whips – that would insure that the delinquent's ability to work was not permanently damaged. Excessive loss of blood was also a concern as it was thought to contribute to the spread of infectious diseases.[40] Emphasis was likewise placed on forms of whipping which would not deeply affect the tormentor himself. A testimonial from a German colonial officer in German Southwest Africa in 1900 established that a whipping carried out by an expert should not have 'any brutish or barbaric character' and be performed as a 'smooth act, soundlessly and without impact on the nerves'.[41] The political and public indignation incurred by the 'colonial scandals' was due at least in part to the fact that they appeared to violate the hygienic economy of punishment. Heinrich Leist, for example, emphatically attempted to dispute the notion that any sadistic motives might have been involved in the whipping of the Dahomeydian women. He insisted that the women were ordered to roll up their loincloths before flogging not for the 'gratification of a sexual thrill',[42] but because this was the common habit in African colonies. Emphasizing the 'hygienic' character of the whipping, he also argued that this measure had led to the discovery of a dangerous skin disease in one of the delinquents. Leist also stressed that 'smooth', rather than 'twisted' whips were used for the flagellation. This distinction seems to have marked the precise boundary between functional, and therefore, normal beatings and excessive, perverted forms of corporeal punishment. Against the background of these debates, Wenden's depiction of Zangen's whipping orgies can be seen as representing a form of punitive practice that does not imply control over the delinquent, but rather the ultimate loss of control on the part of the executioner.

By means of an extensive symbolics of blood, Wenden's text closely connects these sadistic excesses to the crossing of another of sexual boundary that preoccupied contemporary colonial discourse – namely the idea of inter-racial sex and blood-mixing.[43] As Lora Wildenthal argues, the issue of 'miscegenation' (blending of races), far from being a historically stable European phantasm, had gained special political significance in German colonial discourse by the end of the nineteenth century. In her study on the history of the German colonial women's movement, Wildenthal shows that discourses of race and sexuality interacted in quite distinct ways in the early days of the German colonies and in the years around 1900. She convincingly argues that until this time the masculine concept of 'imperial patriarchy',[44] radically embodied in the figures of Leist and Peters, dominated discourses on sexual relations between male colonizers and native women. It sanctioned the wide-ranging personal and sexual autonomy of German men in the colonies, including access to native female concubines as an expression of colonial power. Significantly, for 'imperial patriarchs, racial hierarchy did not require racial purity; sexual relationships with colonized women, far from damaging authority, expressed that authority'.[45] As military occupation gave way to the administrative and juridical integration of the African protectorates within the German political structure in the 1890s, German patriarchal sexual libertinism became problematic. In particular, the political and juridical debate on the citizenship of children produced in colonial unions eventually led to the prohibition of 'racially mixed marriages' (*Rassenmischehen*) in German Southwest Africa (1905), German East Africa (1906) and German Samoa (1912). Acceptance of inter-racial sex was gradually replaced by its criminalisation.[46]

The framing of Tropenkoller as a form of sexual perversion sanctioned this shift towards ideas of racial purity and contributed considerably to the problematization and pathologization of male sexual behaviour in the colonies. Significantly, the political and medical debates that surrounded the syndrome were often focused on questions of racial hygiene. In a 1894 parliamentary debate on the 'colonial scandals', Imperial Chancellor von Caprivi attributed the problem of moral degeneration among the almost exclusively male German colonists in Africa to a lack of available German women abroad.[47] Similarly, the 'doctrine of civilising woman'[48] plays a central role in a 1903 entry in the diary of Ludwig Külz, in which the doctor states that female emigration to Africa would certainly contribute to the 'psychic and physical wellbeing' of the German colonial officers and officials stationed there: 'Many illnesses and disharmonies would not have occurred, many hasty steps would not have been taken if a woman had stood at the man's side.'[49]

Whereas white women were seen as a possible cure for Tropenkoller, their native counterparts figured as its cause. In Paul Kohlstock's *Ratgeber für die Tropen*, one of the most widely circulated German manuals on tropical hygiene at the time, the dangers of inter-racial intercourse are explicitly linked to the emergence of the syndrome. Assuming a close relationship between sexual activity and neurasthenic conditions, Kohlstock asserts that Tropenkoller could be caused by sexual 'excesses' as well as by long periods of abstinence.[50] In the latter case, however, the detrimental effects of 'pollution, masturbation and insomnia' could cause a German man to overcome his possible 'racial aversion' (*Rassenabneigung*) and lead to sexual relations with a native woman. Such relations, he warns, must be undertaken with 'moderation and painstaking cleanliness'.[51] Should, in spite of all precautions, the native concubine become pregnant, Kohlstock suggests that she and the child be disowned since marriage with an African woman would only lead to the *Verkafferung*[52] of the German father. In her novel, von Bülow also casually alludes to the dangerous attraction that black women were said to constitute for German men: With thinly concealed disapproval, Eva notes that her nervous brother seems to be well acquainted with some beautiful native girls who smile coquettishly as they pass.

Centred on the exploration and discursive exposure of male desire, these and many other medical, political, and literary invocations of Tropenkoller fulfilled an important function in the regulation and normalization of gender relations and sexual behaviour in the colonies. Tropenkoller-induced sex was dangerous sex. It threatened to lead to the moral degeneration of German men in the colonies and was seen to have adverse effects on their performance as conscientious trustees of the colonial project. 'Neurasthenics are bad colonisers', as Kohlstock's *Ratgeber* suggestively states.[53] In a Foucauldian and Stolerian sense, Tropenkoller constituted an essential nodal point in discourses on tropical hygiene, and represented a productive form of the pathologization of patterns of behaviour that helped to establish race and gender difference. It produced hygienically and medically legitimated distinctions between the civilizing German and the pernicious native woman; the normal and sick male colonist; as well as necessary punishments and perverted desires.

IV

In this chapter, I hope to have shown that the emergence of Tropenkoller, as one of the most significant and certainly most discussed colonial diseases of the Wilhelmine Empire, was facilitated by the ways in which the syndrome suggestively connected the 'nervous discourse' of the *fin-de-siècle*, with the cultural topos of the degenerating influence of the tropics, ideas of sexual deviancy and colonial violence. The question remains, however, as to whether the syndrome, as a discursive phenomenon, was peculiar to German colonial experience and, if so, why it apparently did not occur in other European colonies. In the realm of European colonial discourse no other pathological syndrome seems to have achieved a comparable cultural career. To be sure, many English, Dutch, and French colonial novels, such as Joseph Conrad's *Heart of Darkness* (1899), Ernest Psichari's *Terres de soleil et de sommeil* (1910) and Louis Couperus' *De stille kracht* (1899), dealt with phenomena that might have been described in Germany as instances of Tropenkoller. There are a number of terms for nervous conditions in European tropical medicine as the French 'caffard', 'soudanité' and 'psychoses tropicales'[54] and the English 'jungle madness' and 'tropical neurasthenia'[55]. However, none of them triggered an interdiscursive explosion equivalent to that one caused by Tropenkoller in the culture of the Wilhelmine Empire around 1900.

It seems reasonable to assume, then, that the national exclusiveness of Tropenkoller is a result of the particularity of the German colonial experience. In his recent analysis of the 'cultivation of colonial desire' in German imperialist imagination, Thomas Schwarz has classified the syndrome as a stopping-off place along a violent *Sonderweg* of German exoticism. Drawing on Russell Berman's debatable assertion that, because of the lack of a stable national identity, German colonialism was characterised by a 'particular openness'[56] towards other cultures, Schwarz interprets the pathologization of racial mixing as a biomedical counteraction or counter-charge that eventually led to national socialist extermination politics.[57] Although I do no totally disagree with this line of reasoning I would like to conclude with a less broad view on Tropenkoller's specific 'Germanness'. Significantly, in Wenden's novel the first symptoms of Zangen's Tropenkoller do not become visible in Africa, but during a military parade held on the metropolitan boulevard Unter den Linden in Berlin on the occasion of the emperor's birthday. Riding a few steps behind Wilhem II, Kurt satisfies his desire to dominate by projecting the public's jubilation for the emperor unto himself and few minutes later his right hand gives a nervous 'twitch' which during the narration becomes a leitmotif of Kurt's deviant desires. While this passage may be interpreted as a subtle comment on the eroticization of power in imperialist culture in general it at the same time also contains a specific allusion to the 'nervousness' of German world politics (*Weltpolitik*). As Joachim Radkau has shown, political language in the Wilhelmine Empire was replete with neurasthenic metaphors that in particular dominated the discourse about the 'nervous irritability' of German foreign politics. The emperor himself was frequently depicted as a megalomaniac and nervous man whose fickle imperial ambitions manifested themselves in a curious mixture of aggressive and defensive elements.[58] From this perspective the prevalence of nervous metaphors in German colonial discourse, culminating in the collective symbol of Tropenkoller, can also appear as the characteristic reaction of a nation that feared to have come late to the colonial distribution of the world but nevertheless dreamt of attaining the imperial composure of its European opponents.

Notes

1. Otto Ladendorff, *Historisches Schlagwörterbuch* (Berlin: Trübner, 1907) 315.
2. Michel Foucault, *The Archaeology of Knowledge and the Discourse of Language*, trans. A. M. Sheridan Smith (London: Tavistock, 1972) 158.
3. Jürgen Link, 'Literaturanalyse als Interdiskursanalyse. Am Beispiel des Ursprungs

318   *Towards a Poetics and Metaphorics of Disease*

literarischer Symbolik in der Kollektivsymbolik', in Jürgen Fohrmann and Harro Müller (eds), *Diskurstheorien und Literaturwissenschaft*, (Frankfurt/M.: Suhrkamp 1988) 288.
4. See Mark Harrison, ' "The Tender Frame of Man": Disease, Climate, and Racial Difference in India and the West Indies, 1760–1860', *Bulletin of the History of Medicine* 70 (1996): 68–93 and Dane Kennedy, 'The Perils of the Midday Sun: Climatic anxieties in the colonial tropics', in John M. MacKenzie (ed.), *Imperialism and the Natural World* (Manchester: Manchester University Press, 1990) 118–40.
5. *Stenographische Berichte über die Verhandlungen des Reichstags* IX. Legislaturperiode, II. Session 1893–94 (Berlin: Norddeutsche Buchdruckerei, 1894) 1315.
6. Heinrich Leist, 'Der Fall Leist', *Die Zukunft* 16 (1896): 271.
7. *Stenographische Berichte über die Verhandlungen des Reichstags* IX. Legislaturperiode, IV. Session 1895–97 (Berlin: Norddeutsche Buchdruckerei, 1897) 1426.
8. 'Sonntagsplauderei', *Vorwärts*, 15 April 1894: 1.
9. *Stenographische Berichte über die Verhandlungen des Reichstags* IX. Legislaturperiode, III. Session 1894–95 (Berlin: Norddeutsche Buchdruckerei, 1895) 1569.
10. 'Der Europakoller', *Vorwärts*, 28 December 1899.
11. Chr. Rasch, 'Über den Einfluss des Tropenklimas auf das Nervensystem', *Allgemeine Zeitschrift für Psychiatrie und psychisch-gerichtliche Medizin* 54 (1898): 752.
12. See Lora Wildenthal, *German Women for Empire, 1884–1945* (Durham: Duke University Press, 2001) 13–54.
13. Frieda von Bülow, *Tropenkoller. Episode aus dem deutschen Kolonialleben*, 2nd edn (1896; Berlin: Fontane, 1897) 19.
14. Ibid., 132.
15. Ibid., 134–5.
16. Ibid., 64.
17. Ibid., 285.
18. Ibid., 64.
19. Russell A. Berman, *Enlightenment or Empire: Colonial Discourse in German Culture* (Lincoln, NE: University of Nebraska Press, 1998) 178.
20. This conclusion could be drawn from Wildenthal's analysis of their relationship (*German Women for Empire*, 69–78).
21. Cited from ibid., 76.
22. Bülow, *Tropenkoller*, 19.
23. Botho Scheube, *Die Krankheiten der warmen Länder*, 3rd edn (Berlin: Thieme, 1903) 771.
24. L. Sofer, 'Tropenbiologie', *Dietrich Reimer's Mitteilungen für Ansiedler, Farmer, Tropenpflanzer, Kolonisten, Forschungsreisende, Kaufleute und Kolonialfreunde* 2.8 (1908): 24.
25. Paul Kohlstock, 'Erfordernisse in gesundheitlicher Hinsicht für Aufenthalt und Tätigkeit in den Tropen', *Dietrich Reimer's Mitteilungen für Ansiedler, Farmer, Tropenpflanzer, Kolonisten, Forschungsreisende, Kaufleute und Kolonialfreunde* 1.3 (1907): 137.
26. See Harrison, ' "The Tender Frame of Man" ' and Kennedy, 'The Perils of the Midday Sun'.
27. See Mitchell G. Weiss, 'The Interrelationship of Tropical Disease and Mental

Disorder: Conceptual Framework and Literature Review', *Culture, Medicine and Psychiatry* 9 (1985), 121–200.

28. See, for example, Scheube, *Die Krankheiten*, 771 and Sofer, 'Tropenbiologie', 24–5.

29. P. C. J. van Brero, 'Die Nerven-und Geisteskrankheiten in den Tropen', in Carl Mense (ed.), *Handbuch der Tropenkrankheiten*, vol. 1 (Leipzig: Barth, 1905) 211. Van Brero's thesis that the tropics do not effect the 'moral feeling' was shared, among others, by Scheube, *Die Krankheiten der warmen Länder*, 771 and Friedrich Plehn, *Die Kamerunküste. Studien zur Klimatologie, Physiologie und Pathologie in den Tropen* (Berlin: Hirschwald) 74. Plehn was one of the first German doctors to use the term 'Tropenneurasthenie' (263).

30. Albert Plehn, 'Über Hirnstörungen in den heissen Ländern und ihre Beurteilung', *Verhandlungen des deutschen Kolonialkongresses 1905* (Berlin: Reimer, 1906) 253.

31. Ludwig Külz, *Blätter und Briefe eines deutschen Arztes aus dem tropischen Deutschafrika*, 2nd edn (1906; Berlin: Süssrott, 1910) 219.

32. Ibid., 219.

33. Ibid., 220.

34. Henry Wenden, *Tropenkoller* (Leipzig: Sattler, 1904) 15.

35. Ibid., 12. See Iwan Bloch, *Beiträge zur Ätiologie der Psychopathia sexualis*, vol. 2 (Dresden: Dohrn 1903) 55.

36. Wenden, *Tropenkoller*, 177.

37. Ibid., 178.

38. Ann Laura Stoler, *Race and the Education of Desire: Foucault's History of Sexuality and the Colonial Order of Things* (Durham: Duke University Press, 1995) 177.

39. Wenden, *Tropenkoller*, 141–2.

40. For a detailed documentation of German whipping regulations see Fritz Ferdinand Müller, *Kolonien unter der Peitsche: Eine Dokumentation* (Berlin: Rütten & Loening 1962).

41. 'Die Exekution vollzieht sich als glatter Akt, lautlos ohne Nerveneindrücke'. Cited from Müller, *Kolonien unter de Peitsche*, 152.

42. Leist, 'Der Fall Leist', 263.

43. See, for example, Robert J. C. Young, *Colonial Desire: Hybridity in Theory, Culture and Race* (London: Routledge, 1995) and Anne McClintock, *Imperial Leather: Race, Gender and Sexuality* (London: Routledge, 1995).

44. Wildenthal, *German Women for Empire*, 80.

45. Ibid., 81.

46. On the issue of the 'Mischehen' see also Pascal Grosse, *Kolonialismus, Eugenik und bürgerliche Gesellschaft in Deutschland 1850–1918* (Frankfurt/M.: Campus, 2000) 145–92.

47. *Stenographische Berichte über die Verhandlungen des Reichstags* IX. Legislaturperiode, II. Session 1893–94 (Berlin: Norddeutsche Buchdruckerei 1894) 1305.

48. John K. Noyes, *The Mastery of Submission: Inventions of Masochism* (Ithaca: Cornell University Press, 1997) 128.

49. Külz, *Blätter und Briefe*, 98.

50. Paul Kohlstock, *Ratgeber für die Tropen: Handbuch für Auswanderer, Ansiedler, Reisende Kaufleute und Missionare über Ausrüstung, Aufenthalt und Behandlung*

von Krankheiten in heißen Ländern, 3rd edn (Stettin: Peters, 1910) 4, 59, 235 and 253.

51. Ibid., 253.
52. Ibid., 120. The word 'Kaffer' is a racist slur on people of colour. The term 'Verkafferung' therefore means 'racial degeneration'.
53. Ibid., 281.
54. Maurice Neveu-Lemaire, *Principes d'hygiène et de médecine coloniales* (Paris: Société d'éditions géographiques, maritimes et coloniales, 1925) 24–6. For 'caffard' and 'soudanité' see Juliano Moreira, 'Die Nerven-und Geisteskrankheiten in den Tropen', *Handbuch der Tropenkrankheiten* ed. Carl Mense, 3rd edn, vol. 4 (Leipzig: Barth 1926) 320–1.
55. Louis H. Fales, 'Tropical Neurasthenia and its Relation to Tropical Acclimation', *The American Journal of the Medical Sciences* 133 (1907): 582–93; Aldo Castellani and Albert J. Chalmers, *Manual of Tropical Medicine* (London: Bailliere, Tindall and Cox, 1910) 1065.
56. Berman, *Enlightenment or Empire*, 18.
57. Thomas Schwarz, 'Die Kultivierung des kolonialen Begehrens: Ein deutscher Sonderweg?', *Kolonialismus und Kultur: Literatur, Medien, Wissenschaft in der deutschen Gründerzeit des Fremden*, ed. Alexander Honold and Oliver Simons (Tübingen: Francke, 2002) 97–100.
58. Joachim Radkau, *Das Zeitalter der Nervosität. Deutschland zwischen Bismarck und Hitler* (München: Hanser, 1998) 275–95.

Index